FY2001 Library Services and Technology
Act (LSTA) Grant titled Collection
Connection administered by the Office
of the Secretary of State/Illinois State
Library.

RECEIVED
MAY 2 2 2001
BY:

HAYNER PUBLIC LIBRARY DISTRICT
ALTON, ILLINOIS

OVERDUES .10 PER DAY. MAXIMUM FINE
COST OF BOOKS LOST OR DAMAGED BOOKS
ADDITIONAL $5.00 SERVICE CHARGE.

Heart Diseases and Disorders
SOURCEBOOK
Second Edition

Health Reference Series

Second Edition

Heart Diseases and Disorders SOURCEBOOK

Basic Consumer Health Information about Heart Attacks, Angina, Rhythm Disorders, Heart Failure, Valve Disease, Congenital Heart Disorders, and More, Including Descriptions of Surgical Procedures and Other Interventions, Medications, Cardiac Rehabilitation, Risk Identification, and Prevention Tips

Along with Statistical Data, Reports on Current Research Initiatives, a Glossary of Cardiovascular Terms, and a Resource Directory

Edited by
Karen Bellenir

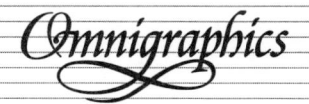

Omnigraphics

615 Griswold Street • Detroit, MI 48226

HAYNER PUBLIC LIBRARY DISTRICT
ALTON, ILLINOIS

Bibliographic Note

Because this page cannot legibly accommodate all the copyright notices, the Bibliographic Note portion of the Preface constitutes an extension of the copyright notice.

Beginning with books published in 1999, each new volume of the *Health Reference Series* will be individually titled and called a "First Edition." Subsequent updates will carry sequential edition numbers. To help avoid confusion and to provide maximum flexibility in our ability to respond to informational needs, the practice of consecutively numbering each volume will be discontinued.

Edited by Karen Bellenir

Health Reference Series

Karen Bellenir, *Series Editor*
Peter D. Dresser, *Managing Editor*
Joan Margeson, *Research Associate*
Dawn Matthews, *Verification Assistant*
Margaret Mary Missar, *Research Coordinator*
Jenifer Swanson, *Research Associate*

Omnigraphics, Inc.

Matthew P. Barbour, *Vice President, Operations*
Laurie Lanzen Harris, *Vice President, Editorial Director*
Kevin Hayes, *Production Coordinator*
Thomas J. Murphy, *Vice President, Finance and Comptroller*
Peter E. Ruffner, *Senior Vice President*
Jane J. Steele, *Marketing Consultant*

Frederick G. Ruffner, Jr., Publisher

© 2000, Omnigraphics, Inc.

All rights reserved. No part of this publication may be reproduced or transmitted in any form or by any means, electronic or mechanical, including photocopy, recording, or any information retrieval system, without permission in writing from the publisher.

Library of Congress Cataloging-in-Publication Data

Heart diseases and disorders sourcebook : basic consumer health information about heart attacks, angina, rhythm disorders, heart failure, valve disease, congenital heart disorders, and more ... / edited by Karen Bellenir.-- 2nd ed.
    p. cm. -- (Health reference series)
    Prev. ed. published with title: Cardiovascular diseases and disorders sourcebook.
    Includes bibliographical references and index.
    ISBN 0-7808-0238-1 (lib. bdg. : alk. paper)
    1. Heart--Diseases--Popular works. I. Bellenir, Karen. II. Health reference series (Unnumbered)

RC672 .H396 1999
616.1'2--dc21

    99-058043

∞

This book is printed on acid-free paper meeting the ANSI Z39.48 Standard. The infinity symbol that appears above indicates that the paper in this book meets that standard.

Printed in the United States

Table of Contents

Preface ix

Part I: Introduction

Chapter 1 — Do You Know the Truth about Heart
                Disease? 3
Chapter 2 — Trends in Ischemic Heart Disease 15
Chapter 3 — Congestive Heart Failure in the United States:
                A New Epidemic 23
Chapter 4 — Gender Differences in Heart Disease 33
Chapter 5 — Cardiac Arrest and the Need for Early
                Defibrillation 53

Part II: Understanding Your Heart

Chapter 6 — The Heart 61
Chapter 7 — The Vascular System 69
Chapter 8 — Understanding Blood Cholesterol 75
Chapter 9 — Insulin Resistance and Heart Disease 103
Chapter 10 — Homocysteine: Does This Amino Acid Play
                 a Role in Heart Disease? 109
Chapter 11 — The Facts about Alcohol and Your Heart 115
Chapter 12 — Common Diagnostic Tests 123

Part III: Preventing Heart Disease

Chapter 13—How to Be Heart Healthy 141
Chapter 14—Identifying Risk Factors for Heart Disease 153
Chapter 15—Stop Smoking 179
Chapter 16—Risks Associated with Second-Hand Smoke 183
Chapter 17—Physical Activity and Cardiovascular
 Health 187
Chapter 18—Energize Yourself: Stay Physically Active 199
Chapter 19—Lose Weight If You Are Overweight 203
Chapter 20—The New Food Label: Help in Preventing
 Heart Disease 209
Chapter 21—Keeping Your Cholesterol Under Control 219
Chapter 22—Get Your Blood Pressure Checked 227
Chapter 23—How to Take Your Own Blood Pressure 233
Chapter 24—Managing Stress 237
Chapter 25—The Effects of Mental Health on Heart
 Health 241
Chapter 26—An Aspirin a Day...Just Another Cliché? 255
Chapter 27—Coenzyme Q10: The Next Aspirin? 261
Chapter 28—Postmenopausal Estrogen/Progestin
 Interventions Trial (PEPI) 265

Part IV: Common Types of Heart Problems

Chapter 29—Angina 273
Chapter 30—Unstable Angina 279
Chapter 31—Arrhythmias/Rhythm Disorders 297
Chapter 32—Heart Attack (Myocardial Infarction) 307
Chapter 33—Heart Failure 313
Chapter 34—Cardiomyopathy (Heart Muscle Disease) 325
Chapter 35—Coronary Artery Disease 339
Chapter 36—Atherosclerosis 343
Chapter 37—Congenital Heart Disorders 345
Chapter 38—Endocarditis 357
Chapter 39—Pericarditis 359
Chapter 40—Valve Disease 363
Chapter 41—Heart Murmur 367
Chapter 42—Heart Palpitations 371
Chapter 43—Fainting Caused by Cardiac Conditions 375

Part V: Medications, Interventions, and Other Treatment Options

Chapter 44—Commonly Prescribed Medications for Heart Patients 381
Chapter 45—The DIG (Digitalis Investigation Group) Trial 401
Chapter 46—Anticoagulants 405
Chapter 47—Blood-Pressure Lowering Drugs 411
Chapter 48—Cholesterol-Lowering Drugs 427
Chapter 49—Heart Catheterization 433
Chapter 50—Procedures for Opening Blocked Arteries 437
Chapter 51—Angioplasty 443
Chapter 52—Coronary Artery Bypass Surgery 447
Chapter 53—A Closer Look at Chelation Therapy: Does It Work? 453
Chapter 54—New Treatments for Rhythm Disorders 457
Chapter 55—Pacemaker Implantation 465
Chapter 56—Implantable Defibrillators 469
Chapter 57—Heart and Heart-Lung Transplants 473

Part VI: Cardiac Rehabilitation

Chapter 58—Recovering from Heart Problems 481
Chapter 59—Lifestyle Changes for Recovering Heart Patients 491
Chapter 60—Emotional Effects of Rehabilitation 495
Chapter 61—Lowering Cholesterol for the Person with Heart Disease 499
Chapter 62—Preventing a Second Heart Attack 531

Part VII: Additional Help and Information

Chapter 63—Glossary of Heart Terms 537
Chapter 64—Heart Healthy Cookbooks 555
Chapter 65—Spanish Language Publications Available from the National Heart, Lung, and Blood Institute 559
Chapter 66—Directory of Resources for Heart Patients 561

Index 573

Preface

About This Book

Heart disease has been the leading cause of death in the United States since 1910. According to estimates made by the Centers for Disease Control and Prevention (CDC), approximately 57 million Americans currently live with some form of cardiovascular disease. Prevention plays an important role in the battle against heart disease. Key elements include education, early recognition of risk factors, lifestyle changes, and treatment.

This *Sourcebook* supplies the tools people need to maintain healthy hearts. It provides basic information about the human heart and how it works, including facts about such common heart disorders as heart attacks, angina, rhythm disorders (arrhythmias), heart failure, valve disease, and congenital heart disorders. It updates the statistics, research, and treatment options presented in *Cardiovascular Diseases and Disorders Sourcebook* (Volume Five of the *Health Reference Series)*. Special sections focus on prevention issues and rehabilitation for cardiac patients. A glossary of important terms, bibliography of heart-healthy cookbooks, and directory of organizations able to provide additional help and information are also featured.

How to Use This Book

This book is divided into parts and chapters. Parts focus on broad areas of interest. Chapters are devoted to single topics within a part.

Part I: Introduction provides basic facts about heart disease, current statistical and trend data, and information about the potential role of automatic external defibrillators in the prevention of sudden cardiac death.

Part II: Understanding Your Heart presents anatomical information about the heart and vascular system. It describes how blood cholesterol, insulin resistance, homocysteine levels, and alcohol can all contribute to heart disease. A chapter describing common tests used to diagnose heart conditions is also included.

Part III: Preventing Heart Disease offers tips and suggestions for maintaining a healthy cardiovascular system.

Part IV: Common Types of Heart Problems describes some of the most common cardiac disorders, including angina, rhythm disorders (arrhythmias), heart attacks (myocardial infarctions), heart failure, heart muscle disease (cardiomyopathy), coronary artery diseases, congenital heart disorders, infectious diseases of the heart lining, valve disease, heart murmurs, palpitations, and cardiac conditions that can cause fainting.

Part V: Medications, Interventions, and Other Treatment Options provides information about commonly prescribed medications to aid heart function, lower blood cholesterol, and regulate blood pressure. Surgical interventions such as catheterization, angioplasty, bypass surgery, pacemaker and defibrillator implantation, and transplants are also described.

Part VI: Cardiac Rehabilitation offers information for patients who are recovering after a first heart attack. It explains what to expect during the rehabilitation period and how to prevent recurrence.

Part VII: Additional Help and Information includes a glossary of heart terms, a bibliography of heart healthy cookbooks, a list of Spanish-language publications available from the National Heart, Lung, and Blood Institute, and a directory of other resources for heart patients.

Bibliographic Note

This volume contains documents and excerpts from publications issued by the following government agencies: Agency for Health Care Policy and Research (AHCPR), Centers for Disease Control and Prevention

(CDC), National Heart, Lung, and Blood Institute (NHLBI), National Institutes of Health (NIH), NIH Consensus Development Program, and the U.S. Food and Drug Administration (FDA).

In addition, this volume contains copyrighted articles produced by the American Heart Association, Cardiovascular Institute of the South, Clinical Reference Systems, Johns Hopkins InteliHealth, Mayo Clinic Health Oasis, MedicineNet, Micromedex, Random House, Springhouse Corp., and the Texas Heart Institute. Copyrighted articles from the following journals are also included: *Harvard Health Letter, Harvard Heart Letter, Harvard Mental Health Letter, Mayo Clinic Health Letter, The Nurse Practitioner,* and *Tufts University Diet and Nutrition Letter.*

Full citation information is provided on the first page of each chapter. Every effort has been made to secure all necessary rights to reprint the copyrighted material. If any omissions have been made, please contact Omnigraphics to make corrections for future editions.

Acknowledgements

In addition to those listed on the copyright page, the editor gratefully acknowledges the important contributions made by the many people who work behind the scenes and who typically receive no recognition. These include: Mary Ann Stavros at the Maswel Group; Rob Rudnick, Edward Prucha, and the rest of the staff at EdIndex; Bonnie Kahler and the staff at Data Reproductions; Bruce Bellenir and his helpers at Wordwright, L.L.C.; and Omnigraphics' wonderful crew in Detroit.

Note from the Editor

This book is part of Omnigraphics' *Health Reference Series*. The series provides basic information about a broad range of medical concerns. It is not intended to serve as a tool for diagnosing illness, in prescribing treatments, or as a substitute for the physician/patient relationship. All persons concerned about medical symptoms or the possibility of disease are encouraged to seek professional care from an appropriate health care provider.

Our Advisory Board

The *Health Reference Series* is reviewed by an Advisory Board comprised of librarians from public, academic, and medical libraries. We would like to thank the following board members for providing guidance to the development of this series:

Dr. Lynda Baker,
Associate Professor of Library and Information Science,
Wayne State University, Detroit, MI

Nancy Bulgarelli,
William Beaumont Hospital Library, Royal Oak, MI

Karen Imarasio,
Bloomfield Township Public Library, Bloomfield Township, MI

Karen Morgan,
Mardigian Library,
University of Michigan-Dearborn, Dearborn, MI

Rosemary Orlando,
St. Clair Shores Public Library, St. Clair Shores, MI

Health Reference Series *Update Policy*

The inaugural book in the *Health Reference Series* was the first edition of *Cancer Sourcebook* published in 1992. Since then, the *Series* has been enthusiastically received by librarians and in the medical community. In order to maintain the standard of providing high-quality health information for the lay person, the editorial staff at Omnigraphics felt it was necessary to implement a policy of updating volumes when warranted.

Medical researchers have been making tremendous strides, and the challenge to stay current with the most recent advances is one our editors take seriously. Each decision to update a volume will be made on an individual basis. Some of the considerations will include how much new information is available and the feedback we receive from people who use the books. If there's a topic you would like to see added to the update list, or an area of medical concern you feel has not been adequately addressed, please write to:

Editor
Health Reference Series
Omnigraphics, Inc.
615 Griswold
Detroit, MI 48226

The commitment to providing on-going coverage of important medical developments has also led to some technical changes in the *Health Reference Series*. Beginning with books published in 1999, each new volume will be individually titled and called a "First Edition." Subsequent updates will carry sequential edition numbers. To help avoid confusion and to provide maximum flexibility in our ability to respond to informational needs, the practice of consecutively numbering each volume will be discontinued.

Part One

Introduction

Chapter 1

Do You Know the Truth about Heart Disease?

Check Your Knowledge about Risk Factors for Heart Disease

The following statements are either true or false. The correct answers are given below.

True or False?

1. The risk factors for heart disease that you can do something about are: high blood pressure, high blood cholesterol, smoking, obesity, and physical inactivity.
2. A stroke is often the first symptom of high blood pressure, and a heart attack is often the first symptom of high blood cholesterol.
3. A blood pressure greater than or equal to 140/90 mm Hg is generally considered to be high.
4. High blood pressure affects the same number of blacks as it does whites.
5. The best ways to treat and control high blood pressure are to control your weight, exercise, eat less salt (sodium), restrict

---

This chapter includes questions and answers taken from National Heart, Lung, and Blood Institute (NHLBI), NIH Pub. Nos. 92-2724, 93-3034, and 96-3795.

your intake of alcohol, and take your high blood pressure medicine, if prescribed by your doctor.

6. A blood cholesterol level of 240 mg/dL is desirable for adults.
7. The most effective dietary way to lower the level of your blood cholesterol is to eat foods low in cholesterol.
8. Lowering blood cholesterol levels can help people who have already had a heart attack.
9. Only children from families at high risk of heart disease need to have their blood cholesterol levels checked.
10. Smoking is a major risk factor for four of the five leading causes of death including heart attack, stroke, cancer, and lung diseases such as emphysema and bronchitis.
11. If you have had a heart attack, quitting smoking can help reduce your chances of having a second attack.
12. Someone who has smoked for 30 to 40 years probably will not be able to quit smoking.
13. Heart disease is the leading killer of men **and** women in the United States.

Answers to Questions in This Section

1. **True.** High blood pressure, smoking, and high blood cholesterol are the three most important risk factors for heart disease. On the average, each one doubles your chance of developing heart disease. So, a person who has all three of these risk factors is 8 times more likely to develop heart disease than someone who has none. Obesity increases the likelihood of developing high blood cholesterol and high blood pressure, which increase your risk for heart disease. Physical inactivity increases your risk of heart attack. Regular exercise and good nutrition are essential to reducing high blood pressure, high blood cholesterol, and overweight. People who exercise are also more likely to cut down or stop smoking.

2. **True.** A person with high blood pressure or high blood cholesterol may feel fine and look great; there are often no signs that anything is wrong until a stroke or heart attack occurs. To find out if you have high blood pressure or high blood cholesterol,

Do You Know the Truth about Heart Disease?

you should be tested by a doctor, nurse, or other health professional.

3. **True.** A blood pressure of 140/90 mm Hg or greater is generally classified as high blood pressure. However, blood pressures that fall below 140/90 mm Hg can some times be a problem. If the diastolic pressure, the second or lower number, is between 85-89, a person is at increased risk for heart disease or stroke and should have his/her blood pressure checked at least once a year by a health professional. The higher your blood pressure, the greater your risk of developing heart disease or stroke. Controlling high blood pressure reduces your risk.

4. **False.** High blood pressure is more common in blacks than in whites. It affects 29 out of every 100 black adults compared to 26 out of every 100 white adults. Also, with aging, high blood pressure is generally more severe among blacks than among whites, and therefore causes more strokes, heart disease, and kidney failure.

5. **True.** Recent studies show that lifestyle changes can help keep blood pressure levels normal even into advanced age and are important in treating and preventing high blood pressure. Limit high-salt foods which include many snack foods, such as potato chips, salted pretzels, and salted crackers; processed foods, such as canned soups; and condiments, such as ketchup and soy sauce. Also, it is **extremely important** to take blood pressure medication, if prescribed by your doctor, to make sure your blood pressure stays under control.

6. **False.** A total blood cholesterol level of under 200 mg/dL is desirable and usually puts you at a lower risk for heart disease. A blood cholesterol level of 240 mg/dL or above is high and increases your risk of heart disease. If your cholesterol level is high, your doctor will want to check your levels of LDL-cholesterol ("bad" cholesterol) and HDL-cholesterol ("good" cholesterol). A **high** level of LDL-cholesterol increases your risk of heart disease, as does a **low** level of HDL-cholesterol. A cholesterol level of 200-239 mg/dL is considered borderline-high and usually increases your risk for heart disease. If your cholesterol is borderline-high, you should speak to your doctor to see if additional cholesterol tests are needed. All adults 20 years of age or older should have their blood cholesterol level checked at least once every 5 years.

7. **False.** Reducing the amount of cholesterol in your diet is important; however, eating foods low in saturated fat is the most effective dietary way to lower blood cholesterol levels, along with eating less total fat and cholesterol. Choose low-saturated fat foods, such as grains, fruits, and vegetables; low-fat or skim milk and milk products; lean cuts of meat; fish; and chicken. Trim fat from meat before cooking; bake or broil meat rather than fry; use less fat and oil; and take the skin off chicken and turkey. Reducing overweight will also help lower your level of LDL-cholesterol as well as increase your level of HDL-cholesterol.

8. **True.** People who have had one heart attack are at much higher risk for a second attack. Reducing blood cholesterol levels can greatly slow down (and, in some people, even reverse) the buildup of cholesterol and fat in the walls of the coronary arteries and significantly reduce the chances of a second heart attack.

9. **True.** Children from "high risk" families, in which a parent has high blood cholesterol (240 mg/dL or above) or in which a parent or grandparent has had heart disease at an early age (at 55 years of age or younger), should have their cholesterol levels tested. If a child from such a family has a cholesterol level that is high, it should be lowered under medical supervision, primarily with diet, to reduce the risk of developing heart disease as an adult. For most children, who are not from high-risk families, the best way to reduce the risk of adult heart disease is to follow a low-saturated fat, low-cholesterol eating pattern. All children over the age of 2 years and all adults should adopt a heart-healthy eating pattern as a principal way of reducing coronary heart disease.

10. **True.** Heavy smokers are 2 to 4 times more likely to have a heart attack than nonsmokers, and the heart attack death rate among all smokers is 70 percent greater than that of nonsmokers. Older male smokers are also nearly twice as likely to die from stroke than older men who do not smoke, and these odds are nearly as high for older female smokers. Further, the risk of dying of lung cancer is 22 times higher for male smokers than male nonsmokers and 12 times higher for female smokers than female nonsmokers. Finally, 80 percent of all deaths from emphysema and bronchitis are directly due to smoking.

Do You Know the Truth about Heart Disease?

11. **True.** One year after quitting, ex-smokers cut their extra risk for heart attack by about half or more, and eventually the risk will return to normal in healthy ex-smokers. Even if you have already had a heart attack, you can reduce your chances of having a second attack if you quit smoking. Ex-smokers can also reduce their risk of stroke and cancer, improve blood flow and lung function, and help stop diseases like emphysema and bronchitis from getting worse.

12. **False.** Older smokers are more likely to succeed at quitting smoking than younger smokers. Quitting helps relieve smoking-related symptoms like shortness of breath, coughing, and chest pain. Many quit to avoid further health problems and take control of their lives.

13. **True.** Coronary heart disease is the #1 killer in the United States. Approximately 489,000 Americans died of coronary heart disease in 1990, and approximately half of these deaths were women.

Check Your Knowledge about Weight and Heart Disease

The following statements are either true or false. The correct answers are given below.

True or False?

1. Being overweight puts you at risk for heart disease.
2. If you are overweight, losing weight helps lower your high blood cholesterol and high blood pressure.
3. Quitting smoking is healthy, but it commonly leads to excessive weight gain which increases your risk for heart disease.
4. An overweight person with high blood pressure should pay more attention to a low-sodium diet than to weight reduction.
5. A reduced intake of sodium or salt does not always lower high blood pressure to normal.
6. The best way to lose weight is to eat fewer calories and exercise.
7. Skipping meals is a good way to cut down on calories.
8. Foods high in complex carbohydrates (starch and fiber) are good choices when you are trying to lose weight.

9. The single most important change most people can make to lose weight is to avoid sugar.

10. Polyunsaturated fat has the same number of calories as saturated fat.

Answers to Questions in This Section

1. **True.** Being overweight increases your risk for high blood cholesterol and high blood pressure, two of the major risk factors for coronary heart disease. Even if you do not have high blood cholesterol or high blood pressure, being overweight may increase your risk for heart disease. Where you carry your extra weight may affect your risk too. Weight carried at your waist or above seems to be associated with an increased risk for heart disease in many people. In addition, being overweight increases your risk for diabetes, gallbladder disease, and some types of cancer.

2. **True.** If you are overweight, even moderate reductions in weight, such as 5 to 10 percent, can produce substantial reductions in blood pressure. You may also be able to reduce your LDL-cholesterol ("bad" cholesterol) and triglycerides and increase your HDL-cholesterol ("good" cholesterol).

3. **False.** The average weight gain after quitting smoking is 5 pounds. The proportion of ex-smokers who gain large amounts of weight (greater than 20 pounds) is relatively small. Even if you gain weight when you stop smoking, change your eating and exercise habits to lose weight rather than starting to smoke again. Smokers who quit smoking decrease their risk for heart disease by about 50 percent compared to those people who do not quit.

4. **False.** Weight loss, if you are overweight, may reduce your blood pressure even if you don't reduce the amount of sodium you eat. Weight loss is recommended for all overweight people who have high blood pressure. Even if weight loss does not reduce your blood pressure to normal, it may help you cut back on your blood pressure medications. Also, losing weight if you are overweight may help you reduce your risk for or control other health problems.

5. **True.** Even though a high sodium or salt intake plays a key role in maintaining high blood pressure in some people, there

is no easy way to determine who will benefit from eating less sodium and salt. Also, a high intake may limit how well certain high blood pressure medications work. Eating a diet with less sodium may help some people reduce their risk of developing high blood pressure. Most Americans eat more salt and other sources of sodium than they need. Therefore, it is prudent for most people to reduce their sodium intake.

6. **True.** Eating fewer calories and exercising more is the best way to lose weight and keep it off. Weight control is a question of balance. You get calories from the food you eat. You burn off calories by exercising. Cutting down on calories, especially calories from fat, is key to losing weight. Combining this with regular exercise program, like walking, bicycling, jogging, or swimming, not only can help in losing weight but also in maintaining the weight loss. A steady weight loss of 1 to 2 pounds a week is safe for most adults, and the weight is more likely to stay off over the long run. Losing weight, if you are overweight, may also help reduce your blood pressure and raise your HDL-cholesterol, the "good" cholesterol.

7. **False.** To cut calories, some people regularly skip meals and have no snacks or caloric drinks in between. If you do this, your body thinks that it is starving even if your intake of calories is not reduced to a very low amount. Your body will try to save energy by slowing its metabolism, that is decreasing the rate at which it burns calories. This makes losing weight even harder and may even add body fat. Try to avoid long periods without eating. Five or six small meals are often preferred to the usual three meals a day for some individuals trying to lose weight.

8. **True.** Contrary to popular belief, foods high in complex carbohydrates (like pasta, rice, potatoes, breads, cereals, grains, dried beans, and peas) are lower in calories than foods high in fat. In addition, they are good sources of vitamins, minerals, and fiber. What adds calories to these foods is the addition of butter, rich sauces, whole milk, cheese, or cream, which are high in fat.

9. **False.** Sugar has not been found to cause obesity; however, many foods high in sugar are also high in fat. Fat has more than twice the calories as the same amount of protein or carbohydrates (sugar and starch). Thus, foods that are high in fat are high in calories. High-sugar foods, like cakes, cookies, candies,

and ice cream, are high in fat and calories and low in vitamins, minerals, and protein.

10. **True.** All fats—polyunsaturated, monounsaturated, and saturated—have the same number of calories. All calories count whether they come from saturated or unsaturated fats. Because fats are the richest sources of calories, eating less total fat will help reduce the number of calories you eat every day. It will also help you reduce your intake of saturated fat. Particular attention to reducing saturated fat is important in lowering your blood cholesterol level.

Check Your Knowledge about Physical Activity and Heart Disease

The following statements are either true or false. The correct answers are given below.

True or False?

1. Regular physical activity can reduce your chances of getting heart disease.
2. Most people get enough physical activity from their normal daily routine.
3. You don't have to train like a marathon runner to become more physically fit.
4. Exercise programs do not require a lot of time to be very effective.
5. People who need to lose some weight are the only ones who will benefit from regular physical activity.
6. All exercises give you the same benefits.
7. The older you are, the less active you need to be.
8. It doesn't take a lot of money or expensive equipment to become physically fit.
9. There are many risks and injuries that can occur with exercise.
10. You should consult a doctor before starting a physical activity program.

Do You Know the Truth about Heart Disease?

11. People who have had a heart attack should not start any physical activity program.
12. To help stay physically active, include a variety of activities.

Answers to Questions in This Section

1. **True.** Heart disease is almost twice as likely to develop in inactive people. Being physically inactive is a risk factor for heart disease along with cigarette smoking, high blood pressure, high blood cholesterol, and being overweight. The more risk factors you have, the greater your chance for heart disease. Regular physical activity (even mild to moderate exercise) can reduce this risk.

2. **False.** Most Americans are very busy but not very active. Every American adult should make a habit of getting 30 minutes of low to moderate levels of physical activity daily. This includes walking, gardening, and walking up stairs. If you are inactive now, begin by doing a few minutes of activity each day. If you only do some activity every once in a while, try to work something into your routine everyday.

3. **True.** Low- to moderate- intensity activities, such as pleasure walking, stair climbing, yardwork, housework, dancing, and home exercises can have both short- and long-term benefits. If you are inactive, the key is to get started. One great way is to take a walk for 10 to 15 minutes during your lunch break, or take your dog for a walk. At least 30 minutes of physical activity everyday can help improve your heart health.

4. **True.** It takes only a few minutes a day to become more physically active. If you don't have 30 minutes in your schedule for an exercise break, find two 15-minute periods or even three 10-minute periods. These exercise breaks will soon become a habit you can't live without.

5. **False.** People who are physically active experience many positive benefits. Regular physical activity gives you more energy, reduces stress, and helps you to sleep better. It helps to lower high blood pressure and improves blood cholesterol levels. Physical activity helps to tone your muscles, burns off calories to help you lose extra pounds or stay at your desirable weight, and helps control your appetite. It can also increase muscle

strength, help your heart and lungs work more efficiently, and let you enjoy your life more fully.

6. **False.** Low-intensity activities—if performed daily—can have some long-term health benefits and can lower your risk of heart disease. Regular, brisk, and sustained exercise for at least 30 minutes, three to four times a week, such as brisk walking, jogging, or swimming, is necessary to improve the efficiency of your heart and lungs and burn off extra calories. These activities are called aerobic—meaning the body uses oxygen to produce the energy needed for the activity. Other activities, depending on the type, may give you other benefits such as increased flexibility or muscle strength.

7. **False.** Although we tend to become less active with age, physical activity is still important. In fact, regular physical activity in older persons increases their capacity to do everyday activities. In general, middle-aged and older people benefit from regular physical activity just as young people do. What is important, at any age, is tailoring the activity program to your own fitness level.

8. **True.** Many activities require little or no equipment. For example, brisk walking only requires a comfortable pair of walking shoes. Many communities offer free or inexpensive recreation facilities and physical activity classes. Check shopping malls, as many of them are open early and late for people who do not wish to walk alone, in the dark, or in bad weather.

9. **False.** The most common risk in exercising is injury to the muscles and joints. Such injuries are usually caused by exercising too hard for too long, particularly if a person has been inactive. To avoid injuries, try to build up your level of activity gradually, listen to your body for warning pains, be aware of possible signs of heart problems (such as pain or pressure in the left or mid-chest area, left neck, shoulder, or arm during or just after exercising, or sudden light-headedness, cold sweat, pallor, or fainting), and be prepared for special weather conditions.

10. **True.** You should ask your doctor before you start (or greatly increase) your physical activity if you have a medical condition such as high blood pressure, have pains or pressure in the chest and shoulder, feel dizzy or faint, get breathless after

Do You Know the Truth about Heart Disease?

mild exertion, are middle-aged or older and have not been physically active, or plan a vigorous activity program. If none of these apply, start slow and get moving.

11. **False.** Regular, physical activity can help reduce your risk of having another heart attack. People who include regular physical activity in their lives after a heart attack improve their chances of survival and can improve how they feel and look. If you have had a heart attack, consult your doctor to be sure you are following a safe and effective exercise program that will help prevent heart pain and further damage from overexertion.

12. **True.** Pick several different activities that you like doing. You will be more likely to stay with it. Plan short-term and long-term goals. Keep a record of your progress, and check it regularly to see the progress you have made. Get your family and friends to join in. They can help keep you going.

Chapter 2

Trends in Ischemic Heart Disease

In 1994, a total of 481,458 persons died as a result of ischemic heart disease (IHD), which comprises two thirds of all heart disease—the leading cause of death in the United States. This report presents trends in IHD mortality in the United States for 1990-1994 (the latest year for which data are available) and compares these trends by race, sex, and state. These findings indicate IHD death rates decreased from 1990 through 1994; however, the rate of decline was slower than rates of previously observed declines.

Age-adjusted IHD death rates for persons aged 35 years or more were calculated using mortality data tapes compiled by CDC and population estimates from the Bureau of the Census. IHD death rates were directly age-adjusted to the 1980 U.S. standard population aged 35 years or more. IHD deaths were defined as those with the underlying cause of death listed on the death certificate as *International Classification of Diseases, Ninth Revision (ICD-9)*, codes 410–414.9. The average annual percentage change in IHD mortality from 1990 through 1994 was calculated as the 1994 rate minus the 1990 rate divided by the 1990 rate divided by 4 multiplied by 100. Data are presented only for blacks and whites because numbers for other racial/ethnic groups were too small for meaningful analysis.

From 1990 through 1994, age-adjusted IHD death rates for the U.S. population aged 35 years or more decreased 10.3%, from 416.3

Centers for Disease Control and Prevention (CDC), *Morbidity and Mortality Weekly Report*, February 21, 1997, vol. 46 no. 7 p. 146(5).

Heart Diseases and Disorders Sourcebook, Second Edition

deaths per 100,000 to 373.6 deaths per 100,000. However, the rate of decrease varied by race and sex; rates of decline were faster for whites than for blacks and for men than for women (Figure 2.1). The largest average annual percentage decrease occurred among white men (2.9%

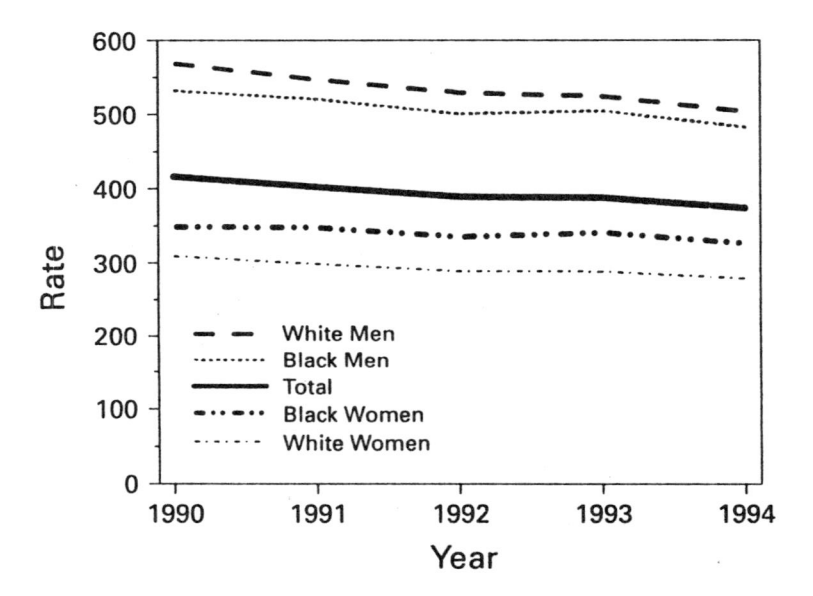

Figure 2.1. Age-adjusted death rate* of ischemic heart disease[†] for adults aged 35 years or more, by race[§] and sex—United States, 1990–1994.

*Per 100,000 population, adjusted to the 1980 U.S. standard population.
[†]International Classification of Diseases, Ninth Revision, codes 410–414.9.
[§]Data are presented only for blacks and whites because numbers for other racial/ethnic groups were too small for meaningful analysis.

per year), followed by white women (2.5%), black men (2.3%), and black women (1.6%).

IHD death rates varied substantially among the states (Table 2.1). In 1994, the rates for both women and men residing in the states with the highest IHD death rates were approximately two times higher than for persons residing in the states with the lowest IHD death rates. For women, IHD death rates in 1994 ranged from 156.7 per 100,000 (Montana) to 406.3 per 100,000 (New York) and, for men, ranged from 289.4 per 100,000 (New Mexico) to 638.8 per 100,000 (New York).

From 1990 through 1994, IHD death rates declined in nearly all 50 states and the District of Columbia (Table 2.1). However, the magnitude of change over time varied widely; some states had small declines (e.g., Nevada, 0.1% per year and Hawaii, 0.9% per year) while other states experienced larger declines (e.g., Alaska, 5.5% per year and Montana, 5.6% per year). Sex-specific IHD death rates for both men and women declined for each state except Idaho and Nevada (small increase for women only) and the District of Columbia (small increase for men only).

Editorial Note [in original]: The findings in this report indicate that, for persons aged 35 years or more, age-adjusted IHD death rates decreased during 1990-1994; however, the magnitude of decline varied by race, sex, and state and was slower than the decline that occurred during the 1980s.[1] During 1980-1988, IHD death rates declined an average of 3.0% per year, and during 1990-1994, declined an average of 2.6%. The slowing of the decline in IHD death rates was first observed in the mid-1970s for black women, black men, and white women.[2] The initial declines in IHD death rates occurred during the 1960s, when rates declined steadily for each racial/sex group. The earliest declines in rates occurred in metropolitan areas, especially those located in the Northeast and Pacific West and in communities with higher levels of socioeconomic development (as reflected by occupational, educational, and income profiles of these communities).[3,4]

Factors contributing to the differential levels and rates of decline in IHD death rates by race, sex, and state may include differences in 1) trends in socioeconomic and behavioral risk factors for IHD, 2) access to quality health care, and 3) geographic and temporal variation in the medical certification of IHD. Previous reports indicate that IHD death rates vary inversely with social, economic, and medical resources.[5,6] Higher levels of community resources contribute to declines in IHD death rates by providing or increasing opportunities for community members to have access to low-fat and high-fiber foods; engage in leisure-time physical activity; quit smoking; and receive medical care for treatment of other conditions and risk factors, including hypertension, hypercholesterolemia, and diabetes. For example, in 1988, the prevalence of leisure-time physical inactivity in 37 states correlated positively with IHD death rates,[7] and in 1960, per capita cigarette sales in 44 states also correlated directly with IHD mortality.[8]

Table 2.1. Age-adjusted death rate* of ischemic heart disease† for adults aged 35 years or more, by year, and average annual percentage change in rate from 1990, to 1994, by sex and state—United States.

State	Women 1990	Women 1994	Women % Change from 1990 to 1994	Men 1990	Men 1994	Men % Change from 1990 to 1994	Total 1990	Total 1994	Total % Change from 1990 to 1994
Alabama	263.8	231.3	-3.1	510.1	448.3	-3.1	366.9	321.9	-3.1
Alaska	197.6	189.3	-1.1	491.5	345.7	-7.4	338.3	263.9	-5.5
Arizona	273.1	237.6	-3.2	504.1	428.5	-3.7	375.7	324.1	-3.4
Arkansas	321.8	304.5	-1.3	592.5	567.7	-1.0	437.8	420.9	-1.0
California	306.4	280.1	-2.1	505.9	456.7	-2.4	392.2	356.5	-2.3
Colorado	246.3	189.6	-5.8	467.8	368.9	-5.3	341.6	266.2	-5.5
Connecticut	262.0	235.1	-2.6	453.6	405.5	-2.7	341.9	306.9	-2.6
Delaware	292.7	253.9	-3.3	493.5	463.2	-1.5	378.0	343.4	-2.3
District of Columbia	199.2	177.8	-2.7	313.6	348.3	2.8	245.6	243.7	-0.2
Florida	288.5	269.5	-1.6	528.7	477.7	-2.4	393.2	361.0	-2.0
Georgia	289.4	254.0	-3.1	548.2	478.9	-3.2	395.0	346.1	-3.1
Hawaii	189.1	173.9	-2.0	307.8	305.5	-0.2	244.6	235.8	-0.9
Idaho	235.3	239.6	0.5	486.4	418.1	-3.5	346.3	320.4	-1.9
Indiana	342.7	315.4	-2.0	581.0	538.0	-1.9	440.9	408.7	-1.8
Illinois	338.4	305.9	-2.4	630.8	555.5	-3.0	459.1	410.2	-2.7
Iowa	271.3	252.2	-1.8	535.9	491.4	-2.1	380.8	353.3	-1.8
Kansas	270.2	234.0	-3.3	529.9	452.5	-3.7	378.6	326.6	-3.4
Kentucky	326.4	300.5	-2.0	635.0	585.0	-2.0	455.3	420.0	-1.9
Louisiana	341.2	276.5	-4.7	597.2	498.4	-4.1	449.3	369.0	-4.5
Maine	294.9	268.0	-2.3	554.8	474.2	-3.6	404.2	356.7	-2.9
Maryland	247.0	226.3	-2.1	430.8	393.0	-2.2	323.4	296.6	-2.1
Massachusetts	282.4	243.6	-3.4	524.6	446.3	-3.7	381.9	327.8	-3.5
Michigan	358.1	316.8	-2.9	612.8	527.2	-3.5	466.0	406.8	-3.2
Minnesota	242.1	194.8	-4.9	518.9	423.8	-4.6	358.3	293.0	-4.6
Mississippi	292.4	281.6	-0.9	557.1	510.7	-2.1	404.2	379.1	-1.6
Missouri	339.4	327.7	-0.9	632.6	569.5	-2.5	460.2	428.9	-1.7
Montana	215.5	156.7	-6.8	454.5	367.2	-4.8	321.3	249.9	-5.6
Nebraska	244.1	208.9	-3.6	501.5	442.0	-3.0	351.2	307.3	-3.1
Nevada	216.8	224.3	0.9	401.8	383.1	-1.2	299.8	299.0	-0.1
New Hampshire	266.8	249.3	-1.6	529.5	461.6	-3.2	376.1	338.2	-2.5

18

Trends in Ischemic Heart Disease

State									
New Jersey	340.7	300.5	-2.9	576.7	514.5	-2.7	439.1	390.6	-2.8
New Mexico	198.5	162.7	-4.5	331.3	289.4	-3.2	258.9	218.3	-3.9
New York	425.0	406.3	-1.1	698.9	638.8	-2.1	537.2	502.0	-1.6
North Carolina	307.1	274.0	-2.7	609.8	544.8	-2.7	431.7	385.4	-2.7
North Dakota	235.9	229.4	-0.7	534.8	484.5	-2.4	367.1	340.2	-1.8
Ohio	344.3	307.8	-2.7	629.7	553.8	-3.0	461.3	410.5	-2.8
Oklahoma	337.6	307.8	-2.2	648.4	602.0	-1.8	468.1	434.0	-1.8
Oregon	264.2	216.2	-4.5	529.9	425.8	-4.9	378.7	307.9	-4.7
Pennsylvania	321.4	296.1	-2.0	577.8	506.9	-3.1	427.5	384.9	-2.5
Rhode Island	323.9	288.4	-2.7	584.4	535.3	-2.1	426.9	391.1	-2.1
South Carolina	315.2	288.3	-2.1	583.1	528.5	-2.3	427.6	388.4	-2.3
South Dakota	283.7	243.3	-3.6	576.3	522.8	-2.3	409.7	366.8	-2.6
Tennessee	326.0	310.6	-1.2	643.0	582.9	-2.3	456.7	422.2	-1.9
Texas	289.8	270.2	-1.7	538.0	482.8	-2.6	394.8	361.0	-2.1
Utah	201.2	175.7	-3.2	377.3	346.2	-2.1	277.6	251.5	-2.4
Vermont	255.4	226.3	-2.8	483.9	468.9	-0.8	354.9	330.5	-1.7
Virginia	275.4	236.9	-3.5	511.1	452.5	-2.9	373.9	326.7	-3.2
Washington	234.6	199.3	-3.8	444.0	388.3	-3.1	325.3	282.7	-3.3
West Virginia	337.8	307.8	-2.2	626.8	537.9	-3.5	458.0	404.7	-2.9
Wisconsin	306.8	255.9	-4.1	579.0	499.5	-3.4	422.8	360.4	-3.7
Wyoming	216.7	208.9	-0.9	495.5	435.4	-3.0	335.3	310.4	-1.9
Total	**311.7**	**281.8**	**-2.4**	**560.4**	**497.8**	**-2.8**	**416.3**	**373.6**	**-2.6**

*Per 100,000 population, adjusted to the 1980 U.S. standard population.
†International Classification of Diseases, Ninth Revision, codes 410–414.9.

These findings indicate the potential for reducing state-specific IHD death rates through statewide promotion of public health policies and legislation that encourages and enables healthy living and working conditions.

Strategies for further reducing the substantial burden of IHD mortality in all states should include improving understanding of the socioeconomic, behavioral, and medical determinants of state variation in IHD death rates. The slowing of declines in IHD death rates underscores the need for innovative approaches to the prevention of IHD, and the intensification of current programs and policies that promote widespread accessibility and adoption of low-fat and high-fiber foods; incentives for smoking cessation; opportunities for leisure-time physical activity/and use of medical-care resources to prevent hypertension, diabetes, and hypercholesterolemia.

References

1. CDC. Trends in ischemic heart disease mortality—United States, 1980-1988. *MMWR* 1992; 41:548-9,555-6.

2. Sempos C, Cooper R, Kovar MG, McMillen M. Divergence of the recent trends in coronary mortality for the four major race-sex groups in the United States. *Am J Public Health* 1988; 78:1422-7.

3. Wing S, Casper M, Riggan W, Hayes C, Tyroler HA. Socioenvironmental characteristics associated with the onset of decline of ischemic heart disease mortality in the United States. *Am J Public Health* 1988; 78:923-6.

4. Wing S, Barnett E, Casper M, Tyroler HA. Geographic and socioeconomic variation in the onset of decline of coronary heart disease mortality in white women. *Am J Public Health* 1992; 82:204-9.

5. Wing S, Dargent-Molina P, Casper M, Riggan W, Hayes C, Tyroler HA. Changing association between community occupational structure and ischaemic heart disease mortality in the United States. *Lancet* 1987; 2:1067-70.

6. Ingram DD, Gillum RF. Regional and urbanization differentials in coronary heart disease mortality in the United States, 1968-85. *J Clin Epidemiol* 1989; 42:857-68.

7. Yeager KK, Anda RF, Macera CA, Donehoo RS, Eaker ED. Sedentary lifestyle and state variation in coronary heart disease mortality. *Public Health Rep* 1995; 110:100-2.

8. Friedman GD. Cigarette smoking an geographic variation in coronary heart disease mortality in the United States. *Journal of Chronic Diseases* 1967; 20:769-79.

Chapter 3

Congestive Heart Failure in the United States: A New Epidemic

An estimated 4.8 million Americans have congestive heart failure (CHF). Increasing prevalence, hospitalizations, and deaths have made CHF a major chronic condition in the United States. It often is the end stage of cardiac disease. Half of the patients diagnosed with CHF will be dead within 5 years.

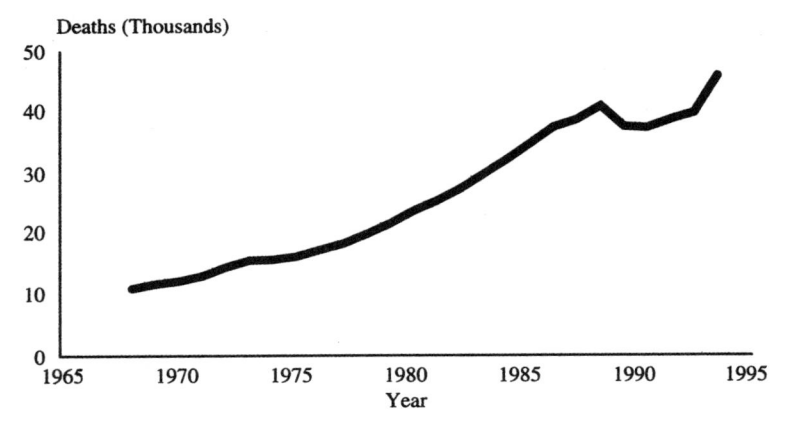

ICD Code 428.0.
The sharp drop occurring in 1989 is attributed to revision of the death certificate.
Source: Vital Statistics of the United States, National Center for Health Statistics.

Figure 3.1. *Deaths From Congestive Heart Failure, 1968 to 1993.*

National Heart, Lung, and Blood Institute (NHLBI), Data Fact Sheet, September 1996.

Heart Diseases and Disorders Sourcebook, Second Edition

Each year, there are an estimated 400,000 new cases. The annual number of deaths directly from CHF increased from 10,000 in 1968 to 42,000 in 1993 (Figure 3.1.), with another 219,000 related to the condition.

CHF is the first-listed diagnosis in 875,000 hospitalizations, and the most common diagnosis in hospital patients age 65 years and older. In that age group, one-fifth of all hospitalizations have a primary or secondary diagnosis of heart failure.

Visits to physicians' offices for CHF increased from 1.7 million in 1980 to 2.9 million in 1993. More than 65,000 persons with CHF receive home care each year. In 1993, an estimated $17.8 billion was spent for the care of CHF patients in hospitals, physicians' offices, home care, and nursing homes as well as for medication.

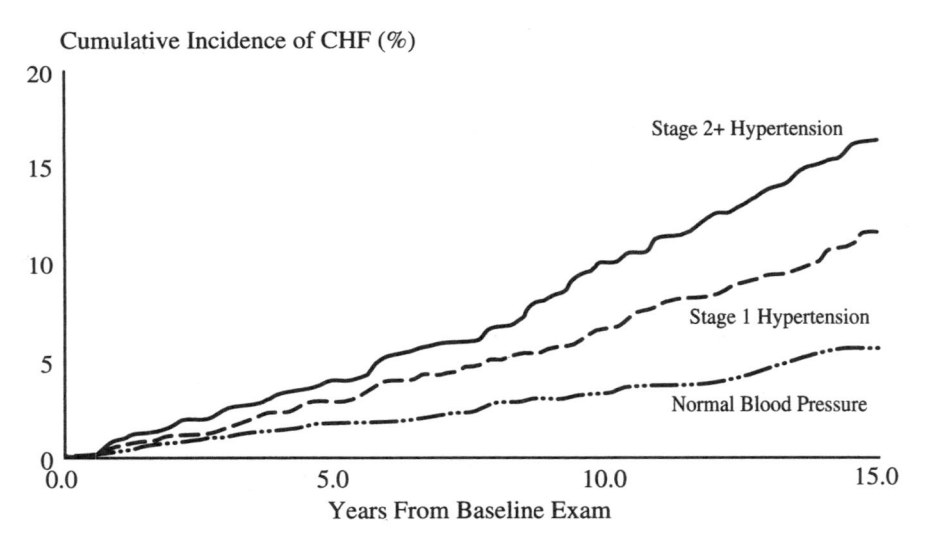

Note: Hypertension is defined as systolic blood pressure (SBP) of 140 mm Hg or greater or diastolic blood pressure (DBP) of 90 mm Hg or greater or taking antihypertensive medication. Stage 1 hypertension is defined as SBP of 140 to 159 mm Hg or DBP of 90 to 99 mm Hg in people not receiving antihypertensive medication; stage 2 or greater hypertension (stage 2+) is defined as SBP of 160 or greater, DBP of 100 or greater, or current use of antihypertensive medication.

Source: Framingham Heart Study, National Heart, Lung, and Blood Institute.

Figure 3.2. Incidence of CHF in Men and Women Age 50 to 79, by Hypertension Status.

Congestive Heart Failure in the United States: A New Epidemic

The financial and other losses of caregivers for these patients are large as well.

The magnitude of the problem of CHF is large now, but it is expected to get much worse because:

- As more and more cardiac patients are able to survive and live longer with their disease, their opportunity for developing CHF increases.
- Future growth in the elderly population will likely result in increasing numbers of persons with this condition regardless of trends in coronary disease morbidity and mortality.

Incidence

Incidence data on congestive heart failure are not available on a national basis. The following estimates are from the study in Framingham, Massachusetts, funded by the National Heart, Lung, and Blood Institute. Incidence of CHF is equally frequent in men and women, and annual incidence approaches 10 per 1,000 population after 65 years of age. Incidence is twice as common in persons with hypertension compared with normotensive persons (Figure 3.2.) and five times greater in persons who have had a heart attack compared to persons who have not (Figure 3.3.).

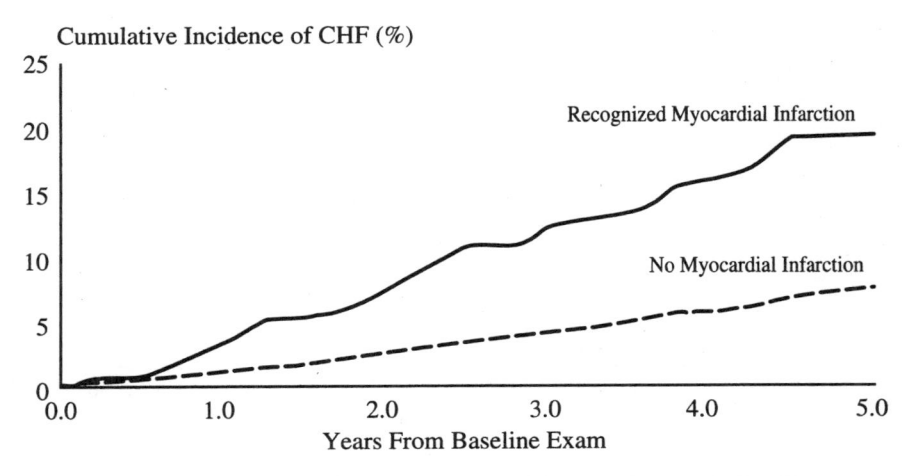

Source: Cardiovascular Health Study, National Heart, Lung, and Blood Institute.

Figure 3.3. *Incidence of CHF, by Myocardial Infarction Status.*

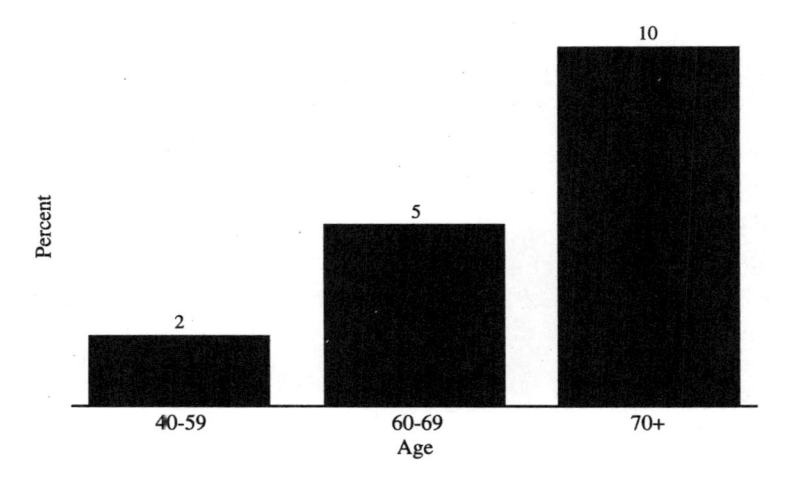

Heart Diseases and Disorders Sourcebook, Second Edition

Source: National Health and Nutrition Examination Survey (1988-91), National Center for Health Statistics.

Figure 3.4. Prevalence of CHF, by Age, 1988-91.

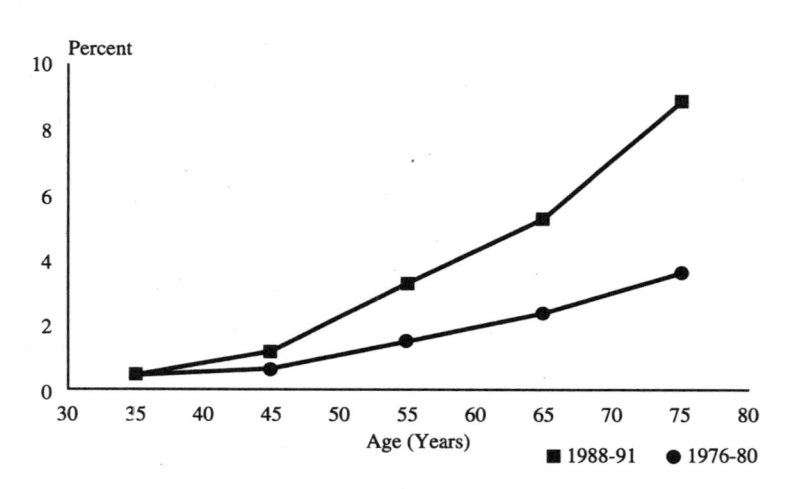

Source: National Health and Nutrition Examination Survey (1976-80 and 1988-91), National Center for Health Statistics.

Figure 3.5. Prevalence of CHF, by Age, 1976-80 and 1988-91.

Congestive Heart Failure in the United States: A New Epidemic

Prevalence

According to the National Health and Nutrition Examination Surveys, an estimated 4.8 million Americans have congestive heart failure, with approximately equal numbers of men and women. Almost 1.4 million are under 60 years of age. CHF is present in 2 percent of persons age 40 to 59, more than 5 percent of persons age 60 to 69, and 10 percent of persons age 70 and older (Figure 3.4.). Prevalence is at least 25 percent greater among the black population than among the white population. Prevalence at each age increased substantially between two periods surveyed nationally: 1976-80 and 1988-91 (Figure 3.5.).

Hospitalizations

The rate of hospitalizations for heart failure increased more than three times between 1970 and 1994 at age 45 to 64 and age 65 and older, with a large absolute increase in the older age group (Figure 3.6). In 1994, CHF was the first-listed discharge diagnosis in 874,000 hospital discharges (alive or dead) and a secondary diagnosis in another 1.8 million discharges. One in five of all discharged patients age 65 and older had CHF as a primary or secondary diagnosis. The percent-

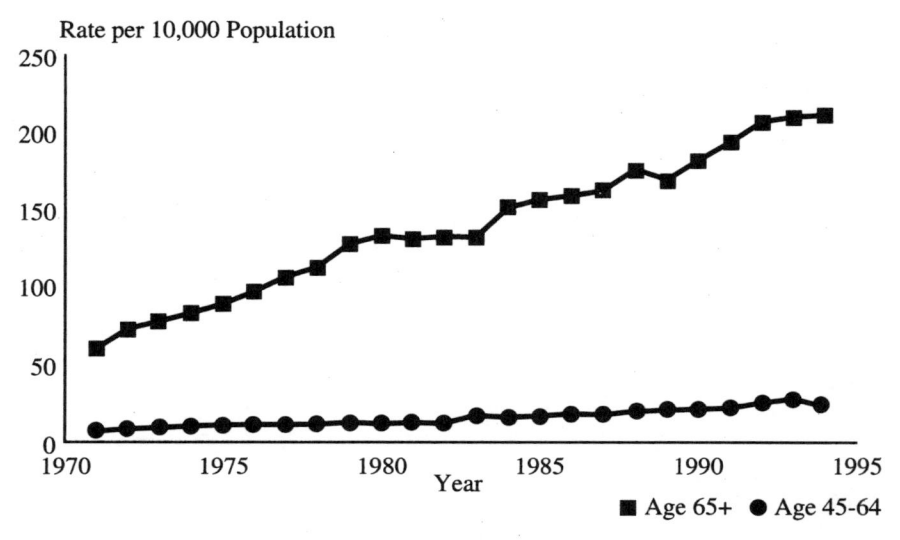

Source: National Hospital Discharge Survey, National Center for Health Statistics.

Figure 3.6. Hospitalization Rates for CHF, by Age, 1971 to 1994.

age of CHF patients discharged dead from hospitals, however, decreased from 11.3 percent in 1981 to 6.1 percent in 1993. This trend is seen for persons age 45 to 64 and for those age 65 and older (Figure 3.7.).

Prognosis

Survival following diagnosis of congestive heart failure is worse in men than women, but even in women, only about 20 percent survive much longer than 8 to 12 years. The outlook is not much better than for most forms of cancer. The fatality rate for CHF is high, with one in five persons dying within 1 year. Sudden death is common in these patients, occurring at a rate of six to nine times that of the general population. Thus, CHF remains a highly lethal condition. With the use of angiotensin-converting enzyme (ACE) inhibitors as a possible exception, advances in the treatment of hypertension, myocardial ischemia, and valvular heart disease have not resulted in substantial improvements in survival once CHF ensues.

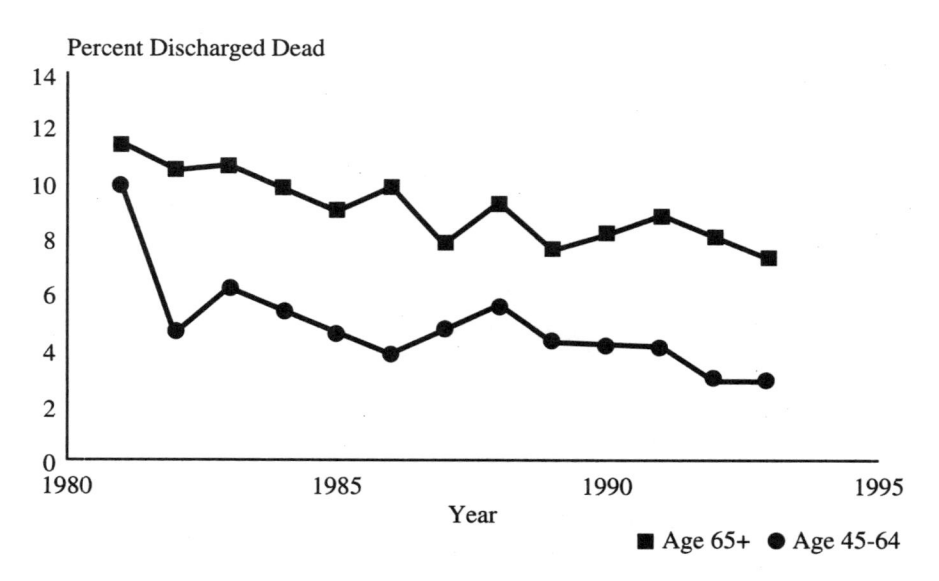

Source: National Hospital Discharge Survey, National Center for Health Statistics.

Figure 3.7. Percent of Hospitalized CHF Patients Discharged Dead, by Age, 1981 to 1993.

Congestive Heart Failure in the United States: A New Epidemic

Mortality

The death rate for congestive heart failure increased most years between 1968 and 1993 (Figure 3.1.). These increases are in contrast to mortality declines for most heart and blood vessel diseases. In 1993, there were 42,000 deaths where CHF was identified as the primary cause of death and another 219,000 deaths where it was listed as a secondary cause on the death certificate. The death rate for CHF in 1993 was nearly 1.5 times higher in black men and women than in white men and women (Figure 3.8.).

Research

The National Heart, Lung, and Blood Institute (NHLBI) supports a wide range of basic, clinical, and epidemiological research to better understand the causes and improve the prevention, diagnosis, and treatment of CHF. The studies include investigations of how the heart contracts normally and what goes wrong in CHF, the development of new drug therapies and other innovative treatments of CHF, and ways to better detect the condition in those at a high risk of CHF.

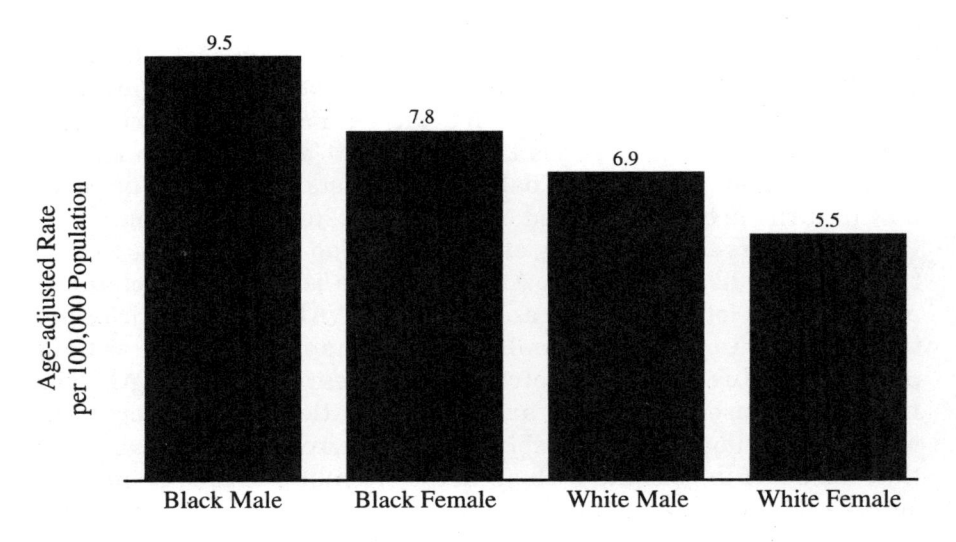

Source: Vital Statistics of the United States, National Center for Health Statistics.

Figure 3.8. *Death Rates for CHF, by Race and Sex, 1993.*

Some studies are trying to stop the loss of cell function that happens in CHF. Muscle cells die or no longer function properly, which causes the heart to lose its ability to pump blood. In studies on animals, researchers have begun inserting healthy muscle cells into a failing heart to replace damaged cells. Results so far have been promising: The grafted cells appear to thrive and function normally. This animal research has shown that the grafted cells can even come from muscles other than the heart, such as muscles of the leg. Furthermore, it may be possible to genetically engineer grafted cells to make them stronger.

Other studies are developing drugs with multiple actions to treat CHF. Such a drug would have several effects. For example, a drug might improve the heart's pumping ability, open clogged arteries, and prevent tissue damage from free radicals, a by product of the body's metabolic processes. Free radicals are thought to contribute to the development of atherosclerosis. One of these multiple-acting drugs has already been tested and appears not only to lengthen survival but also to improve symptoms for those with CHF.

Investigations also are being done to improve heart transplantation for CHF patients. In some cases, a heart transplant is the only possible treatment. However, such patients face a shortage of donor hearts. A possible solution to this critical shortage may be the use of a heart from other animals. Called xenotransplantation, this procedure once was made difficult because of the rejection of the heart by the CHF patient's immune system. However, new technologies have been forged that can overcome such a barrier. For example, scientists have been able to alter genes in the heart of a pig to diminish the immune system reaction in a baboon. Scientists still need to discover how to turn such genes on and off to prevent human rejection.

Researchers are continuing efforts to develop better devices to help the damaged heart function. Already in use is a small mechanical pump called a left ventricular assist device (LVAD). The ventricles are the heart's main pumping chambers. These chambers enlarge as CHF progresses. Muscle fibers stretch, and the heart loses strength. The LVAD is now used as a temporary assist for patients with severe CHF who are awaiting a heart transplant. However, researchers have found that the heart in patients with an LVAD often improves after months of use—so much that a transplant is no longer needed. Thus, efforts are under way to identify patients who may benefit from a longer-term LVAD.

Through its national education efforts, the NHLBI is working to prevent CHF too, especially through the early detection and aggressive

Congestive Heart Failure in the United States: A New Epidemic

treatment of high blood pressure and heart attack—the two leading causes of CHF. New drug therapies, better diagnosis, speedier therapies are lessening those conditions' impact on the heart.

Additional Information

For more information, contact:

NHLBI Information Center
P.O. Box 30105
Bethesda, MD 20824-0105
(301) 251-1222

Chapter 4

Gender Differences in Heart Disease

Despite the common view that it is a male health problem, heart disease kills more women than men in America.[1] As a woman ages, the risk of heart attack increases as does the likelihood of death and disability from heart attack. The advances in prevention, diagnosis, treatment, and rehabilitation associated with better outcomes have been developed on research whose sampling bias has favored male subjects. Although the disease is an equal opportunity killer, women may not equally have access to or benefit from the prevention, early diagnosis, treatment, and rehabilitation strategies that have helped so many men.[2]

Primary care practitioners can reduce the needless death and disability that result from this traditional gender bias. Health promotion interventions geared toward risk identification, awareness, and reduction are at least as important as the routine screening tests.[3-4] Astute practitioners can recognize subtle changes in the presentation of angina, or atypical symptoms that signal a myocardial infarction (MI) or unstable angina in women. Further, primary care practitioners are in a position to help women gain access to the same appropriate testing, referrals, treatment, and follow-up care that men receive.

Original title: "Women and Heart Attacks: Prevention, Diagnosis, and Care." Used with permission from P.M. Arnstein, E.F. Busselli, and S.H. Rankin, *The Nurse Practitioner*, May 1996, Volume 21, Number 5, page 57-69. © Springhouse Corporation.

Magnitude of the Problem

Cardiovascular disease is the leading cause of death in America, regardless of gender. For women, it accounts for 2.5 million hospitalizations and half a million deaths a year.[2] There is growing evidence that once in the hospital, women receive substandard care more often than men.[5-7] Women can suffer an MI at any stage of adult life, although on average they are 10 years older than their male counterparts. Women narrow the gap after menopause, and by age 75 the incidence of coronary heart disease in women exceeds that of men.[1,6]

Part of the reason women are believed to have fewer heart attacks is that they are often not diagnosed when an MI has occurred. Of those in the Framingham Study who have had heart attacks, 38% of women (compared with 27% of men) had an MI that went unrecognized.[3] The predictive value of the standard diagnostic tests are lower in women[2] and once diagnosed, they are often treated less aggressively.[8] Death rates for women after MI are higher than for men, whether the death occurs in the hospital,[7,9] within 6 months,[10-11] at 1 year,[12] or in the years that follow.[13-14] These studies indicate that women have a three-times higher death rate than men both in the hospital and at 1 year after an MI. Those women who do survive are more likely to be disabled or unable to participate in cardiac rehabilitation programs.[2]

Primary Prevention

Nonmodifiable Risks

Advancing age, race, and family history are considered nonmodifiable risk factors. The current cardiopulmonary resuscitation (CPR) courses that are widely taught to lay and professional groups still list the male gender as a nonmodifiable risk factor;[15] this may foster an unwarranted sense of security in women.

Age is considered a powerful independent risk factor for the increased incidence, morbidity, and mortality associated with MI, regardless of gender.[5,10,12-13, 16-17] In fact, many investigators have discounted the presence of a gender bias because, when the influence of age is removed, the differences between men and women are reportedly insignificant.[10,12,17-18] Other investigators confirm that despite differences in age, the female gender is a significant predictor of death and disability from heart attacks.[5,9,13,16]

Race has been associated with relative risk of heart disease prevalence and mortality. African-Americans have a higher prevalence of heart disease than whites. African-American women have the highest rate of nonfatal types of coronary disease, with twice the rate of angina as white women and five times that of white men.[19] African-American women have close to a 50% mortality rate from MI, nearly double that of African-American men, compared with 32% for white women and 23% mortally for white men.[20] Among Asian-Americans, South Asians have a higher relative risk (3.7 times), and Chinese have a lower (0.6 times) relative risk of ischemic heart disease when compared with whites. However, after emigrating to America, Japanese, Filipinos, and other Asian-Americans had comparable risks of ischemic heart disease as whites.[21] This raises questions whether this risk is related to race, ethnicity, culture, or diet.

Family history of an MI by a first-degree relative is considered an important risk factor.[15] A large-scale longitudinal study indicated that this risk is significant only as a predictor of premature (before age 55) coronary heart disease, and is a stronger predictor among women than men.[22] First-degree relatives of women who died from coronary heart disease before age 55 were more than five times as likely to have early coronary disease than control family members. Their daughters incurred nearly twice the risk of coronary heart disease than their sons.[23] Despite knowledge of familial risks, their progeny have failed to engage in risk-reduction behavior.[24]

Modifiable Risk Factors

Primary care practitioners can positively influence health in the area of modifiable risk factors, including lifestyle changes, cholesterol reduction, co-morbidity management, and attention to psychosocial factors.

Lifestyle. Lifestyle modification of risks (e.g., diet, exercise, and smoking) is considered to be as important as the dramatic treatment advances during the 1970s in explaining the decline of morbidity and mortality from MIs in the past 2 decades.[25] Cigarette smoking (including passive smoking), however, is the greatest single cause of preventable death in America.[15] Women who have heart attacks before age 40 are almost always smokers and older women who smoke are at five-times greater risk for sudden death than women who don't smoke.[6] Women who stop smoking can realize a 50% to 80% reduction in their risk of coronary disease within 5 years of quitting.[26]

Smoking-related risks are compounded for young women when other risk factors (e.g., obesity or sedentary lifestyle) are present or when estrogen is being used for contraception.[27-29] The effects of smoking, which increases platelet aggregability, fibrinogen activity,[30] cholesterol levels, and triglyceride levels,[31] increase the woman's risk of both heart attack and stroke. Despite the known risks associated with cigarette smoke, more young women smoke today than young men, possibly because smoking is used to control weight.[6]

Women with more upper body fat (as measured by waist to hip ratio) are at greater risk for heart disease. Wing and associates question whether this is a direct effect or related to other known risk factors.[28] High correlations were found between women with more upper body fat and such factors as higher blood pressure, cholesterol, anxiety, anger, depression, and smoking. Upper body fat is also associated with lower levels of high-density lipoprotein and less perceived social support. These factors remain significant even after controlling for body mass.[28] The primary care practitioner should discuss the known risks with all women, regardless of their "apple, pear, or carrot shape," to identify opportunities for improvement, set goals, and reinforce healthy lifestyle patterns. Weight loss, a low-fat diet, smoking cessation, stress management, and regular exercise make up the healthy lifestyle that is believed to reduce cardiac risk, primarily by significantly reducing serum cholesterol.[32]

Cholesterol. Lipid abnormalities influence coronary artery disease development in both men and women. Holme analyzed 19 research reports, each with 100 to 50,000 people studied. His analysis found that each 1% reduction in cholesterol corresponded to a 2% reduction in the risk of cardiac disease.[32] More than two-thirds of those studies excluded women despite known gender differences, and thus the extent of benefit women realize by reducing their cholesterol remains unclear. Of the observational studies done on women, 90% indicate that as total cholesterol rises, so does the risk of coronary heart disease,[26] supporting the importance of managing cholesterol levels in women.

Early in life women have higher high-density lipoprotein (HDL) levels and lower low-density lipoprotein (LDL) levels than men, both of which are strongly associated with a lower risk of heart attacks.[26,33] At menopause, however, women's LDLs and triglyceride levels generally increase, so that by age 55 they exceed those of men. These increases are strong independent risk factors for heart attacks in women.[26,34]

Menopause is believed to affect lipids by decreasing circulation of women's own estrogens. Before menopause however, estrogen-containing oral contraceptives raise cholesterol, LDLs, and triglycerides while lowering HDLs.[33,35] These undesired effects are similar to changes in lipids noted by premenopausal smokers.[31] The relative risk of having a heart attack as the result of taking oral contraceptives is believed insignificant, unless the women also smoke.[26] After menopause, oral estrogen has the desired effect of raising HDLs and lowering LDLs.[33] Hormone replacement therapy using estrogen, with or without added progestin, has been shown to significantly reduce the risk of coronary disease in large-scale studies representing geographically and culturally diverse groups of postmenopausal women.[27,36-39] A review of over 30 observational studies suggests that replacement estrogen increases HDLs and reduces LDLs by as much as 15%, resulting in a 44% reduction in the risk of coronary heart disease in women after menopause.[26]

Studies done predominantly on men suggest that serum cholesterol levels can be reduced by as much as 20% by diet, weight loss, and exercise.[40] These methods are less effective in lowering cholesterol for women than men;[41] thus estrogen replacement therapy may be used in combination with these lifestyle changes to reduce or delay the need for lipid-lowering drugs.

Co-morbidities. Co-morbidities that increase the risk of MI in women include hypertension, hyperlipidemia, diabetes, congestive heart failure, and obesity.[6,14,16] Although the risks of developing coronary artery disease with hyperthyroidism have not been calculated, generalized cardiac effects of this primarily female disease are known. Co-morbidities such as arthritis, peptic ulcer, or chronic lung disease do not have known relationships to heart disease; however, their symptoms may contribute to delays or a missed diagnosis when a heart attack has occurred.

Hypertension and hyperlipidemia are the most consistent risk factors for predicting cardiovascular diseases in women over 35 years old.[14] Of the women who had heart attacks, 29% were found to have preexisting angina, diabetes, or hypertension. Those with diabetes are at particularly high risk for dying if they do have a heart attack.[25] This association with preexisting heart disease or other co-morbidities is significantly stronger in women than men.[6,17-18,42-43] It is assumed that effective management (secondary prevention) of these disorders will reduce the related risk.

Psychosocial factors. Psychosocial factors are believed to contribute to heart disease. The extent that stress contributes to heart disease in women is not currently clear. The psychosocial profile for women is not the high-status, high-stress picture normally associated with cardiovascular risk in men. Women employed in pink-collar occupations, with low control and little power (e.g., secretaries and clerks), are twice as likely to develop coronary artery disease than women working in white-collar jobs.[44] Women who have careers and maintain the role of wife and mother have better cardiac health than those who occupy fewer roles.[45] Another interesting contrast is that stress is significantly elevated in women who work more than 10 hours a week in overtime and reduced in men.[46]

Factors Affecting Morbidity and Mortality

Women have more complications and higher mortality rates than their male counterparts from the time they are diagnosed with coronary heart disease until several years after their MI. The reasons for this are not clear. However, the current delays in seeking care, misdiagnosis, and the less-aggressive treatment of women probably contribute to these higher rates. These need to be corrected before other strategies can be investigated.

Morbidity

Angina is the first symptom of heart disease in 56% of women compared with 43% of men. African-American women have an even higher prevalence of angina than Anglo-American women.[47] Women are more likely to experience nonobstructive variant angina (at rest with reversible ST-segment elevation) than men.[48-49] This nonobstructive form of angina has the advantage of lower associated mortality rates but the disadvantage of more false-negative diagnostic tests and less responsiveness to pain relief treatments.[48] The rate of women with unstable angina or silent ischemia also exceeds that of men. Still, some professionals fail to believe women's reports of pain even though 75% of women with angina have evidence of significant myocardial ischemia when tested.[48]

Women also have non-Q wave (subendocardial) MIs more often than men, which puts them at risk for a higher rate of re-infarction.[20,50] This may explain why 29% of women have a second heart attack during hospitalization, compared with a 12% re-infarction rate in men. This trend continues during the first postinfarction year when 40% of women, compared with 13% of men have re-infarctions.[20] These nonobstructive, non-Q wave MIs may contribute to the undertreatment or under-representation of women in research protocols as they fail to meet the eligibility criteria.

Mortality

Fewer women (34% versus 50% in men) present with MI as the first symptom of heart disease. However, 68% of women (compared with 49% of men) have a fatal MI without prior symptoms of heart disease. More women ages 35-44 and substantially more women over 75 years die from heart disease than men of the same age.[48]

The most significant predictors of death in both men and women are the extent of heart damage as measured by the degree of heart failure by Killip class (1=no failure to 4=cardiogenic shock), ejection fractions (less than 35%), and the presence of co-morbidities.[10] Additional factors associated with higher mortality rates that are more prevalent in women include such complications as stroke, heart failure, cardiac rupture, depression, and less social support.[10,51-52] In fact, patients with two or more sources of emotional support (e.g., spouse or confidant) were three times more likely to survive 5 years than those who had no one. Women who are alone, are confined to home, have persistent unrelieved symptoms, and have difficulty with household tasks are most vulnerable.[53] Provisions for outside support made by the practitioner may enhance survival.

Practitioners can perhaps have the greatest impact on mortality by reducing the time from the onset of symptoms to effective treatment by convincing women that they are at risk and that it is important to seek help expediently.

In Rankin's study of African-American and Anglo-American women, there was an average delay of 10 hours from the presentation of symptoms to arrival at the emergency department.[54] Thus many were not eligible for thrombolysis. The absence of classical chest pain in these women contributed to missed diagnosis, which then contributed to the tragic disability and needless death of women with heart attacks.[54-55]

Pathophysiology

The process of coronary artery damage, thrombosis, and platelet aggregation often progresses until there is a total occlusion of one or more coronary arteries. The expanding area of ischemia, injury, and necrosis results in irreversible myocardial damage within 6 hours. This process is believed to be the same regardless of gender;[50,56] however, women do have more nonocclusive forms of the disease.

Since women are often elderly when they experience an MI, age-related physiology may be relevant. Increased density, sclerosis, or calcification of the blood vessels, myocardium, and heart valves reduces the responsiveness and efficiency of the cardiovascular system. Heart murmurs, abnormal heart rates, irregular rhythms, and reduction in cardiac output often occur.[57-58] Angina in the elderly is less typically in the substernal location, often nonexertional, less severe in intensity, and not as responsive to nitroglycerin when compared with the younger population.[59] Nonangina symptoms, such as indigestion, dyspnea, exacerbation of congestive heart failure, and confusion, may signal an MI in the elderly population.[59]

Anatomically, women generally have smaller rib cages, heart muscles, and coronary lumens than men.[60] Osteoporosis and kyphosis change the shape of the thorax and may produce an anatomic emphysema.[58] Women's breast tissue may further add complexity to diagnosis by serving as the site for referred pain, or interfere with assessment and diagnostic procedures. These changes make evaluating the subtle (but significant) physical changes challenging to even the best diagnostician.

The pain associated with angina pectoris is believed due to the production of lactic acid by ischemic muscle, which chemically stimulates pain fibers.[56] This description may be challenged because the heart is innervated by the glossopharyngeal and the vagus nerve (9th and 10th cranial nerves), which are neither designed to carry messages of pain, nor connect directly with pain pathways in the spine or brain.[61] This form of "visceral pain" is by nature vague, sickening and difficult to describe or locate.[62] Since visceral pain is not yet understood completely in the animal model, it will likely be several years before the differences between male and female patterns of angina can be satisfactorily explained.

Symptoms

Although physical, emotional, and environmental stress are often considered factors that can precipitate an MI, 83% of women develop infarctions while at rest.[6] The typical presentation of angina in men is described as a pressure, heaviness, or tightness in the chest that radiates to the neck, jaw, or arm. It is usually relieved by rest and sublingual nitroglycerin. Only 24% of women with MI in a recent study presented with this classic description of chest pain.[54] Table 4.1 lists the atypical presenting symptoms as described by women in interviews after their MI. Other symptoms, such as nausea, diaphoresis, weakness, fatigue, and blood pressure aberrations, may signal an MI with or without angina.[16] This suggests that primary care practitioners should consider the diagnosis of MI in women even when chest pain is not present. It also demands that practitioners listen carefully to what women say as well as clarify what is implied but not said. Table 4.2 delineates functional health patterns that are relevant to a woman's cardiovascular health and should be considered while obtaining a history.

Table 4.1. Atypical Presenting Symptoms Reported by Women and the Onset of a Heart Attack(*).

- Epigastric pain
- Chest cramping
- Flutters without pain
- Shortness of breath
- Lower abdominal pain
- Severe fatigue
- Tiredness, depression
- Epigastric burning
- Dull pain between breasts
- Bilateral arm pain half an hour before chest pain
- Sudden shortness of breath, unable to talk move or breathe
- Bilateral posterior shoulder pain
- Ankle edema, rapid weight gain
- Thoughts of death

(*) Examples of MI presenting symptoms were reported in interviews of Anglo-American and African-American women participating in Dr. S. Rankin's study (R55 NR02617).

Table 4.2. History by Functional Health Patterns. (continued on next page)

Health Perception/Health Management
Chief concern. Past history and history of current problem. Medications and pattern of use. Perceived cardiac risk factors. COLDERR assessment (Character, Onset, Location, Duration, Exacerbation, Relief, Radiation) of discomforts. Intensity (0=none, 10=worst) of discomfort.

Nutrition/Metabolic
Type of diet. Association of discomfort to eating. Volume and frequency of alcohol or caffeinated beverage consumption. Nutritional problems (including being overweight or undernourished) and knowledge of desirable nutrition. Thyroid or other metabolic disorders.

Table 4.2. History by Functional Health Patterns. (continued)

Elimination
Frequency of urination. Ankle edema or dyspnea. Symptoms during bowel movements.

Activity/Exercise
Types, frequency, duration, and tolerance of activities. Symptoms before, during, or after activities. Regularity of exercise or activities. Physical setup of home (e.g., stairs).

Sleep/Rest
Usual sleep pattern. Presence of daytime fatigue, nocturnal dyspnea, or orthopnea. Preferred method of relaxation.

Cognitive/Perceptual
Patient's perception of what the problem is and what is needed. Knowledge of presenting symptoms and importance of seeking help expediently. Information desired about cardiac health.

Roles/Relationships
Living situation and important people in their current life (e.g., spouse, children, neighbors, friends). Satisfaction with support received. Need for additional support or counseling.

Sexual/Reproductive
Current level of sexual activity. Symptoms during sex. Hormone replacement therapy.

Stress/Coping
Rate intensity of current stress (0=none, 10=worst). Symptoms associated with stress. Stress-reduction techniques. Thinks of people that help when stressed. Sources of stress.

Self-Perception/Self-Concept
Recent changes in mood or personality. Perceived reason for change.

Values/Beliefs
Objects of meaning and value in life. Beliefs about what is needed to be in a satisfactory health state. Motivators to change health behavior.

Suspicious Signs
Short of obvious signs of distress (e.g., pain behaviors, dyspnea, or unresponsiveness), there are some subtle signs that may be indicative of cardiac ischemia that the astute practitioner can perceive. Confusion, fatigue, anxiety, or agitation are easily discounted as associated with emotional state, personality trait, or simply related to old age. Table 4.3 lists additional signs of MI[63] with special considerations for women.

Gender Differences in Heart Disease

Table 4.3. Suspicious Signs Indicate of MI with Special Consideration for Women.

Assessment	Signs	Considerations for Women
Inspection	Pallor, jugular venous distension, dyspnea and edema. Point of maximal impulse (PMI) may reveal a dyskinetic precordial heave.	Breast tissue may preclude visualization of the PMI.
Percussion	Percussion of the cardiac borders may reveal an enlarged heart or mass, but contributes little to the evaluation of coronary artery patency.	Breast tissue interference. Women have smaller hearts than men when healthy and less hypertrophy when ill.
Palpation	Right ventricular precordial impulse in late diastole is the only palpable sign of cardiac disease. Palpation of peripheral pulses indirectly assesses hardening of arteries, but doesn't accurately advise the practitioner of lumen patency.	Breast tissue may render trills or pulses less palpable.
Auscultation	A fourth heart sound (S_4) is audible in almost all patients with acute ischemia. The third acute ischemia. The third heart sound (S_3), like the fourth, is best heard at apex during inspiration. S_3 is usually associated with a massive MI. New heart murmur signals heart disease. Pericardial friction rub at the sternal border. Bibasilar crackles with abnormal heart sounds favors the diagnosis of coronary heart disease.	May result from normal aging heart. Breast tissue may interfere with auscultation. Thoracic change associated with aging may also interfere. Women are less likely to develop a pericardial friction rub than men post-MI.

Making the Diagnosis

The presence of any suspicious signs and symptoms (see Tables 4.1. and 4.3.) compels the practitioner to rule out MI. In addition to documenting baseline and repeat measures of vital signs (including a pain assessment), a 12-lead electrocardiogram (ECG) should be done as soon as possible. If the condition warrants, emergency treatment and continuous monitoring are initiated per local protocol.

During the diagnostic workup, the practitioner should recall that any symptom or noninvasive test has less predictive value in women than men.[48] Further, women tend to have: non-Q wave infarctions;[9] more atrial fibrillation, supraventricular tachycardia and heart blocks; less ventricular ectopy;[64] and false-positive ECG exercise tests (very few false-negatives). Many of the newer radionuclide studies need to be further analyzed to clarify their usefulness in women; however the exercise radionuclide ventriculography test has poor diagnostic value in women and should be avoided.[48]

Implications for Practice

Implications for practice include primary prevention-oriented interventions, diagnostic considerations, and rehabilitation guidelines. Each is discussed in the following section with particular attention given to differences between men and women.

Primary Prevention

Utilization of primary prevention principles involves health teaching for all age-groups. Since women are the chief health educators in households, young women need instruction regarding the importance of low-fat, low-calorie diets after their children are 2 years old. At the same time, they need to be advised of their own future risk of coronary artery disease (CAD) in much the same way that young women are taught to consider risk factors for breast cancer. The importance of exercise as a means of decreasing obesity and stress is also within the purview of the practitioner's teaching regarding CAD.

Rankin's recent article may explain why the current group of older women experiencing MI are least likely to have engaged in health promotion activities earlier in life.[54] For example, information regarding cigarette smoking and appropriate dietary information was not available to women when they were young and establishing health-related lifestyles. Thus today's women with CAD and MI may have amended their eating patterns but prior behavior may have already established atherosclerosis. Likewise, the women who are now suffering CAD and MI were less likely to engage in vigorous exercise when they were younger when compared with the young women of today. Therefore, older women may not profit from primary prevention interventions to the same extent as younger women. Younger women, and their offspring, will benefit, however, if primary health care providers can educate them about the importance of smoking cessation, limiting fat intake, and regular aerobic exercise.

Diagnostic Considerations

Once women have been apprised of their risk of CAD and MI they need to be taught the symptoms that signify the need for medical attention. In addition to the symptoms commonly experienced by men, women may have accompanying shortness of breath, nonclassic chest pain, or epigastric distress.[54] The importance of considering other than midsternal discomfort as symptomatic of CAD and MI is underlined by the long delay before women present for treatment. Women should be taught that the faster they report their symptoms to their provider, the greater the possibility of limiting cardiac damage.

Because health care providers have disregarded women's symptoms in the past, it is crucial that the practitioner teach women to advocate for themselves in medical situations, and, if necessary, assist in the advocacy process. Women need to know that many health care providers will take their complaints seriously and not write them off as hypochondriacs as has been noted in past research.[65]

If women are at risk for MI because of modifiable and nonmodifiable risk factors, family members, significant others and paraprofessional health care providers, such as emergency medical technicians, should also be included in teaching related to symptomatology. Women experiencing acute MI accompanied by epigastric pain, nausea and vomiting, and shortness of breath are not in a good position to advocate for themselves.

Rehabilitation

The practitioner must be aggressive in suggesting rehabilitation activities. Only a very small percentage of women experiencing MI are likely to engage in structured cardiac rehabilitative exercise for health restoration, a fact that most likely results from cohort influences in the group of women currently experiencing MI. These women were not socialized to competitive activities, exercising in the company of men, or to "working up a sweat," thus they are frequently uncomfortable in standard cardiac rehabilitation services.

Rankin's work demonstrates that women are slower to return to physical activity than men.[54] For example, at 6 weeks post-MI only 57% were walking two level blocks outdoors. The slower return to activity levels may be related to their preexisting co-morbidities, which limit activity levels. On the other hand, women may not receive specific information that is tailored to their own exercise tolerance levels or to realistic exercise performance and preferences. Women often have less transportation, encouragement, and support from their spouses than men after MI, which further contributes to their higher dropout rate. Given the higher demands to fulfill household and caregiver roles, women may lack the motivation or energy necessary to participate fully in rehabilitation programs.[66]

Other factors that should be considered during the recovery period from acute MI include psychosocial stressors, such as limited income and lack of a partner. That women post-MI are likely to be widowed or retired and living on a fixed income may make socioeconomic status (SES) a greater source of stress for women, especially older women, than men. The acknowledged discrepancy in incomes between U.S. males and females and limited access to health insurance following the death of a spouse suggest that SES is a more potent source of stress for women with CAD than men.

Even when women have partners, the partners are often ill or in need of care and unable to offer care-giving assistance. Indeed, widowed, single, or divorced women may be advantaged in not having to worry about the care of a sick spouse. Recovering women may need a chance to discuss the emotional burdens with a nurse practitioner and may also need encouragement to ask others for help. Frasure-Smith demonstrated that an average of 6 hours of emotional and social support provided by a nurse was correlated with a 50% reduction in subsequent deaths following an MI.[67]

Caring for women at risk for CAD or recovering from MI is a challenge to the practitioner who must constantly be aware that women may have physiological and psychological needs different from those of men. Searching for treatment methods that are specific to women's health care demands thoughtfulness, surveillance, and perseverance.

References

1. U.S. Bureau of the Census: *Statistical Abstracts of the United States: 1994* (114th edition). Washington, DC, 1994:95.

2. Wenger NK, Speroff L, Packard B: Cardiovascular health & disease in females. *N Engl J Med* July 22, 1993;329(4):247-56.

3. Kannell WB, Abbott RD: Incidence and prognosis of unrecognized MI: An update on the Framingham study. *N Engl J Med* 1984;311:1144-47.

4. Selig, PM: The prevention and screening of cardiovascular disease: An up date. *Nurs Pract Forum* 1991;2(1):14-18.

5. Lincoff AM, Califf RM, Ellis SG, et al: Thrombolytic therapy for females with MI: Is there a gender gap? *J Am Col Cardiol* 1993;22(7):1780-87.

6. Murdaugh C: Coronary artery disease in women. *J Cardiovasc Nurs* 1994;4(4):35-50.

7. Maynard C, Litwin PE, Marun JS, et al: Gender differences in the treatment and outcome of acute MI. *Arch Intern Med* 1992;152(5):972-76.

8. Steingart RM, Packer M, Hamm P, et al: Sex differences in the management of coronary artery disease. *New Engl J Med* 1991;325:226-30.

9. Kahn SS, Nessim S, Gray R, et al: Increased mortality of women in coronary artery bypass surgery: Evidence of referral bias. *Ann Intern Med* 1990; 1 12:561-67.

10. Berkman LF, Leo-Summers L, Horwitz RL: Emotional support and survival after myocardial infarction. A prospective, population-based study of the elderly. *Ann Intern Med* 1992:117(12):1003-9.

11. Wilkinson P, Ranjadayalaak L, Parsons L, et al: Acute Ml in females: survival analysis in the first 6 months. *Br Med J* 1994;309(6954):566-69.

12. Karlson BW, Herlitz J, Hartford M: Prognosis in MI in relation to gender. *Am Heart J* 1994;128(3):477-83.

13. Tsuyuki RT, Teo KK, Ikuta RM, et al: Mortality risk and patterns of practice in 2,070 patients with acute myocardial infarction 1987-1992: Relative importance of age set and medical therapy *Chest* 1994;105(6):1687-92.

14. Shaw LJ, Miller D, Romeis JC, et al: Gender differences in the noninvasive evaluation and management of patients with suspected coronary artery disease. *Ann Intern Med* 1994; 120(7):559-66.

15. Emergency Cardiac Care Committee and Subcommittees, American Heart Association. Guidelines for the cardiopulmonary resuscitation and emergency cardiac care. *JAMA* 1992;268:2175.

16. U.S. Department of Health Clinical Practice Guideline: *Unstable angina: Diagnosis and management.* AHCPR Publication No. 94-0602, May 1994.

17. Pagley PR, Yarzebski J, Goldberg R, et al: Gender differences in the treatment of patients with acute MI. *Arch Intern Med* 1993;625-29.

18. Fiebach NH, Viscoli CM, Hornitz RI: Differences between women and men in survival after myocardial infarction: Biology or methodology? *JAMA* 1990;263(8):1092-96.

19. Keller C, Fleury J, Bergstrom DL: Risk factors for coronary heart disease in African-American women. *Cardiovasc Nurs* 1995;31(2):9-14.

20. Tofler GH, Stone PH, Muller JE, et al: Effects of gender and race on prognosis after myocardial infarction: Adverse prognosis for women, particularly black women. *J Am Col Cardiol* 1987;9:473.

21. Klatsky AL, Tekawa I, Armstrong MA, et al: The risk of hospitalization for ischemic heart disease among Asian Americans in northern California. *Am J Public Health* 1994;84(10):1672-75.

22. Marenberg ME, Risch N, Berkman LF, et al: Genetic susceptibility to death from coronary heart disease in a study of twins. *N Engl J Med* 1994; 330(15):1041-46.

23. Hunt S, Blickenstaff K, Hopkins PN, et al: Coronary disease risk factors in close relatives of Utah women with early coronary death. *West J Med* 1986;145(3):329-34.

24. Langner NR, Rowe PC, Davies R: The next generation: poor compliance with risk factor guidelines in the children of parents

with premature coronary heart disease. *Am J Public Health* 1994;84(1):68-71.

25. Donahue RP, Goldberg RT, Chen Z, et al: The influence of sex and diabetes mellitus on survival following acute myocardial infarction: A community prospective. *J Clinical Epidem* 1993;46(3):245-52.

26. Rich-Edwards JW, Manson JE, Hennekens CH, et al: The primary prevention of coronary heart disease in women. *N Engl J Med* 1995;332(26)175866.

27. Wilson PWF, Garrison RJ, Castelli WP: Postmenopausal estrogen use, cigarette smoking & cardiovascular morbidity in women over 50. The Framingham study. *N Engl J Med* 1985;313:1038-43.

28. Wing RR, Matthews KA, Kuller LH, et al: Waist to hip ratio in middle aged women. Associations with behavioral and psychosocial factors and changes in cardiovascular risk factors. *Arteriosclerosis & Thrombosis* 1991;11(5)125057.

29. Sherman SE, D'Agostino RB, Cobb JL, et al: Physical activity and mortality in females in the Framingham Heart Study *Am Heart J* 1994;128:879-84.

30. Hawkins RI: Smoking platelets and thrombosis. *Nature* 1972;236:450-52.

31. Willet W, Hennekens CH, Castelli W, et al: Effects of cigarette smoking on fasting triglycerides total cholesterol, HDL, and cholesterol in women. *Am Heart J* 1983;105:4i7-21.

32. Holme I: An analysis of randomized trials evaluating the effect of cholesterol reduction on total mortality and coronary heart disease incidence. *Circulation* 1990;82:1916-24.

33. Miller VT: Lipids, lipoproteins women and cardiovascular disease. *Atherosclerosis* 1994;1 08(supp):S73-82.

34. Castelli WP: A triglyceride issue: A view from Framingham. *Am Heart J* 1986;112:432-37.

35. Notelovitz M, Feldman EB, Gillespy M, et al: Lipid and lipoprotein change in women taking low dose, triphasic oral contraceptives: A controlled comparative 12 month clinical trial. *Am J Obstet Gyn* 1989;160:1269-80.

36. Stampfer M, Colditz G, Willet W, et al: Post menopausal estrogen therapy and cardiovascular disease. *N Engl J Med* 1991;325:756-62.

37. Mason JE: Postmenopausal hormone therapy and atherosclerotic disease. *Am Heart J* 1994;128:1337-43.

38. Psaty BM, Heckbert SR, Atkins D, et al: The risk of myocardial infarction associated with the combined use of estrogens and progestins in postmenopausal women. *Arch Intern Med* 1994;154(12):1333-39.

39. PEPI Trial writing group: Effects of estrogen/progestin regimens on heart disease risk factors in postmenopausal women. The Postmenopausal Estrogen/Progestin Interventions (PEPI) Trial. *JAMA* 1995;273(3):199-208.

40. Amsterdam EA, Hyson D, Kappagoda CT: Nonpharmacologic therapy for coronary artery atherosclerosis: Result of primary and secondary prevention trials. *Am Heart J* 1994;128:1344-52.

41. Lokey EA, Tran ZV: Effect of exercise training on serum tepid and lipoprotein concentrations in women: A meta-analysis. *Int J Sports Med* 1989;10:424-29.

42. Cochrane BL: Acute myocardial infarction in women. *Crit Care Clin North Am* 1992; 4(2):279-89.

43. Bell MR, Holmes DR Jr, Berger PB, et al: The changing in hospital mortality rates of women undergoing percutaneous transluminal coronary angioplasty. *JAMA* 1993;269(16):2091-95.

44. Haynes SG, Feinleib M: Women, work and coronary heart disease. *Am J Public Health* 1980;70:133-40.

45. La Rosa JH: Women, work and health: Employment as a risk factor for coronary heart disease. *Am J Obstet Gyn* 1988;158:1597-1602.

46. Theorell T: Psychosocial cardiovascular risks on the double loads in women. *Psychother Psychosom* 1991;55:81-89.

47. Keil JE, Loadholt CB, Weinrich MC, et al: Incidence of coronary heart disease in blacks in Charleston, South Carolina. *Am Heart J* 1984;108:779.

48. Wenger NK: Coronary heart disease: Diagnostic decision making. In: Douglas P, ed. *Cardiovascular Health and Disease in Women*. Philadelphia: W.B. Saunders, 1993:22-42.

49. Selzer A, Langston M, Ruggeroli C: Clinical syndrome of variant angina with normal coronary arteriogram. *N Engl J Med* 1976;295:1343.

50. Hendel RC: Myocardial infarction in women. *Cardiology* 1990;77(supp 2):4157.

51. Frasure-Smith N, Lesperance F, Talajic M: Depression and 18 months prognosis after myocardial infarction. *Circulation* 1995;91:999-1005.

52. Williams RB: Prognostic importance of social and economic resources among medically treated patients with angiographically documented CAD. *JAMA* 1992;267(4):520-24.

53. Friedman MM: Stressor and perceived stress in older females with heart disease. *Cardiovasc Nurs* 1993;29(4):25-29.

54. Rankin SH: Going it alone: Female managing recovery from acute MI. *Fam Community Health* 1995;17(4):50-62.

55. Moser DK, Dracup K: Gender differences in treatment-seeking delay in acute myocardial infarction. *Prog Cardiovasc Nurs* 1993;8(1):6-12.

56. Smith, MA, Johnson DG: Evaluation & management of coronary artery disease: Guidelines for the primary care nurse practitioner. *Nurs Pract Forum* 1993;2(1):14-26.

57. Bennett AF, Save HC: Special considerations in cardiovascular assessment of the aged. *Nurs Pract Forum* 1991;2(1):55-60.

58. Dubin S: The physiologic changes of aging. *Orthopedic Nurs* 1992;11(3):45

59. Mukerji V, Holman AJ, Alport MA: The clinical description of angina pectoris in the elderly Am Heart 1989;117:705.

60. Klapholz M, Buttrick P: Myocardial function and cardiomyopathy. In Douglas P, ed. *Cardiovascular Health and Disease in Women*. Philadelphia: W.B. Saunders, 1993:105-6.

61. Grays H: *Anatomy: Descriptive and Surgical, 5th ed*. New York: Bounty Books, 1977.

62. de Groot J, Chusid JG: *Correlative Neuroanatomy, 21st ed.* Norwalk: Appleton & Lange, 1991:195-200.

63. Craddock LD: Physical Signs of acute myocardial events. *Emerg Med* 1991;8(15):23-37.

64. Moss AJ, Carleen E, and the Multi-center Postinfarction Research Group: Gender differences in the mortality risk associated with ventricular arrhythmias after myocardial infarction. In: Eaker ED, Packard B, Wenger NK, et al, eds. *Coronary Heart Disease in Women.* New York: Haymarket Doyma 1987:204.

65. Tobin JN, Wassertheil-Smoller S, Wexler JP: Sex bias in considering coronary bypass surgery. *Ann Intern Med* 1987; 107:19-25.

66. Hamilton GA, Seidman RN: A comparison of the recovery period for women and men after an acute myocardial infarction. *Heart Lung* 1993;22(4):308-15.

67. Frasure-Smith N: Long-term follow-up of ischemic heart disease: Life-style monitoring program. *Psychosom Med* 1991;51:485-512.

Acknowledgments

This project was supported in part by the Boston College University Fellowship Program and a National Institute of Nursing Research Grant R55 NR02617. The authors wish to thank Ann Rolfe for her assistance with an early draft of this manuscript.

Paul M. Arnstein, RN,CS, NP-C, MS,is a family nurse practitioner and a doctoral student at Boston College School of Nursing in Massachusetts.

Elizabeth Florentino Buselli, RN,C, MS, is an adult nurse practitioner doctoral student at Boston College School of Nursing.

Sally H. Rankin, RN, C-NP, PhD, FAAN, is a family nurse practitioner and an associate professor, Nursing, at Boston College School of Nursing.

Chapter 5

Cardiac Arrest and the Need for Early Defibrillation

Without warning, while enjoying a round of golf, an elderly man with no known heart disease collapses from sudden cardiac arrest. Fire department personnel respond in less than eight minutes. But they have no automatic external defibrillator (AED). They initiate CPR. Twenty-two minutes later, paramedics arrive with a defibrillator to shock the man several times. But it's too late. He's dead.

A young man, just 34-years-old, complains of shortness of breath and chest pains. Paramedics arrive quickly, giving him oxygen. That made him feel better. But seconds later, he suffers a sudden cardiac arrest, his head slumping forward. With electrodes already attached to his chest to monitor his heart rhythm, paramedics immediately defibrillate him. He's alive today.

In most cases, it's all but impossible to predict who will have a sudden cardiac arrest, or where and when it will happen.

What we do know is that each day nearly 1,000 Americans suffer from sudden cardiac arrest—usually away from a hospital. More than 95 percent of them die, in many cases because life-saving defibrillators arrive on the scene too late, if at all.

The American Heart Association estimates that 20,000 or more deaths could be prevented each year if AEDs were more widely available to first-line responders such as police officers and fire department personnel.

Reproduced with permission of American Heart Association World Wide Web site. Copyright 1998 American Heart Association.

Sudden Cardiac Arrest: A Major Cause of Death

Sudden cardiac arrest, also known as sudden cardiac death, is a major cause of death in the United States. It claims an estimated 250,000 lives each year.

Abnormal heart rhythms called arrhythmias cause most sudden cardiac arrests. Ventricular fibrillation (VF) is the most common arrhythmia that causes cardiac arrest. It's a condition in which the heart's electrical impulses suddenly become chaotic, often without warning. This causes the heart to stop abruptly. Victims collapse and quickly lose consciousness. Death usually follows unless responders restore a normal heart rhythm within 5-7 minutes.

However, people who survive a sudden cardiac arrest have a good long-term outlook. About 80 percent are alive at one year and as many as 57 percent are alive at five years.

The basic cause of sudden cardiac arrest is not well understood. Many victims have no history of heart disease, or the underlying heart disease has not affected their lives. It may even happen to people in the prime of their lives—like Hank Gathers, the Loyola Marymount University basketball star who collapsed and died during a game several years ago.

Unlike other life-threatening conditions such as cancer or AIDS, there is a definitive therapy for sudden cardiac arrest: defibrillation (de-fib"rah-LA'shun). As dramatized in many television shows, paddles are placed on the unconscious person's chest and the doctor yells, "Clear!" Then, an electric shock is delivered to the heart. This shock stops the abnormal rhythm and allows a coordinated rhythm and normal pumping action to resume.

The Chain Of Survival

The American Heart Association advocates using the "chain of survival," which refers to the four crucial links in the emergency treatment of sudden cardiac arrest. Starting these procedures quickly may determine whether one lives or dies.

1. **Early Access to Care:** In most communities, dialing 911 activates the emergency medical system, which dispatches the appropriate emergency personnel to the scene.

2. **Early Cardiopulmonary Resuscitation:** If performed properly, CPR can add a few minutes to the time available for successful defibrillation. Millions of people have learned the

Cardiac Arrest and the Need for Early Defibrillation

breathing and chest compression techniques of CPR, but it does not replace defibrillation in saving lives.

3. **Early Defibrillation:** The critical link in treating victims in VF is delivery of an electrical shock. Each minute of delay in returning the heart to its normal pattern of beating decreases the chance of survival by 10 percent. After as little as 10 minutes, very few resuscitation attempts are successful.

4. **Early Advanced Care:** After successful defibrillation, some patients require more advanced treatments, such as airway control or intravenous drugs, on the way to the hospital.

Early Defibrillation: Key to Survival

Communities around the country have invested in the chain of survival by instituting 911 systems, training personnel, and buying police, fire and ambulance vehicles. Yet, many of these communities have failed to provide enough defibrillators.

The chain of survival is only as strong as its most critical link—which in most cases of cardiac arrest is early defibrillation.

For example, in New York City, where it takes an average of more than 12 minutes for emergency vehicles to arrive at the scene of a sudden cardiac arrest, the survival rate is less than 2 percent. In Seattle, the average time to defibrillation is less than seven minutes, resulting in a survival rate for VF of almost 30 percent. If a similar survival rate could be achieved nationally, it would result in nearly 250 lives saved each day.

To accomplish this life-saving goal, a defibrillator should be carried in any vehicle or be available to any person likely to arrive first at an emergency scene. Any person trained in a program using the U.S. Department of Transportation's National Highway Traffic Safety Administration First Responder National Curriculum is considered a first responder. A broad range of people can be first responders, including EMTs, police officers, fire department personnel, security personnel, and flight attendants.

First responders use a limited amount of equipment to perform an initial assessment and intervention. They are trained to assist other EMS providers. First-responder training and designation should be extended to all who respond to emergencies.

Currently, about 50 percent of ambulances and a smaller percentage of fire department vehicles used for emergencies have portable external defibrillators. That's way too low, considering the number of cardiac-related emergencies handled by first responders and the critical impact of early defibrillation.

As Dr. Joseph P. Ornato of the Medical College of Virginia said in a New York Times article: "Sending an emergency vehicle to a cardiac arrest without a defibrillator is like having policemen with guns but no bullets."

AEDs: New Technology for Widespread Deployment

AEDs were developed in the 1980s after advances in solid-state circuitry and micro-computers allowed defibrillators to recognize VF. These AEDs were the first to identify VF, advise the operator that a shock was indicated, and deliver the shock. Safety records for the patient and operator are excellent.

However, AEDs have not been deployed widely to many groups of emergency responders. The barriers include cost, size, maintenance needs, and integration into existing EMS systems.

Recent breakthroughs in technology will mean AEDs are:

- easier to use and maintain;
- smaller, lightweight and rugged; and
- lower in cost.

The new generation of AEDs will make it more practical to train and equip a wider range of responders, including fire department personnel, police officers, lifeguards, flight attendants, security guards, and others responsible for public safety.

"Anyone who can learn CPR can learn to use AEDs," says Dr. Richard Cummins, a pioneer in the treatment of out-of-hospital sudden cardiac arrest.

Public Access Defibrillation is the ultimate goal as a result of this new technology. This will mean the general public will have access to defibrillators in highly populated areas such as office buildings, stadiums, and airplanes, where survival rates from sudden cardiac arrest are less than 1 percent.

A next step will be to place AEDs in the homes of high-risk patients and to train family members to use them. Other citizens will also be trained to use AEDs to extend bystander-initiated defibrillation in rural and congested urban areas. These settings often have low survival rates because defibrillators do not reach victims in time.

We know that definitive therapy exists to treat sudden cardiac arrest. New technology is available that addresses the barriers to widespread deployment of AEDs.

Cardiac Arrest and the Need for Early Defibrillation

You Can Make a Difference

So what can you do to help improve access to AEDs in your community?

- Find out if the first-responder vehicles (ambulances, police cars, and fire department vehicles) in your community are equipped with AEDs. If they are not, ask why.
- Speak to members of city councils, county boards and state legislatures. Advocate starting an early defibrillation program in your community, including equipping all first responders with AEDs.
- Support allocating funds to establish an early defibrillation program and to equip all first responders with AEDs in your community.
- Advocate and support regulatory changes in your state that expand the use of AEDs by a broader range of first responders.

To learn more about sudden cardiac arrest and what you can do to bring early defibrillation to your community, contact your nearest American Heart Association or call 1-800-AHA-USA1 (1-800-242-8721).

Part Two

Understanding Your Heart

Chapter 6

The Heart

The heart is a muscular structure about the size of your fist, connected to the rest of your body by a 60,000-mile network of blood vessels. Shaped more like a cone than the Valentine we picture, the heart lies slightly to the left of the center of your chest, protected by the breastbone (sternum) in front, the spinal column in back, and the lungs and ribs on both sides. The heart is positioned so that the tip of the cone points toward your left hip.

In a lifetime, the human heart will typically beat 2.5 billion times. That amounts to about once a second, every minute of your life—considerably faster during exercise and slower when you sleep. Although the heart only weighs between 7 and 15 ounces (depending on your size and weight), it can pump five or more quarts of blood a minute. Each day, your heart pumps about 2,000 gallons of blood throughout your body—enough blood in a lifetime to fill more than three supertankers—and is strong enough to drive a single drop of blood throughout your entire body in about 24 seconds.

The heart's pumping action consists of squeezing blood out of its chambers (contracting), and then expanding to allow blood to flow back in (relaxation). The action is as simple as squeezing water out of a soft plastic bottle while holding it under water and then releasing your grasp so water is sucked back into the bottle as it expands.

Johns Hopkins InteliHealth (www.intelihealth.com), © 1997 The Johns Hopkins University; reprinted with permission of InteliHealth. Illustrations are from "The Human Heart: A Living Pump," National Heart, Lung, and Blood Institute, NIH Pub. No. 95-1059.

Heart Diseases and Disorders Sourcebook, Second Edition

This cycle of contraction and relaxation, the heartbeat, creates the pulse you can feel in your wrist. Doctors look at two measures to determine the strength of the heart muscle: ejection fraction and cardiac output.

Ejection fraction: No matter how forceful your heart's contraction, it doesn't pump all the blood out of the ventricles with each beat. The portion of blood pumped out of a filled ventricle is referred to as the ejection fraction. A normal ejection fraction of about 60 to 65 percent means that about two-thirds of the blood in the ventricles is pumped out with each beat. The ejection fraction is a good indicator of the overall function of the heart. In a healthy person, the ejection fraction increases about 5 percent with exercise. However, when the ventricles are diseased, as a result of a heart attack or other heart disorders, the ejection fraction can fall to 30 percent.

Cardiac output: The actual amount of blood pumped by the left ventricle during one contraction is called the stroke volume. The stroke volume and the heart rate determine the cardiac output, which is the amount of blood the heart pumps through the entire circulatory system in one minute.

Parts of the heart include:

- Chambers
- Protective Membranes
- Valves
- The Conduction System
- The Cardiac Cycle

Chambers

The heart is divided into four chambers—the right atrium, the left atrium, the right ventricle and the left ventricle. The upper chambers (the atria) receive blood, while the lower chambers (ventricles) pump blood. The left and right atria and the left and right ventricles are separated from each other by a wall of muscle called the septum.

Blood returning from the rest of the body enters the heart through the right atrium, which acts as something of a storage bin. After collecting in the right atrium, blood enters the right ventricle. As the right ventricle contracts, it pumps the blood into the lungs, where it is enriched with oxygen. Pulmonary veins in the lungs then bring the oxygen-enriched blood to the left atrium, where it collects until it is

The Heart

pushed into the left ventricle, the main pumping chamber of the heart. The left ventricle pumps the blood through the aorta and into the circulatory system, where it is distributed to the entire body.

In a healthy heart, blood cannot flow between the right and left sides. The atria are separated by a wall called the atrial septum, and the ventricles by the ventricular septum.

Protective Membranes

The outside surface of the heart is covered by a thin, glossy membrane called the epicardium. Another smooth, glossy membrane, the endocardium, covers the inside surfaces of the four heart chambers, plus the valves and the muscles that attach to the valves. The entire heart is enveloped in two sacs called the pericardium. A small amount

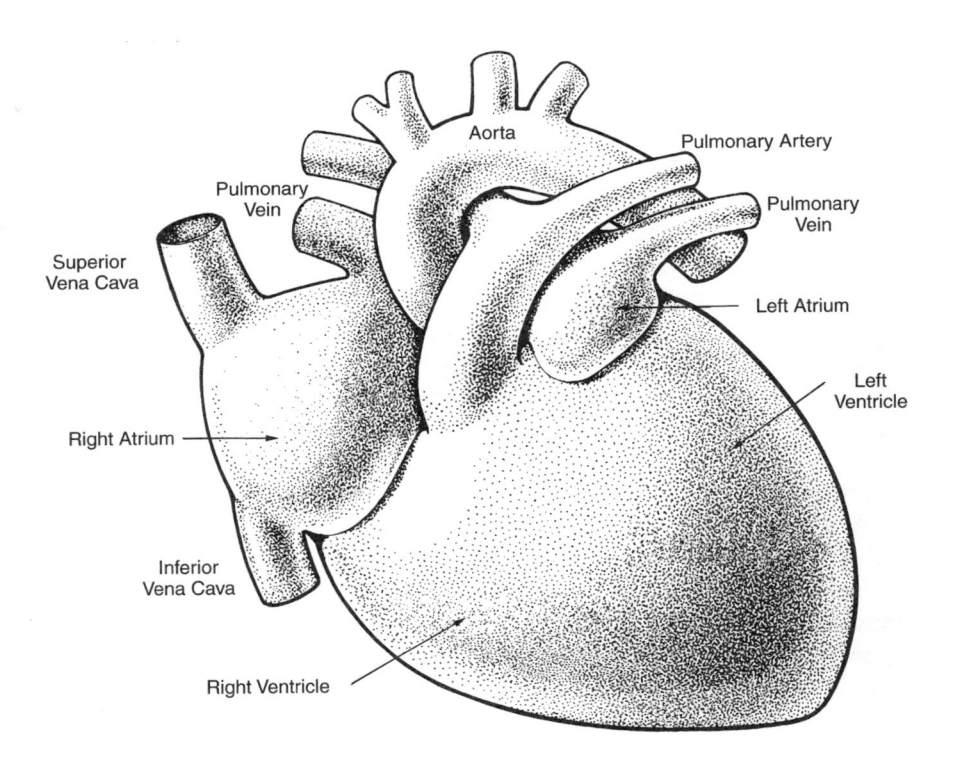

Figure 6.1. The heart is a hollow, muscular organ with four chambers. The upper two are blood-receiving chambers called atria. The lower two are blood-pumping chambers called ventricles.

of fluid between the two sacs acts as a lubricant, allowing the heart to beat with minimal friction. The inner sac of the pericardium is a thin, moist membrane, which cushions the heart. The tough outer layer attaches to several areas in the chest to anchor the heart in place. When the heart muscle contracts, the pumping chambers become smaller, squeezing blood out of the heart. When the heart muscle relaxes, the pumping chambers expand and blood flows back into the heart.

Valves

Although the pumping action of your heart is certainly effective at ejecting blood from its chambers, it also needs a method to guarantee that the pumped blood goes only in the desired direction. This task falls to four heart valves: the tricuspid, mitral, pulmonary, and aortic. The valves are strong, thin leaflets of tissue anchored to the myocardium. The flaps consist of single sheets of fibrous tissue covered by endocardial cells. At the base of each valve leaflet, the fibrous layer merges with the myocardium to form a flexible hinge.

The tricuspid valve (on the right side of the heart) and the mitral valve (on the left side) regulate blood flow from the atria to the ventricles. The aortic and pulmonary valves guard the openings from the ventricles to the aortic and pulmonary arteries, respectively. The valves are designed to allow blood to pass in only one direction. The valves don't automatically open when blood is approaching. Instead, they function like a gate that opens only when it's pushed and is designed so that it can swing open in only one direction. The valves open and close due to the natural pressure differences that build up within the heart's chambers during the systolic and diastolic portions of each cardiac cycle [see "The Cardiac Cycle" below].

For example, the aortic valve opens to allow blood to eject from the left ventricle into the aorta, because during systole (contraction) the pressure in the left ventricle is higher than in the aorta. This pressure difference forces the valve to open and allows blood to flow through it. During diastole, when the left ventricle relaxes, the pressure in the left ventricle becomes low again while the pressure in the aorta remains high. The valve is pushed closed by the pressure, and blood is prevented from leaking back into the heart.

The familiar sound of the heartbeat is caused by the heart valves slamming shut. The first thump is heard when the valves between the atria and ventricles close; the second when the valves between the ventricles and arteries close.

The Heart

The Conduction System

The intricate timing system that controls the rhythmic beating of your heart is handled by the heart's electrical, or conduction system. This system is the circuitry that conducts electrical impulses throughout the muscle of the heart. These electrical impulses stimulate the heart muscle to contract and squeeze blood out of the heart and into the arteries.

The sinus node, the heart's natural pacemaker, consists of a group of cells in the upper part of the right atrium. Also called the sinoatrial node, it's the normal point of origin of the electrical impulses.

Once the electrical signal is generated by the sinus node, it moves from cell to cell down through the heart until it reaches the atrioventricular (AV) node, a cluster of cells in the center of the heart between

Heart Valves:

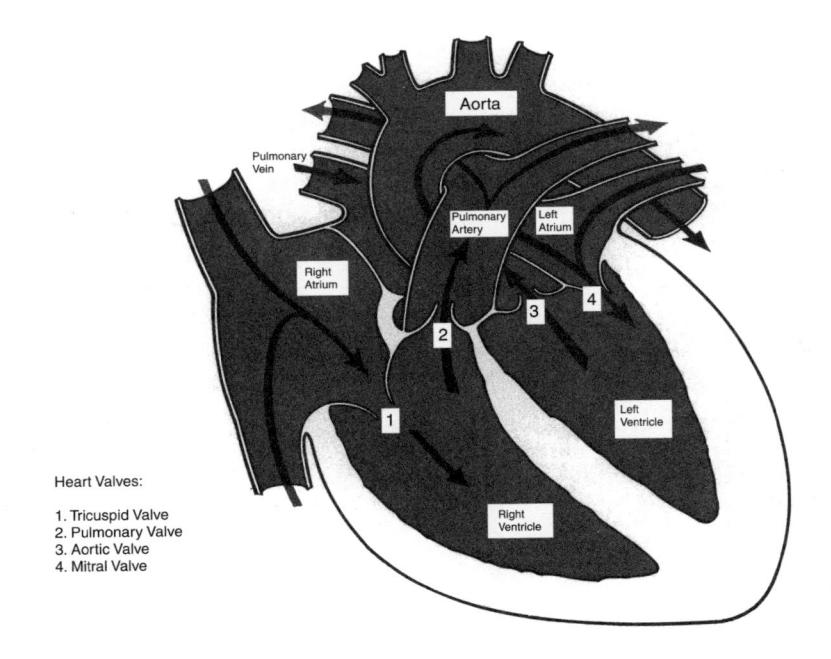

1. Tricuspid Valve
2. Pulmonary Valve
3. Aortic Valve
4. Mitral Valve

Figure 6.2. *Oxygen-poor blood from the body flows down through the right atrium to fill the right ventricle which pumps the blood out through the pulmonary artery to the lungs. Oxygen-rich blood from the lungs flows down through the left atrium to fill the left ventricle which pumps it into the aorta, the main artery to the body. The four heart valves: the tricuspid, mitral, pulmonary, and aortic, regulate the direction of blood flow.*

the atria and ventricles. The AV node acts as a gate that slows the electrical current before it's allowed to pass through to the ventricles. This delay ensures that the atria have had a chance to fully contract before the ventricles are stimulated.

After clearing the AV node, the electrical current is channeled to the ventricles by special fibers embedded in the walls of the lower parts of the heart. It's this transfer of electrical impulses that doctors measure when they take an electrocardiogram to measure how well a heart is beating.

The autonomic nervous system, the same system that automatically controls blood pressure, breathing and excretion, for example, controls the firing of the sinus node, which triggers the start of the cardiac cycle. This system can make snap decisions, causing the sinus node to increase the heart rate to twice normal within only 3 to 5 seconds. This flexibility is important during exercise, when the heart must rapidly increase its beating speed to keep up with the body's increased demand for oxygen.

As you age, your heart rate slows. The decrease is not noticeable during everyday activities, but your maximal heart rate during exercise decreases as you grow older. For example, your maximal heart

Table 6.1. Heart Rates for Different Ages

Normal Heart Rates at Rest

Age Group	Beats per Minute
Newborn	140
Young Child	100-120
Adult	60-100

Maximal Attainable Heart Rates

Age in Years	Beats per Minute
25	200
35	188
45	176
55	165
65	155

rate at age 25 is about 200 beats per minute; by age 65, it has dropped to about 155 beats per minute.

The Cardiac Cycle

The pathway of the electrical impulses can best be seen by looking in detail at a single heart cycle. The period from the beginning of one heartbeat to the next is called the cardiac cycle. The cardiac cycle consists of a period of contraction, called systole, followed by a period of relaxation, called diastole. During the diastole phase, your heart relaxes and allows blood to flow into the two ventricles; during the systole phase, the ventricles contract, driving blood to the lungs and throughout the body. In a healthy, resting adult, the heart beats about 70 to 75 times a minute, so that the cardiac cycle lasts only about .8 seconds.

Chapter 7

The Vascular System

Spreading out from your heart, a network of arteries, veins, and tiny capillaries delivers oxygen and nutrients to every cell in the body, while veins return carbon dioxide and waste materials to the heart. The circulatory system was first described in the 17th century by British physician William Harvey, who concluded that blood flows through the body in a continuous circuit. Prior to that it was believed that the blood, produced in the liver, was dispatched by the heart to reservoirs, where it waited until it was needed.

While the main function of blood is to act as the body's transport system, it also plays a major role in the defense against infections.

The circulatory system (heart and blood vessels) consists of two main parts: the systemic circulation, which comprises the blood supply to the entire body except the lungs, and the pulmonary circulation to the lungs, which is responsible for reoxygenating the blood and removing carbon dioxide.

You have three types of blood vessels in your body: arteries, veins and capillaries.

Arteries

The heart supplies blood to itself through two coronary arteries and to parts throughout the body through 20 major arteries. These arteries

---

Johns Hopkins InteliHealth (www.intelihealth.com), © 1997 The Johns Hopkins University; reprinted with permission of InteliHealth. Illustrations are from "The Human Heart: A Living Pump," National Heart, Lung, and Blood Institute, NIH Pub. No. 95-1059.

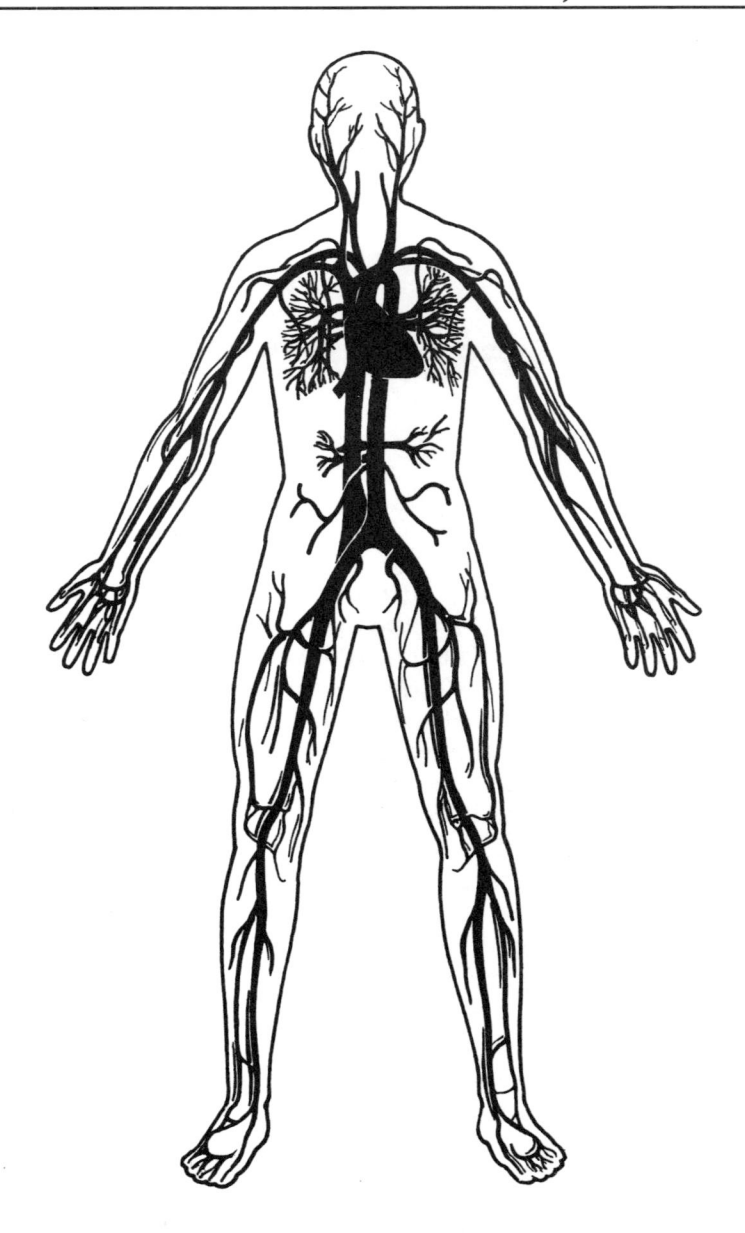

Heart Diseases and Disorders Sourcebook, Second Edition

Figure 7.1. A vast web of blood vessels supplies all areas of the body with blood. Some blood vessels carry fresh, oxygen-rich blood; some carry used, oxygen-poor blood. The pumping heart keeps the blood moving through the vessels—so that blood in the heart can travel to the big toe and back in less than 60 seconds.

The Vascular System

are pliable tubes with thick walls that enable them to withstand the high blood pressure they endure each time the heart beats. This structure helps even out the peaks and troughs of blood pressure caused by the heartbeat, so that blood flows at a relatively constant pressure by the time it reaches the smaller blood vessels. An artery's walls consist of three layers: a smooth inner lining that allows blood to flow easily; a muscular elastic middle layer; and a tough fibrous outer coating to protect the artery from damage.

When the heart is working hard—such as during exercise—the coronary arteries dilate or widen to increase oxygen supply to the heart. Sometimes, arteries widen as much as six times their normal size. Arteries can be thought of as a tree in which the trunk splits into smaller and small branches and twigs. The main artery, the aorta, arches from the left ventricle with oxygen-rich blood, runs down through the chest and into the abdomen. Major arteries branch off from the aorta; they split into smaller and smaller arteries, then to still smaller vessels called arterioles, and finally into tiny capillaries.

Veins

The seven major veins in the body bring blood back toward the heart. From the capillaries blood enters small veins, called venules, that merge into larger and larger veins, until they finally join the body's largest vein, the vena cava, returning the oxygen-poor blood to the right atrium of the heart. The vena cava actually has two branches: the lower branch brings blood from the lower part of the body, while the upper branch carries blood from the upper part of the body and the brain.

On its journey from the heart to the tissues, blood is forced through the arteries at high pressure. But on the return journey through the veins and back to the heart, the blood flows at low pressure. It's kept moving by the muscles in the arms and legs that compress the walls of the veins, and by valves in the veins that prevent the blood from flowing backward. Because each type of blood vessel performs a different job under very different pressure, the structures of the arteries, veins, and capillaries are quite different.

Veins also have three layers, but since the blood pressure in the veins is much lower than in the arteries, the vein walls are thinner, less elastic, less muscular and weaker than arteries. The inner linings of many veins contain folds, which act as valves, ensuring that blood flows only toward the heart.

Capillaries

These are the tiny vessels—only slightly wider than a single blood cell—that carry blood between the smallest arteries and the smallest veins. Capillaries form a fine network throughout the body's organs and tissues. It's through the thin capillary walls that blood and its constituent cells pass oxygen and nutrients to tissues and receive carbon dioxide and other waste products for excretion. Capillaries are not open to blood flow all the time; they open and close according to each individual organ's requirements for oxygen and nutrients.

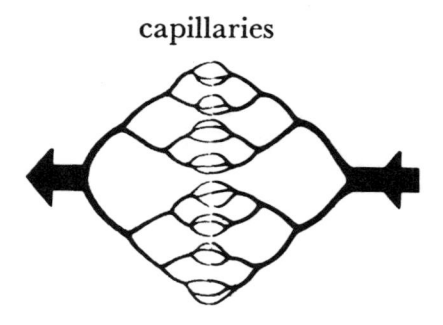

Figure 7.2. *From the arterioles, blood flows into dense networks of tiny, thin-walled blood vessels called capillaries. Oxygen and nutrients in the blood easily pass through the thin capillary walls to the cells, and carbon dioxide and other cellular waste products can pass back through the walls into the blood to be carried away.*

Blood

The average-sized adult has about 10 pints of blood, called "units" by blood banks. At rest, that entire quantity is pumped by the heart via the arteries to the lungs and all other tissues every minute. Almost half the volume of blood consists of cells, which include red blood cells, white blood cells and platelets. The remainder is a watery fluid called serum, which contains dissolved proteins, sugars, fats, minerals, and other chemicals.

Trillions of red blood cells (erythrocytes) carry oxygen from the lungs to the tissues, where it's exchanged for the waste product carbon dioxide. Red blood cells get their color from the iron-containing

The Vascular System

protein called hemoglobin, which carts oxygen and carbon dioxide through the blood. The flexibility of red cells, which are thin in the center and thick at the edges, makes it possible for them to fit through even the narrowest blood vessel. Red cells survive about three to four months, but are rapidly replaced.

White blood cells (leukocytes) play an important role in defending the body against infection by viruses, bacteria, fungi, and parasites. The five types of white cells, which multiply as needed, can pass through the capillary walls to pursue invading organisms within the body's tissues.

Platelets (thrombocytes) are essential for arresting bleeding and repairing damaged blood vessels. They are formed in the bone marrow and survive for about 10 days in the blood.

Blood plasma is a straw-colored fluid, consisting mainly of water (95 percent) with a salt content similar to seawater. Plasma also serves to transport nutrients, waste products, proteins and hormones throughout the body.

Clotting is the process by which blood becomes solid. Clotting starts almost immediately at the site of a cut and helps limit blood loss by sealing damaged blood vessels. However, if abnormal clotting occurs in a major blood vessel, it may trigger a heart attack, stroke or other major disorder.

The clotting process has two main parts: platelet activation and the formation of fibrin filaments.

Platelets are activated by coming into contact with damaged blood vessel walls, where they become sticky and then clump together to block small holes. These clumps release chemicals that begin the process of clotting by forming filaments of fibrin at the site of injury. The fibrin filaments enmesh the platelets along with red and white blood cells. Once the cut blood vessel is plugged by the mass of fibrin, platelets and red and white blood cells, the fibrin filaments contract to form a solid clot.

Chapter 8

Understanding Blood Cholesterol

Why Blood Cholesterol Matters

Blood cholesterol plays an important part in deciding a person's chance or risk of getting coronary heart disease (CHD). The higher your blood cholesterol level, the greater your risk. That's why high blood cholesterol is called a risk factor for heart disease. Did you know that heart disease is the number one killer of men and of women in the United States? About a half million people die each year from heart attacks caused by CHD. Altogether 1.25 million heart attacks occur each year in the United States.

Even if your blood cholesterol level is close to the desirable range (see Tables 8.1. and 8.2.), you can lower it and reduce your risk of getting heart disease. Eating in a heart-healthy way, being physically active, and losing weight if you are overweight are things everyone can do to help lower their levels. This chapter will show you how. But first, a few things you ought to know.

The Blood Cholesterol—Heart Disease Connection

When you have too much cholesterol in your blood, the excess builds up on the walls of the arteries that carry blood to the heart. This buildup is called "atherosclerosis" or "hardening of the arteries." It narrows the arteries and can slow down or block blood flow to the

---

National Heart, Lung, and Blood Institute (NHLBI), NIH Pub. No. 96-2696, August 1996.

heart. With less blood, the heart gets less oxygen. With not enough oxygen to the heart, there may be chest pain ("angina" or "angina pectoris"), heart attack ("myocardial infarction"), or even death. Cholesterol buildup is the most common cause of heart disease, and it happens so slowly that you are not even aware of it. The higher your blood cholesterol, the greater your chance of this buildup.

Other Risk Factors for Heart Disease

A high blood cholesterol level is not the only thing that increases your chance of getting heart disease. Here is a list of known risk factors:

Factors You Can Do Something about

- Cigarette smoking
- High blood cholesterol (high total and LDL-cholesterol)
- Low HDL-cholesterol
- High blood pressure
- Diabetes
- Obesity/overweight
- Physical inactivity

Factors You Cannot Control

- Age:
    - 45 years or older for men
    - 55 years or older for women
- Family history of early heart disease (heart attack or sudden death):
    - father or brother stricken before the age of 55
    - mother or sister stricken before the age of 65

The more risk factors you have, the greater your chance of heart disease. Fortunately, most of these risk factors are things you can do something about.

Who Can Benefit From Lowering Blood Cholesterol?

Almost everyone can benefit from lowering his or her blood cholesterol. Lowering cholesterol slows the fatty buildup in the arteries, and in some cases can help reduce the buildup already there. And, if you have two or more other risk factors for heart disease or already

Understanding Blood Cholesterol

have heart disease, you have a great deal to gain from lowering your high blood cholesterol. In this case, lowering your level may greatly reduce your risk of any more heart problems.

Many Americans have had success in lowering their blood cholesterol levels. From 1978 to 1990, the average blood cholesterol level in the U.S. dropped from 213 mg/dL to 205 mg/dL.

Cholesterol—In Your Blood, In Your Diet

Cholesterol is a waxy substance found in all parts of your body. It helps make cell membranes, some hormones, and vitamin D. Cholesterol comes from two sources: your body and the foods you eat. Blood cholesterol is made in your liver. Your liver makes all the cholesterol your body needs. Dietary cholesterol comes from animal foods like meats, whole milk dairy foods, egg yolks, poultry, and fish. Eating too much dietary cholesterol can make your blood cholesterol go up. Foods from plants, like vegetables, fruits, grains, and cereals, do not have any dietary cholesterol.

LDL- and HDL-cholesterol: The Bad and the Good

Just like oil and water, cholesterol and blood do not mix. So, for cholesterol to travel through your blood, it is coated with a layer of protein to make a "lipoprotein." Two lipoproteins you may have heard about are low density lipoprotein (LDL) and high density lipoprotein (HDL). LDL-cholesterol carries most of the cholesterol in the blood. Remember, when too much LDL-cholesterol is in the blood, it can lead to cholesterol buildup in the arteries. That is why LDL cholesterol is called the "bad" cholesterol. HDL-cholesterol helps remove cholesterol from the blood and helps prevent the fatty buildup. So HDL-cholesterol is called the "good" cholesterol.

Things That Affect Blood Cholesterol

Your blood cholesterol is influenced by many factors. These include:

- **What you eat:** High intake of saturated fat, dietary cholesterol, and excess calories leading to overweight can increase blood cholesterol levels. Americans eat an average of 12 percent of their calories from saturated fit, and 34 percent of their calories from total fat. These intakes are higher than what is recommended for the health of your heart. The average daily intake of dietary cholesterol is 220-260 mg for women and 360 mg for men.

- **Overweight:** Being overweight can make your LDL-cholesterol level go up and your HDL-cholesterol level go down.

- **Physical activity:** Increased physical activity lowers LDL-cholesterol and raises HDL-cholesterol levels.

- **Heredity:** Your genes partly influence how your body makes and handles cholesterol.

- **Age/Sex:** Blood cholesterol levels in both men and women begin to go up around age 20. Women before menopause have levels that are lower than men of the same age. After menopause, a woman's LDL-cholesterol level goes up—and so her risk for heart disease increases.

Have Your Blood Cholesterol Checked

All adults age 20 and over should have their blood cholesterol (also called "total" blood cholesterol) checked at least once every 5 years. If an accurate HDL-cholesterol measurement is available, HDL should be checked at the same time. If you do not know your total and HDL levels, ask your doctor to measure them at your next visit.

Total and HDL-cholesterol measurements require a blood sample that is taken from your arm or finger. You do not have to fast for this test. If you have had your total and HDL-cholesterol checked, check the Table 8.1 to see how they measure up.

Blood cholesterol levels of under 200 mg/dL are called "desirable" and put you at lower risk for heart disease. Any cholesterol level of 200 mg/dL or more increases your risk; over half the adults in the United States have levels of 200 mg/dL or greater. Levels between 200 and 239 mg/dL are "borderline-high." A level of 240 mg/dL or greater is "high" blood cholesterol. A person with this level has more than twice the risk of heart disease compared to someone whose cholesterol is 200 mg/dL. About one out of every five American adults has a high blood cholesterol level of 240 mg/dL or greater.

Unlike total cholesterol, the lower your HDL, the higher your risk for heart disease. An HDL level less than 35 mg/dL increases your risk for heart disease. The higher your HDL level, the better.

In certain cases, it may be necessary to have your LDL-cholesterol checked, too, because it is a better predictor of heart disease risk than your total blood cholesterol. You will need to fast. That means you can have nothing to eat or drink but water, coffee, or tea, with no cream or sugar, for 9 to 12 hours before the test.

Understanding Blood Cholesterol

If your doctor has checked your LDL level, use the chart in Table 8.2. to see how it measures up.

Table 8.1. Total Blood Cholesterol and HDL-Cholesterol Categories.

Total Cholesterol
- Less then 200 mg/dL — Desirable
- 200 to 239 mg/dL — Borderline-High
- 240 mg/dL or greater — High

HDL-cholesterol
- Less than 35 mg/dL — Low HDL-cholesterol

Note: These categories apply to adults age 20 and above.

Table 8.2. LDL-Cholesterol Categories.

- Less than 130 mg/dL — Desirable
- 130 to 159 mg/dL — Borderline-High Risk
- 160 mg/dL and above — High Risk

Note: These categories apply to adults age 20 and above.

If your LDL-cholesterol level is high or borderline-high and you have other risk factors for heart disease, your doctor will likely plan a treatment program for you. Following an eating plan low in saturated fat and cholesterol and increasing your physical activity is usually the first and main step of treatment. Some people will also need to take medicine.

Guidelines for Heart-Healthy Living

Whatever your blood cholesterol level, you can make changes to help lower it or keep it low and reduce your risk for heart disease. These are guidelines for heart-healthy living that the whole family (including children ages 2 and above) can follow:

Choose Foods Low in Saturated Fat

All foods that contain fat are made up of a mixture of saturated and unsaturated fats. Saturated fat raises your blood cholesterol level more than anything else you eat. The best way to reduce blood cholesterol is to choose foods lower in saturated fat. One way to help your family do this is by choosing foods lower in saturated fat such as fruits, vegetables, and whole grains—foods naturally low total fat and high in starch and fiber.

Choose Foods Low Total Fat

Since many foods high in total fat are also high in saturated fat, eating foods low in total fat will help your family eat less saturated fat. When you do eat fat, substitute unsaturated fat—either polyunsaturated or monounsaturated—for saturated fat. Fat is a rich source of calories, so eating foods low in fat will also help you eat fewer calories. Eating fewer calories can help you lose weight—and, if you are overweight, losing weight is an important part of lowering your blood cholesterol. (Consult your family doctor if you have a concern about your child's weight.)

Choose Foods High in Starch and Fiber

Foods high in starch and fiber are excellent substitutes for foods high in saturated fat. These foods—breads, cereals, pasta, grains, fruits, and vegetables—are low in saturated fat and cholesterol. They are also lower in calories than foods that are high in fat. But limit fatty toppings and spreads like butter and sauces made with cream and whole milk dairy products. Foods high in starch and fiber are also good sources of vitamins and minerals.

When eaten as part of a diet low in saturated fat and cholesterol, foods with soluble fiber—like oat and barley bran and dry peas and beans—may help to lower blood cholesterol.

Choose Foods Low in Cholesterol

Remember, dietary cholesterol can raise blood cholesterol, although usually not as much as saturated fat. So it's important for your family to choose foods low in dietary cholesterol.

Dietary cholesterol is found only in foods that come from animals. And even if an animal food is low in saturated fat, it may be high in cholesterol; for instance, organ meats like liver and egg yolks are low in saturated fat but high in cholesterol. Egg whites and foods from plant sources do not have cholesterol.

Table 8.3. The National Cholesterol Education Program Recommendations.

The National Cholesterol Education Program (NCEP) recommends that all healthy Americans ages 2 and above adopt an eating pattern lower in saturated fat and cholesterol to lower their blood cholesterol. The recommended eating pattern for everyone in the family over 2 years old is:

- Less than 10 percent of calories from saturated fat.
- An average of 30 percent of calories or less from total fat.
- Less than 300 mg a day of dietary cholesterol.

These goals are to be averaged over several days. Refer to Table 8.8. for guidance on the recommended intakes of saturated fat and cholesterol.

Be More Physically Active

Being physically active helps improve blood cholesterol levels: it can raise HDL and lower LDL. Being more active also can help you lose weight, lower your blood pressure, improve the fitness of your heart and blood vessels, and reduce stress. And being active together is great for the entire family.

Maintain a Healthy Weight, and Lose Weight if You Are Overweight

People who are overweight tend to have higher blood cholesterol levels than people of a healthy weight. Overweight adults with an "apple" shape—bigger (pot) belly—tend to have a higher risk for heart disease than those with a "pear" shape—bigger hips and thighs. Whatever your body shape, when you cut the fat in your diet, you cut down on the richest source of calories. A family eating pattern high in starch and fiber instead of fat is a good way to help control weight. Do not go on crash diets that are very low in calories since they can be harmful to your health. If you are overweight, losing even a little weight can help to lower LDL-cholesterol and raise HDL-cholesterol.

Making the Guidelines Work: Eat the Heart-Healthy Way

Look at how your family eats now and begin to plan. You don't have to cut out all high saturated fat, high cholesterol foods, just substitute one or two low saturated fat or low cholesterol foods each day, and soon you will reach your goal of heart-healthy eating for you and your family. By making the changes slowly, you are more likely to stick with your new eating plan.

Choose heart-healthy foods from different food groups—meat, poultry, fish, and shellfish; dairy foods; eggs; fruits and vegetables; breads, cereals, pasta, rice and other grains, and dry peas and beans; fats and oils; and sweets and snacks. Choose the number and size of portions to help you reach and stay at your desirable weight. Eating a variety of foods each day will help your whole family get the nutrients you need. Use these tips to choose foods low in saturated fat and cholesterol:

Meat, Poultry, Fish, and Shellfish

Buying Tips:

- Choose lean cuts of meat. Choose fish and skinless poultry more often; they are generally lower in saturated fat than meat. Eat moderate portions—no more than about 6 ounces a day (a 3-ounce portion is about the size of a deck of cards).

- Look for meats labeled "lean" or "extra lean."

- Limit organ meats like liver, sweetbreads, and kidneys. Organ meats are high in cholesterol, even though they are fairly low in fat.

- Limit high fat processed meats like bacon, bologna, salami, hot dogs, and sausage.

- Remember that some chicken and turkey hot dogs are lower in saturated fat and total fat than pork and beef hot dogs. There are also "lean" beef hot dogs that are low in fat and saturated fat. Usually, processed poultry products have more fat and cholesterol than fresh poultry. To be sure, check the nutrition label on deli products such as hot dogs and luncheon meats to find those that are lowest in fat and saturated fat.

- Try fresh ground turkey or chicken made from white meat, like the breast.
- Limit use of goose and duck. They are higher in saturated fat, even with the skin removed.
- Choose shellfish occasionally. Shellfish has little saturated fat in general, but its cholesterol content varies—some (like squid, shrimp, and oysters) are fairly high while others (like scallops, mussels, and clams) are low.
- Buy canned fish packed in water, not oil.
- You may have heard that a type of unsaturated fat called "omega-3 fatty acids" found in fish and shellfish is good for your heart. Health benefits have not been proven. Still, any fresh or frozen fish is a good food choice because it is low in saturated fat. Avoid fish oil pills because they are high in fat and calories, and they may have long-term side effects.

Table 8.4. Lean* Cuts of Meat

Beef	Eye of the round, Top round
Veal	Shoulder, Ground veal, Cutlets, Sirloin
Pork	Tenderloin, Sirloin, Top loin
Lamb	Leg, Shank

*Lean defined as less than 10 grams of fat and 4.5 grams or less of saturated fat in 3 cooked ounces, as currently used on food labels.

Preparation Tips:

- Trim fat from meat and remove skin from poultry before eating.
- Bake, broil, microwave, poach, or roast instead of frying. When you do fry, use a nonstick pan and nonstick cooking spray or a small amount of vegetable oil to reduce the fat.
- When you roast, place the meat on a rack so the fat can drip away.
- Brown ground meat and drain well before adding other ingredients.

- Use fat free ingredients like fruit juice, wine, or defatted broth to baste meats and poultry.

Dairy Foods

Buying Tips:

- Drink skim or 1 percent milk rather than 2 percent and whole milk.
- When looking for hard cheeses, go for versions that are "fat free," "reduced fat," "low fat," "light," or "part-skim." These have less fat per ounce than the regular versions.
- When shopping for soft cheeses, choose low fat (1 percent) or nonfat cottage cheese, farmer cheese, pot cheese, or part-skim or "light" ricotta. These cheeses have less fat per ounce than the whole milk versions.
- Use low fat or nonfat yogurt; try it in recipes or as a topping.
- Try low fat or nonfat sour cream or cream cheese blends for spreads, toppings, or in recipes.

Preparation Tips:

- Try low fat cheese in casseroles, or try a sharp-flavored regular cheese and use less than the recipe calls for. Save most of the cheese for the top.
- Use skim, 1 percent, or evaporated skim milk for creamed soups or white sauces.

Eggs

Buying Tips:

- Eggs are included in many processed foods and baked goods. Look at the nutrition label to check the cholesterol content.
- Try egg substitutes.

Preparation Tips:

- Egg whites have no cholesterol, so try substituting them for whole eggs in recipes; two egg whites are equal to one whole egg. Or, use egg substitutes.

Fruits and Vegetables

Buying Tips:

- Buy fruits and vegetables often fresh, frozen, or canned. They have no cholesterol and most are low in saturated fat. Also, most fruits and vegetables, except avocados, coconut, and olives are low in total fat.

Preparation Tips:

- Use fruits as a snack or dessert.
- Prepare vegetables as snacks, side dishes, and salads. Season with herbs, spices, lemon juice, or fat free or low fat mayonnaise. Limit use of regular mayonnaise, salad dressings, and cream, cheese, or other fatty sauces.

Breads, Cereals, Pasta, Rice and Other Grains, and Dry Peas and Beans

Buying Tips:

- Use whole-grain breads, rolls, and cereals often.
- Limit baked goods like these that are made with large amounts of fat, especially saturated fat:
    - Croissants
    - Biscuits
    - Doughnuts
    - Butter rolls
    - Muffins
    - Coffee cake
    - Danish pastry

    Be aware that some baked goods contain palm, palm kernel, and coconut oils. These oils are high in saturated fats, even though they are vegetable oils.

- Choose ready-to-eat cereals often. Most are low in saturated fat, except for granola, muesli, or oat bran types made with coconut or coconut oil.
- Buy dry peas and beans often. They are low in saturated fat and total fat and high in fiber.

Preparation Tips:

- Try pasta or rice in soups, or with low fat sauces as main dishes or casseroles.
- Stretch meat dishes with pasta or vegetables for hearty meals. You can use less meat this way and still have the flavor.
- Bake your own muffins and quick breads using unsaturated vegetable oils; substitute two egg whites for each egg yolk, or use egg substitutes. Experiment with substituting applesauce for oil or cut back the amount of oil in the recipe. For each two cups of flour, you only need 1/4 cup of vegetable oil.
- Use dry peas and beans as the main ingredient in casseroles, soups, or other one dish meals. They are excellent sources of protein and fiber.

Fats and Oils

Buying Tips:

- Choose liquid vegetable oils high in unsaturated fat for cooking and in salad dressings. Examples are canola, corn, olive, peanut, safflower, sesame, soybean, and sunflower oils.
- Buy light or nonfat mayonnaise instead of the regular kinds that are high in fat.

Preparation Tips:

- In cooking, limit butter, lard, fatback, and solid vegetable shortenings.
- When using fats and oils, use only small amounts and substitute those high in unsaturated fat for those high in saturated fat.
- For a spread, use tub or liquid margarine, or vegetable oil spread instead of butter.
- Flavor cooked vegetables with herbs or butter-flavored seasoning.
- You may have heard that margarine has a type of unsaturated fat called "trans" fat. "Trans" fats appear to raise blood cholesterol more than other unsaturated fats, but not as much as saturated fats. "Trans" fats are formed when vegetable oil is hardened or "hydrogenated" to make margarine or shortening.

Understanding Blood Cholesterol

The harder the margarine or shortening, the more likely it is to certain more "trans" fat. Read the ingredient label to choose margarines containing liquid vegetable oil as the first ingredient rather than hydrogenated or partially hydrogenated oil. Use the nutrition label to choose margarines with the least amount of saturated fat.

Sweets and Snacks (Have Only Now and Then)

Buying Tips:

- Choose these low fat sweets for a special treat:
  - Brownies, cakes, cheesecakes, cupcakes, and pastries labeled "fat free" or "low fat." Even though they have less fat, they still may be just as high in calories. If you are trying to lose weight, read the label to compare;
  - Animal crackers, devil's food cookies, fig and other fruit bars, ginger snaps, graham crackers, and vanilla or lemon wafers;
  - Frozen low fat or nonfat yogurt, fruit ices, ice milk, popsicles, sherbet, and sorbet; and
  - Gelatin desserts.
- Try these low fat snacks:
  - Bagels, bread sticks, melba toast, rice cakes, rye crisp, and soda crackers;
  - Unsweetened, ready-to-eat cereals;
  - Fresh fruit, fruit leather, or other dried fruit;
  - Pretzels, no-oil baked tortilla chips; and
  - Plain, air-popped popcorn.

Preparation Tips:

- Freeze grapes or banana slices for treats.
- Make puddings with skim or 1 percent milk.
- Top angel food cake with fruit puree or fresh fruit slices.
- Cut up raw vegetables and serve with a low fat dip.
- Make air-popped or "light" microwave popcorn.

Read Food Labels

Reading food labels can help you and your family eat the heart-healthy way. Food labels have two important parts: the nutrition label and the ingredients list. Also, some labels have claims like "low fat" or "light."

Look on the nutrition label for the amount of saturated fat, total fat, cholesterol, and total calories in a serving of the product. Use this information to compare similar products and find the ones with the smallest amounts.

If there is no nutrition label, look for the list of ingredients. Here, the ingredient in the greatest amount is shown first and the ingredient in the least amount is shown last. So, to choose foods low in saturated fat or total fat, go easy on products that list fats or oil first—or that list many fat and oil ingredients.

In addition to the nutrition information and ingredients list, some food packages have claims like "low fat," "light," or "fat free." (See the section, "The Low-Down on Food Label Claims" later in this chapter for a list of these claims and what they mean.) And for more detailed information on reading labels, order Step by Step: Eating to Lower Your High Blood Cholesterol (For ordering information, see "How to Find out More" near the end of this chapter).

Eat Out the Heart-Healthy Way

Whether your family is eating on the run or sitting down together to a full course meal, you can make choices that are low in saturated fat and cholesterol. These tips will help:

- Choose restaurants that have low fat, low cholesterol menu items. Don't be afraid to ask for foods that follow your eating pattern: It's your right as a paying customer.

- Select poultry, fish, or meat that is broiled, grilled, baked, steamed, or poached rather than fried. Choose lean deli meats like fresh turkey or lean roast beef instead of higher fat cuts like salami or bologna.

- Look for vegetables seasoned with herbs or spices rather than butter, sour cream, or cheese. Ask for sauces on the side.

- Order a low fat dessert like sherbet, fruit ice, sorbet, or low fat frozen yogurt.

- Control serving sizes by asking for a small serving, sharing a dish, or taking some home.

- At fast food restaurants, go for grilled chicken, and lean roast beef sandwiches or lean plain hamburgers (but remember to hold the fatty sauces), salads with low fat salad dressing, low fat milk, and low fat frozen yogurt. Pizza topped with vegetables is another good choice. Eat these less often: combination burgers, fried chicken and fish, french fries, milkshakes, and regular salad dressings.

Make Physical Activity Part of Your Routine

Regular physical activity improves cholesterol levels: It helps to lower LDL and raise HDL. it can also help you lose weight, if you are overweight. But you don't have to train like a long distance runner to benefit: Even doing any physical activity for just a few minutes each day is better than none at all. Try to build physical activity into your daily routine in ways like these:

- Take a walk at lunch time or after dinner.
- Use the stairs instead of the elevator.
- Get off the bus one or two stops early and walk the rest of the way.
- Park farther away from the store.
- Ride a bike.
- Work in the yard or garden.
- Go dancing.

Try to be active as a family: Take trips that include hiking, swimming, or skiing. Use your back yard or the park for games like badminton, basketball, football, or volleyball. Vigorous activities like brisk walking, running, swimming, or jumping rope are called "aerobic." They are especially good for the health of your heart and can burn off extra calories. Aerobic activities can condition your heart if you do them for at least 30 minutes, three to four times a week. But even if you don't have 30 minutes, three to four times a week, try to find two 15-minute periods or even three 10-minute periods. Most people do not need to see a doctor before they start being active, especially if they start off slowly and work up gradually to a sensible plan. But you should get advice from your doctor beforehand if any of these conditions apply to you: If you have a medical condition; if you have pains or pressure in the chest or shoulder area; if you tend to feel dizzy or faint; if you get very breathless after a mild workout; and if you are middle-aged or older, have not been physically active, and plan a fairly strenuous exercise program.

Lose Weight Sensibly

If you are overweight, losing even 5 to 10 pounds can improve your blood cholesterol levels. But don't go on a crash diet: The healthiest and longest-lasting weight loss happens when you take it slowly, losing ½ to 1 pound a week. If you cut 500 calories a day by eating less and being more active, you should lose 1 pound (which amounts to about 3,500 calories) in a week. (Overweight children and adolescents should not be put on strict weight loss diets; consult your family doctor if this is a concern.)

A heart-healthy eating plan can help you lose weight because cutting down on fat is a good way to cut down on calories. And, if you are overweight, you should take care to eat foods high in starch and fiber (like vegetables, fruits, and breads and cereals) instead of high fat foods. Choose low fat and low calorie items from each food group; the food chart in the back will help. Finally, you'll need to limit the amount—or serving sizes—as well.

But there's more to losing weight than just eating less. The most successful weight-loss programs are those that combine diet and increased physical activity. A low fat, low calorie way of eating combined with increased physical activity can help you lose more weight and keep it off longer than either way can achieve alone.

Lose Weight by Keeping Track

Here's a tip to help you control or change you eating habits: Keep track of what you eat, when you eat, and why, by writhing it down. Note whether you snack on high fat, high calorie foods in front of the TV, or if you skip breakfast and then eat a large lunch. Once you see your habits, you can set goals for yourself: Cut back on TV snacks and, when you do snack, have low fat ones. If there's no time for breakfast at home, take a bagel, fruit, or cereal with you to eat at work. Changing your behavior will help you change your weight for the better.

In Case You Were Wondering

What about Cholesterol Levels in Children?

Most children do not need to have their blood cholesterol checked. But, all children should be encouraged to eat in a heart-healthy way

Understanding Blood Cholesterol

Table 8.5. Calories Burned During Physical Activities*

Activity	Calories Burned in an Hour*	
	Man**	Woman**
Light activity: Cleaning house Office work Playing baseball Playing golf	300	240
Moderate activity: Walking briskly (3.5 mph) Gardening Cycling (5.5 mph) Dancing Playing basketball	460	370
Strenuous activity: Jogging (9 min./mile) Playing football Swimming	730	580
Very strenuous activity: Running (7 min./mile) Racquetball Skiing	920	740

*May vary depending on a variety of factors including environmental conditions.
**Healthy man, 175 pounds, healthy woman, 140 pounds.

Source: Dietary Guidelines for Americans, U.S. Department of Agriculture, U.S. Department of Health and Human Services, third edition, 1990 (adapted from McArdle, et al., "Exercise Physiology," 1986).

along with the rest of the family. Children who should be tested at age 2 or older include those who have any of these conditions:

- at least one parent who has been found to have high blood cholesterol (240 mg/dL or greater), or

- a family history of early heart disease (before age 55 in a parent or grandparent).

Also, if the parent's medical history is not known, the doctor may want to check the child's blood cholesterol level, especially in children with other risk factors like obesity.

How High Is a Child's "High" Blood Cholesterol?

If your child does need to have a cholesterol test, it can be part of a regular doctor's visit. Your doctor will likely measure your child's total cholesterol level first. However, if your family has a history of early heart disease, the doctor may measure the LDL-cholesterol level right from the start. Otherwise, your child's LDL-cholesterol level should be, measured if his or her total cholesterol level was checked and found to be 170 mg/dL or greater. The blood cholesterol categories for children from families with high blood cholesterol or early heart disease are shown in the box below.

Table 8.6. Total and LDL-cholesterol Levels in Children and Teenagers from Families with High Blood Cholesterol or Early Heart Disease

	Total Cholesterol	LDL-cholesterol
Acceptable	Less than 170 mg/dL	Less than 110 mg/dL
Borderline	170 to 199 mg/dL	110-129 mg/dL
High	200 mg/dL or greater	130 mg/dL or greater

Note: These blood cholesterol levels apply to children 2 to 19 years old.

Should You Know Your Cholesterol Ratio?

When you have your cholesterol checked, some laboratories may give you a number called a cholesterol ratio. This number is your total cholesterol or LDL level divided by your HDL level. The idea is that combining the levels into one number gives you an overall view of your risk for heart disease. But the ratio is too general: It is more important to know the value for each level separately because LDL- and HDL-cholesterol both predict your risk of heart disease.

Understanding Blood Cholesterol

What Are Triglycerides?

Triglycerides are the form in which fat is carried through your blood to the tissues. The bulk of your body fat tissue is in the form of triglycerides. Your triglycerides are measured whenever your LDL-cholesterol is checked. Triglyceride levels less than 200 mg/dL are considered normal.

It is not clear whether high triglycerides alone increase your risk of heart disease. But many people with, high triglycerides also have high LDL or low HDL levels, which do increase the risk of heart disease.

Will Lowering My Blood Cholesterol Help Me Live Longer?

Many studies show that lowering cholesterol levels reduces the risk of illness or death from heart disease, which kills more men and women each year than any other illness. If you have heart disease, lowering your cholesterol level will probably help you to live longer. If you don't have heart disease, the studies so far do not show that you, will live longer, but you will definitely reduce your risk of illness and death from heart attack.

Is It Safe To Eat In a Heart-Healthy Way?

Eating in a way that is lower in saturated fat and cholesterol is safe and can be more nutritious than an eating plan higher in saturated fat and cholesterol. It will even meet the higher needs that women, children, and teenagers have for nutrients like calcium, iron, and zinc, and an eating pattern lower in total fat will reduce the risk for other chronic diseases, such as cancer. And an eating pattern lower in saturated fat, total fat, and cholesterol can still provide enough calories for the proper growth and development of children ages 2 and above. Children younger than 2 years have special nutrient needs for fat.

How Much Will Your Cholesterol Levels Change?

Generally your blood cholesterol level should begin to drop a few weeks after you start eating the heart-healthy way. How much it drops depends on the amount of saturated fat you used to eat, how high your high blood cholesterol is, how much weight you lose if you are overweight and how your body responds to the changes you make. Over time, you may reduce your cholesterol level by 5 to 35 mg/dL or even more.

Heart Diseases and Disorders Sourcebook, Second Edition

Table 8.7. A Comparison of Saturated Fat, Total Fat, Cholesterol, Calories, and Sodium in Foods.

This table gives the saturated fat, total fat, cholesterol, calories, and sodium for some basic foods. Remember, there are 9 calories in each gram of fat. The foods within each group are ranked from low-to-high

Product	Saturated Fat (grams)	Cholesterol (mgs)	Total Fat (grams)	Total Calories	Sodium (mgs)
Meat Poultry, Fish, and Shellfish (3 0z., cooked)					
Beef (Fat trimmed to 1/8 in. unless otherwise noted)					
Liver, beef, braised*	2	331	4	137	60
Eye of round, roasted	3	60	8	171	52
Top round, broiled	3	73	8	185	51
Top sirloin, broiled	5	77	13	204	52
Ground, extra lean, broiled medium	6	71	14	217	59
Ground, lean, broiled medium	7	74	16	231	65
Salami, cooked (3 oz. is about 4 slices, 4-in. around, 1/8 in. thick)	7	51	17	216	984
Chuck, arm pot roast, braised	8	86	19	277	52
Short loin, T-bone steak, broiled (1/4 in. trim)	9	70	18	253	52
Chuck, blade roast, braised	9	88	23	308	56

*Liver and most organ meats are low in fat but high in cholesterol

Lamb (Fat trimmed to 1/8 in.)					
Leg, whole, roasted	5	79	12	207	58
Loin, broiled	7	81	16	229	71
Shoulder, arm, braised	8	103	19	289	62
Pork (fresh unless noted otherwise) (Fat trimmed to 1/4 in.)					
Cured, ham steak, boneless, extra lean, cooked, served cold	1	39	4	105	1,080
Loin, tenderloin, roasted	2	67	5	147	47
Leg (ham), rump half, roasted	5	81	12	214	52
Cured, shoulder, arm picnic, roasted	7	49	18	238	912
Ground pork, cooked	7	80	18	252	62
Chicken					
Chicken, roasting, light meat without skin, roasted	1	64	4	130	43
Breast, without skin (3 oz. is about 1/2)	1	72	3	140	63
Chicken roll, light meat, about 2 slices or 2 oz.	1	27	4	87	321
Drumstick, without skin (3 oz. is about 2)	2	79	5	146	81
Breast, with skin (3 oz. is about 1/2)	2	71	7	168	60
Wing, without skin (3 oz. is about 4)	2	72	7	173	78
Chicken, roasting, dark meat without skin, roasted	3	63	7	152	81
Drumstick, with skin (3 oz. is about 1 1/2)	3	77	10	184	77
Thigh, without skin (3 oz. is about 1 1/2)	3	81	9	178	75
Chicken hot dog, about 1	3	55	11	142	754
Thigh, with skin (3 oz. is about 1 1/2)	4	79	13	210	71
Wing, with skin (3 oz. is about 2 1/2)	5	71	17	247	70
Turkey					
Breast, without skin	<1	71	<1	115	44
Breast, with skin	<1	77	3	130	45

Table 8.7. A Comparison of Saturated Fat, Total Fat, Cholesterol, Calories, and Sodium in Foods. (continued)

saturated fat. Choose most often the foods from the top part of each group; they are lower in saturated fat and cholesterol. The examples are meant to show the difference in fat and cholesterol in select foods.

Product	Saturated Fat (grams)	Cholesterol (mgs)	Total Fat (grams)	Total Calories	Sodium (mgs)
Wing, without skin	1	87	3	139	66
Leg, without skin	1	101	3	135	69
Turkey roll, light meat, about 2 slices or 2 oz.	1	23	4	81	269
Leg, with skin	1	60	5	145	68
Wing, with skin	2	98	8	176	62
Ground turkey, meat and skin, cooked	3	87	11	200	90
Turkey bologna, about 2 slices or 2 oz.	n/a	54	8	110	483
Turkey hot dog, about 1	n/a	59	10	125	785
Fish (baked, broiled, or microwaved)					
Haddock	<1	63	<1	95	74
Halibut	<1	35	3	119	59
Bluefin tuna, fresh	1	42	5	157	43
Sockeye salmon	2	74	9	183	56
Shellfish (steamed, poached, or boiled)					
Northern lobster	<1	61	<1	83	323
Clams	<1	57	2	126	95
Clams, canned, drained solids	<1	57	2	126	95
Shrimp	<1	167	1	85	192
Oyster	1	89	4	116	359

Dairy Foods

Milk (1 cup)

Skim milk	<1	4	<1	86	126
Buttermilk	1	9	2	99	257
Low fat milk, 1% fat	2	10	3	102	123
Low fat milk, 2% fat	3	18	5	121	122
Whole milk, 3.3% fat	5	33	8	150	120

Yogurt (1 cup)

Plain yogurt, nonfat	<1	4	<1	127	174
Plain yogurt, low fat	2	14	4	144	160
Plain yogurt, whole milk	5	29	7	139	105

Soft cheeses (1 oz.)

Pot cheese or uncreamed dry curd cottage cheese, 1/3 cup	<1	3	<1	41	189
Cottage cheese, low fat (1%), 1/2 cup	<1	5	1	82	459
Ricotta, part-skim (1/4 cup)	3	19	5	86	78
Cottage cheese, creamed, 1/2 cup	3	17	5	117	457
Ricotta, whole milk, 1/4 cup	5	32	8	108	52

Hard cheeses (1 oz.)

Fat free, low cholesterol imitation cheese	<1	1	<1	41	439
Swiss cheese, reduced fat	3	9	4	70	35

Heart Diseases and Disorders Sourcebook, Second Edition

Table 8.7. A Comparison of Saturated Fat, Total Fat, Cholesterol, Calories, and Sodium in Foods. (continued)

Product	Saturated Fat (grams)	Cholesterol (mgs)	Total Fat (grams)	Total Calories	Sodium (mgs)
Reduced fat and low sodium cheese—American, cheddar, colby, monterey jack, muenster, or provolone**	3	18	4	71	88
Mozzarella, part-skim	3	16	5	72	132
Reduced fat cheese—American, cheddar, colby, monterey jack, muenster, provolone, or string cheese**	3	15	5	79	150
Mozzarella	4	22	6	80	106
Swiss	5	26	8	107	74
American processed cheese, pasteurized	6	27	9	106	406
Cheddar	6	30	9	114	176

** The nutrient values shown for these cheeses are averages of the different types and brands.

Eggs

Egg white (1)	0	0	0	17	55
Egg yolk (1)	2	213	5	59	7

Nuts and Seeds (1 ounce—about 1/4 cup—unless noted otherwise)
(Note: All nuts and seeds are unsalted)

Almonds	1	0	15	167	3
Sunflower seed kernels, roasted	2	0	14	165	1
Pecans	2	0	19	190	0
English walnuts	2	0	17	182	3
Pistachio nuts	2	0	14	164	2
Peanuts	2	0	14	159	5
Peanut butter, smooth, made with added salt, 2 Tbsp.	3	0	16	190	149
Brazil nuts	5	0	19	186	0

Breads, Cereals, Pasta, Rice, and Dry Peas and Beans

Breads

Corn tortilla, 1 (6-7 in. around)	<1	0	<1	56	40
English muffin, 1 muffin	<1	0	1	134	265
Bagel, plain, 1 (3 1/2 in.)	<1	0	1	195	379
Whole wheat bread, 1 slice	<1	0	1	70	149
Hamburger or hotdog bun, plain, 1	<1	0	2	123	241
Croissant, butter, 1 medium (4 1/2 x 4 x 1 3/4 in.)	7	0	12	232	424

Cereals

Oatmeal, instant, (1 packet, 3/4 cup)	<1	0	2	108	180
Oatmeal, quick, cooked without salt, 1 cup	<1	0	2	145	1
Corn flakes, 1 cup	n/a	0	<1	98	240
Granola, 1/2 cup	3	0	17	298	6

Pasta (1 cup cooked)

Spaghetti or macaroni	<1	0	1	197	1***
Egg noodles	<1	53	2	212	11***

Understanding Blood Cholesterol

Table 8.7. A Comparison of Saturated Fat, Total Fat, Cholesterol, Calories, and Sodium in Foods. (continued)

Product	Saturated Fat (grams)	Cholesterol (mgs)	Total Fat (grams)	Total Calories	Sodium (mgs)
Grains (1 cup cooked)					
White rice	<1	0	<1	205	1
Brown rice	<1	0	2	216	9
Dry Peas and Beans (1/2 cup cooked)					
Kidney beans, canned, solids, and liquid	<1	0	<1	104	445****
Kidney beans, dry	<1	0	1	112	2
Garbanzo beans/chickpeas, canned, solids, and liquid	<1	0	1	143	359****
Black-eyed peas, canned, solids, and liquid	<1	0	<1	92	359****

*** Pasta cooked without salt.
****Rinsing canned beans and peas with water will reduce the sodium content.

Fruits and Vegetables

Fruit, raw

Product	Saturated Fat (grams)	Cholesterol (mgs)	Total Fat (grams)	Total Calories	Sodium (mgs)
Peach, 1	<1	0	<1	37	0
Orange, 1	<1	0	<1	62	0
Apple, 1	<1	0	<1	81	1
Banana, 1	<1	0	<1	105	1
Avocado, 1/6 (or 2 Tbsp.)	<1	0	5	54	4

Vegetable, cooked (1/2 cup)

Product	Saturated Fat (grams)	Cholesterol (mgs)	Total Fat (grams)	Total Calories	Sodium (mgs)
Potato	<1	0	<1	68	3
Corn	<1	0	1	89	14
Carrot	<1	0	<1	35	52
Broccoli	<1	0	<1	23	8

Sweets and Snacks

Product	Saturated Fat (grams)	Cholesterol (mgs)	Total Fat (grams)	Total Calories	Sodium (mgs)
Hard candy (1 oz.)	0	0	0	106	11
Angel food cake, purchased, 1/12 of 9 in. cake	0	0	<1	73	212
Ginger snap, 1 (about 1/4 oz.)	<1	0	<1	29	46
Frozen yogurt, fruit or vanilla, nonfat (1/2 cup)	<1	2	<1	82	39
Vanilla wafer, 1	<1	2	<1	18	12
Fig bar, 1 (about 1/2 oz.)	<1	0	1	56	56
Pretzels, salted (1 ounce, about 5 twists, 3 1/4 x 2 1/4 x1/4 in.)	<1	0	1	108	486
Popcorn, air popped without salt (1 oz. is about 3 1/2 cups)	<1	0	1	108	1
Chocolate chip cookie, 1 (2 1/4 in. around)	<1	0	2	48	32
Sherbet, orange, (1/2 cup)	1	5	2	132	44
Ice milk, vanilla, hard, (1/2 cup)	2	9	3	92	56
Potato chips (1 oz.)	3	0	10	152	168
Pound cake, purchased, 1/10 of 10.75 oz. cake	3	66	6	117	119
Ice cream, vanilla, regular, (1/2 cup)	5	29	7	132	53

Heart Diseases and Disorders Sourcebook, Second Edition

Table 8.7. A Comparison of Saturated Fat, Total Fat, Cholesterol, Calories, and Sodium in Foods. (continued)

Product	Saturated Fat (grams)	Cholesterol (mgs)	Total Fat (grams)	Total Calories	Sodium (mgs)
Fast Foods					
Tossed salad, no dressing, 1 1/2 cup	0	0	<1	32	53
Grilled chicken sandwich	1	60	7	288	758
Cheese pizza, 1/8 of 12 in. pizza	2	9	3	140	336
Roast beef sandwich, plain	4	52	14	346	792
French fries, regular order	4	0	12	235	124
Hamburger, plain	4	36	12	275	387
Hot dog	5	44	15	242	671
Fish sandwich with tartar sauce	5	55	23	431	615
Chicken, breaded and fried, boneless pieces, 6	6	62	18	290	542
Cheeseburger, plain, single patty	7	50	15	320	500
Chicken fillet sandwich, plain	9	60	30	515	957
Egg & bacon biscuit, 1	10	353	31	457	999
Cheeseburger, large, double patty with condiments	18	141	44	706	1,149

Product	Saturated Fat (grams)	Cholesterol (mgs)	Polyunsaturated Fat (grams)	Monounsaturated Fat (grams)
Fats and Oils (1 Tbsp.)				
Margarine, diet	1	0	2	3
Canola oil	1	0	4	9
Safflower oil	1	0	11	2
Corn oil	2	0	8	4
Olive oil	2	0	1	10
Margarine, soft, tub	2	0	5	4
Margarine, liquid, bottled	2	0	5	4
Margarine, stick	2	0	4	5
Lard	5	12	2	6
Butter	7	28	<1	3

in. = inches < = less than
oz. = ounces n/a = not available
Tbsp. = tablespoon

Sources:

Composition of Foods - Raw-Processed-Prepared, Agriculture Handbook 8. Series and Supplements. United States Department of Agriculture, Human Nutrition Information Service.

New beef and lamb nutrient data for cuts trimmed to 1/8 in. external fat. United States Department of Agriculture, Human Nutrition Information Service, unpublished data, 1994.

Minnesota Nutrition Data System (NDS) software, developed by the Nutrition Coordinating Center, University of Minnesota, Minneapolis, MN. Food Database version 5A, Nutrient Database version 20.

How To Find out More

The National Cholesterol Education Program (NCEP) has other booklets for the public and health professionals on lowering blood cholesterol. Most are free of charge. The NCEP has booklets for adults with high blood cholesterol, age-specific booklets for children and adolescents with high blood cholesterol and their parents, and a pamphlet on physical activity and how to get started. To order publications on cholesterol, weight and physical activity or request a catalog, write to the address below:

NHLBI Information Center
P.O. Box 30105
Bethesda, MD
20824-0105

The Low-Down on Food Label Claims

Here are the main label claims used on food packages and what they mean:

Saturated Fat

- Saturated fat free: Less than ½ gram saturated fat in a serving; levels of trans fatty acids must be not more than 1 percent of total fat.
- Low saturated fat: 1 gram saturated fat or less in a serving and 15 percent or less of calories from saturated fat. For a meal or main dish (like a frozen dinner): 1 gram saturated fat or less in 100 grams of food and less than 10 percent of calories from saturated fat.

Cholesterol

- Cholesterol free: Less than 2 milligrams (mg) cholesterol in a serving; saturated fat content must be 2 grams or less in a serving.
- Low cholesterol: 20 mg cholesterol or less in a serving; saturated fat content must be 2 grams or less in a serving. For a meal or main dish: 20 mg cholesterol or less in 100 grams of food, with saturated fat content less than 2 grams in 100 grams of food.

Fat

- Fat free: Less than ½ gram fat in a serving.
- Low fat: 3 grams total fat or less in a serving. For a meal or main dish: 3 grams total fat or less in 100 grams of food and not more than 30 percent calories from fat.
- Percent fat free—A food with this claim must also meet the low fat claim.

Calories

- Calorie free: Less than 5 calories in a serving.
- Low calorie: 40 calories or less in a serving.

Sodium

- Sodium free: Less than 5 mg sodium in a serving.
- Low sodium: 140 mg sodium or less in a serving. For a meal or main dish: 140 mg sodium or less in 100 grams of food.
- Very low sodium: 35 mg sodium or less in a serving.

Vocabulary

- Words that mean the same thing as free: "no," "zero," "without," "trivial source of," "negligible source of," and "dietarily insignificant source of."
- Words that mean the some thing as low: "contains a small amount of" and "low source of."
- Light: A product has been changed to have half the fat or one-third fewer calories than the regular product; or the sodium in a low calorie, low fat food has been cut by 50 percent, or a meal or main dish is low fat or low calorie.
- "Light" also may be used to describe things like the color or texture of a food, as long as the label explains this: for example, "light brown sugar" or, "light and fluffy."
- Reduced/Less/Lower/Fewer: A food (like a lower-fat hot dog or a lower-sodium cracker) has at least 25 percent less of something like calories, fat, saturated fat, cholesterol, or sodium than the regular food or a similar food to which it is compared.

Understanding Blood Cholesterol

- Lean and Extra Lean: Two terms—"lean," and "extra lean,"—are used to describe the fat content of meat, poultry, fish, and shellfish:
    - Lean: Less than 10 grams fat, 4.5 grams or less of saturated fat, and less than 95 mg cholesterol in a serving.
    - Extra lean: Less than 5 grams fat, less than 2 grams saturated fat, and less than 95 mg cholesterol in a serving.

Table 8.8. Recommended Amounts of Saturated Fat and Total Fat.

If you eat this many calories a day...

Calories	1,200	1,500	1,800	2,000	2,500

...This is the recommended amount of fat for each day:

Saturated Fat*, in grams	12	15	18	20	25
Total Fat**, in grams	40	50	60	65	80

*Amounts are equal to 9 percent of total calories; the recommendation is to eat less than 10 percent of total calories as saturated fat. Remember, 1 gram of fat is equal to 9 calories.

**Amounts are equal to 30 percent of total calories (rounded down to the nearest 5), the recommendation is to eat this much or less.

Note: On average, women consume about 1,800 calories a day and men consume about 2,500 calories a day.

Chapter 9

Insulin Resistance and Heart Disease

For years, doctors have known that people with diabetes mellitus — a condition that causes high blood sugar — are at increased risk for heart disease and heart attack. Despite the association of diabetes with damage to the nerves and other organs, the main causes of death for people with this condition are heart attack and stroke.

Why are these problems so common in people with diabetes? The conventional wisdom used to attribute this to the high rates of high blood pressure and cholesterol abnormalities in people with diabetes. However, recent research suggests that diabetes may work its ills in other ways — including direct effects on the inner lining of blood vessels, the endothelium.

Although diabetes is usually defined by the detection of high blood sugar levels, it seems unlikely that the sugar levels themselves are totally responsible for diabetes' cardiovascular effects. Another likely culprit is insulin, the hormone secreted by the pancreas to help control sugar levels.

Insulin levels are rarely measured in the course of routine patient care today. However, some experts believe that, in the next decade, measuring insulin levels may well emerge as an important tool for detecting people at increased risk for heart disease — even among those without a formal diagnosis of diabetes.

Excerpted from November 1998 issue of *Harvard Heart Letter*, © 1998, President and Fellows of Harvard College; reprinted with permission.

Checks and Balances

Insulin is a hormone that helps sugar move from the bloodstream into the body's cells. This process is pivotal in a fine balancing act that is crucial to the body's use of energy. The body constantly monitors the amount of sugar in the blood. When blood sugar rises after a meal, the pancreas (a small organ that lies between the stomach and the spinal column) releases insulin into the bloodstream. In addition to helping sugar get inside the cells, where it is used for fuel, insulin helps prevent the body from losing high levels of glucose (sugar) via the kidneys into urine.

Between meals, when blood sugar levels fall, the pancreas slows down insulin production and produces another hormone, glucagon. Glucagon causes the liver and other tissues to release stored glucose. This helps maintain a constant supply of energy for the other cells in the body. All told, the pancreas does an amazing job—it keeps blood levels of glucose within a tight range so that none is wasted, yet ensures that there is always enough of this nutrient between meals.

Out of Whack

This system of checks and balances can go wrong in several ways—and the result can be the disease called diabetes mellitus. One form of diabetes mellitus is due to destruction of the cells in the pancreas that produce insulin. Without insulin, glucose quickly "piles up" in the bloodstream.

This form of the disease is called "insulin-dependent" diabetes mellitus (IDDM), or Type I diabetes. It must be treated with regular injections of insulin. The high glucose levels cause sugar and water to spill into the urine, so people develop an incredible thirst—the body's way of getting large amounts of fluid to prevent dehydration. This symptom is often the first sign of diabetes. This form of diabetes typically begins during childhood or early adulthood. Until insulin therapy became available in 1922, this form of diabetes was usually fatal.

A second, more common form of diabetes usually begins in middle age or later in life. In this type of diabetes, the pancreas usually produces plenty of insulin, so the disease is called "non-insulin-dependent" diabetes mellitus (NIDDM), or Type II diabetes. Here, the problem is that the cells in the body do not respond normally—in other words, they become resistant to insulin's effects.

Insulin Resistance and Heart Disease

Insulin resistance develops slowly, and initially the pancreas tries to compensate and control blood sugar by pumping out more and more insulin.

However, eventually the pancreas just cannot keep up, and blood-sugar levels rise, despite high levels of insulin in the blood. For some people, losing weight and changing the diet can often control this form of diabetes. Doctors also may treat this condition with pills that stimulate the release of yet more insulin from the pancreas or that increase the sensitivity of the body's cells to insulin. In some people, pills are not enough, and insulin injections are required to bring the blood-sugar level under control.

When Does It Begin?

One of the more important insights emerging from recent research is that the real link between diabetes and heart disease begins well before high blood sugars are detected. In fact, there seems to be a collection of risk factors for atherosclerosis that run together—including elevated insulin levels, hypertension, and abnormal lipid profiles.

One factor that may connect these conditions is obesity. Research has demonstrated that weight loss and physical activity can help the body to become more responsive to insulin—and also has beneficial effects on hypertension and elevated cholesterol levels. But what happens in the body that links these conditions and heart disease? The common factor may lie in the inner lining of the blood vessels, the endothelium.

Controlling the Flow

The endothelium is a thin layer of cells that lines the inside of the arteries of the body. For many years, scientists viewed blood vessel endothelium as no more significant than the veneer on furniture. However, we now know that the cells of the endothelium produce many chemical factors that help to control blood flow within an artery. These chemicals markedly influence changes in the size of arteries with and without atherosclerosis build-up. When the function of the endothelium is impaired, the arteries are particularly prone to the development of complete blockages—blockages that can cause heart attacks and strokes.

One of the most important substances produced by the endothelium is nitric oxide. When nitric oxide is released into a healthy blood-vessel wall, it causes the vessel to relax. The artery expands, which increases blood flow to the tissues supplied by that artery.

Nitric oxide also may reduce the inflammation that occurs when cholesterol builds up in the walls of arteries. Reducing inflammation may help to prevent these fatty deposits from becoming unstable and prone to rupturing, a significant cause of heart attacks.

The amount of nitric oxide in the artery wall seems to decline in the presence of several risk factors for heart disease, including high cholesterol, high blood pressure, smoking, and diabetes. These conditions either reduce the production of nitric oxide, hasten its breakdown, or both.

Insulin Resistance and Risk Factors

One of the reasons that insulin resistance is attracting so much interest these days is that high insulin levels have been found in many people who do not have diabetes. Over time, many of these people go on to develop diabetes, but even if they do not, people with high insulin levels appear to be prone to hypertension and heart disease.

Researchers examining the impact of insulin resistance on the blood vessels have found that people with elevated insulin often have abnormal responses to nitric oxide. Some data suggest that insulin resistance impairs the effects of dilating factors on blood vessels, thereby allowing the constricting factors to predominate. This imbalance could make it difficult for the blood vessels to deliver additional oxygen and nutrients when the body is placing high demands on an organ—for example, it might impair needed blood flow to the heart when a person is exercising.

Most likely, insulin has additional effects on blood vessels that could contribute to the development of heart disease. This hormone also appears to increase the growth of certain cells in the blood-vessel wall, which may contribute to atherosclerosis. Elevated insulin levels also may decrease the breakdown of blood clots. Thus, high insulin levels could have an "anti-aspirin" effect, which also could increase a person's heart-attack risk.

Bitter Sweet

In the early stages, the only way to detect this condition would be to test the blood levels of this hormone. Ultimately, though, insulin resistance usually progresses, leading to a tendency for blood sugar levels to rise.

Insulin Resistance and Heart Disease

This is a gradual process in adult-onset diabetes, so people may have insulin resistance with slightly high blood sugar for years—without having diabetes. Once the blood sugar reaches a certain level, the person is officially diagnosed with diabetes. By this time, critical damage to the blood vessels may have occurred.

Recent research results point toward the possibility that measuring insulin levels may soon become a standard test to evaluate a person's risk of developing diabetes and heart disease. While not yet routinely available, someday this test might be used to identify people who should make special efforts to lose weight and increase physical activity in an attempt to control their risk factors, including insulin resistance. In the meantime, people concerned about their risk for heart attack do not need to wait for a test of insulin levels to know that it is a good idea to maintain a healthy weight and implement a regular exercise program.

Chapter 10

Homocysteine: Does This Amino Acid Play a Role in Heart Disease?

Homocysteine (pronounced homo-SIS-teen) is an amino acid and is found normally in the body. Its metabolism is linked to that of several vitamins, especially folic acid, B6, and B12. Deficiencies of those vitamins may cause elevated levels of homocysteine.

In recent years, studies have accumulated suggesting that a high level of homocysteine increases a person's chance of developing heart disease, stroke, and peripheral vascular disease (a reduced blood flow to the hands and feet).

In September 1995, the National Heart, Lung, and Blood Institute (NHLBI) convened a special panel to review the scientific evidence about homocysteine's possible link to heart disease. The information that follows is based on the panel's conclusions.

Briefly, the panel said that an elevated homocysteine level appears to increase the risk of heart disease, stroke, and peripheral vascular disease. However, no studies have been done to show that lowering the homocysteine level reduces the risk of heart disease. The panel stressed that more research, especially a clinical trial, must be done to understand the possible association between the level of homocysteine and heart and related diseases.

Honocysteine and Heart Disease

Various studies have found that persons with elevated levels of homocysteine in their blood are at an increased risk of heart and vessel

National Heart, Lung, and Blood Institute (NHLBI), March 13,1996.

disease. These studies include the Physicians' Health Study, the Tromso Study from Norway, the Framingham Heart Study, and a meta-analysis of nearly 40 studies.

Some studies indicate that persons with elevated homocysteine levels tend to also have other risk factors for heart disease, especially smoking, high blood pressure, and high blood cholesterol.

So far, no clinical trial has been done to show that lowering homocysteine levels alters the progression of heart disease, or prevents heart attacks or strokes.

Why Homocysteine?

Much more basic research must be done before scientists understand how an elevated homocysteine level affects the development and progression of heart disease. However, scientists have several theories: First, a high level of homocysteine may be involved with the process called atherosclerosis, the gradual buildup of fatty substances in arteries. Homocysteine also may make blood more likely to clot by increasing the stickiness of blood platelets. Clots can block blood flow, causing a heart attack or stroke. Increased homocysteine may affect other substances involved in clotting too. Finally, higher homocysteine levels may make blood vessels less flexible—and so less able to widen to increase blood flow. However, none of theories has so far been proven.

What Determines Homocysteine Levels?

Individuals differ in their levels of homocysteine. Two key factors affect a person's homocysteine level—genetics and environment.

Genetics

Genetic factors help regulate the level of homocysteine in the blood. For instance, genetic flaws (mutations) can affect homocysteine's metabolism. The NHLBI Family Heart Study found families with genetic mutations in the enzymes involved in homocysteine metabolism.

The NHLBI Framingham Heart Study and other investigations have found a relationship between elevated homocysteine levels and families with early heart disease.

Homocysteine

Environment

The level of homocysteine in the blood also is affected by the consumption of vitamins, especially folic acid, B6, and B12.

Data from the Framingham Heart Study show that only 30-40 percent of the population was getting 200 or more micrograms of folic acid in their diet. The data indicated that for many persons an intake of at least 400 micrograms was needed to keep homocysteine levels from becoming elevated.

Data also indicate that homocysteine levels are higher in older persons than younger ones, and in women after menopause than in those before. But more research is needed to confirm and explain these differences.

Sources of Folic Acid, B6, and B12

Americans who follow a well-balanced diet should get enough vitamins, including folic acid, B6, and B12. There are no data to support the benefit of taking a folic acid supplement for heart and vessel diseases.

Some food sources of folic acid, B6, and B12 are given below. The list includes sample percentages of the recommended daily value (RDV) for each vitamin. These RDVs are: 400 micrograms for folic acid, 2 milligrams for B6, and 6 micrograms for B12.

Folic Acid, Also Called Folate

More than a third of the folic acid in most Americans' diet comes from citrus fruits, tomatoes, and vegetables. Grain products also are an important source of folic acid.

For example, ½ cup of spinach gives at least a third of the RDV for folic acid. A ½ cup of asparagus, broccoli, or green peas gives 10-24 percent of the RDV. An 8-ounce glass of orange juice and ½ cup of asparagus each has about a quarter of RDV.

Americans also can use beans and lentils as sources of folic acid. A ½ cup of black-eyed peas, lentils, lima beans, pinto beans, or navy beans gives at least a third of the RDV for folic acid.

Vitamin B6

Americans' major sources of vitamin B6 are meat, poultry, fish, fruits, vegetables, and grain products.

For example, 1 banana has up to 40 percent of the RDV for B6. One baked potato, a 1 3/4-cup serving of watermelon, or a 3-ounce serving of salmon or turkey gives up to a quarter of the RDV for B6.

Vitamin B12

Americans' major sources of vitamin B12 are meat, poultry, fish, and milk and milk products. B12 is not found in fruits, vegetables, beans, grains, nuts, or seeds.

For example, a 3-ounce serving of mackerel or trout has more than 40 percent of the RDV for B12. A 3-ounce serving of tuna has up to 40 percent of the RDV for B12. One cup of nonfat plain yogurt has about a quarter of the RDV for B12.

Some foods, such as breakfast cereals, have folic acid and other nutrients added to them. Check the food label for the RDV for folic acid.

Beginning in January 1998, certain foods will be required by the U.S. Food and Drug Administration to add folic acid in order to help prevent birth defects, such as spina bifida. These foods include enriched breads and rolls, all enriched flours, corn meals, all enriched macaroni and noodle products, and breakfast cereals. Food labels may say the product has been fortified with folic acid.

What Lies Ahead?

It is not yet definitely known if elevated homocysteine is a risk factor for heart disease—that is, if it really increases a person's chance of developing heart disease. Known risk factors for heart disease are age (being 45 or older for men; 55 or older for women), a family history of early heart disease, high blood pressure, high blood cholesterol, smoking, obesity, physical inactivity, and diabetes.

Until more research is done, Americans can protect their health by following a heart-healthy food plan. Those concerned about homocysteine should talk to their doctor.

The September NHLBI panel called for more research to help answer the many questions about homocysteine's possible role in the development and progression of heart disease and stroke. These questions include:

- Does homocysteine damage blood vessel walls?
- What regulates the level of homocysteine in the blood and how?
- What happens to heart disease when homocysteine levels drop?

- What are the differences in homocysteine levels among men and pre- and post-menopausal women? If significant differences exist, why?
- Can keeping homocysteine levels low prevent heart disease and stroke?
- Can reducing homocysteine levels prevent repeat heart attacks?
- What is the best amount and of which vitamins to prevent heart attack and stroke?
- Does the homocysteine level interact with known modifiable risk factors for heart disease?

For More Information

A healthy eating plan supplies enough folic acid, B6, and B12. For more information about healthy eating, write to:

NHLBI Information Center
P.O. Box 30105
Bethesda, MD
20824-0105.

Another source of information about healthy eating is: "Nutrition and Your Health: Dietary Guidelines for Americans." To get a copy, send $0.50 by check or money order made payable to the "Superintendent of Documents" to the Consumer Information Center, Department 378-C, Pueblo, CO 81009. The guidelines also are available for free from the Department of Health and Human Services Home Page on the World Wide Web at: http://www.os.dhhs.gov.

Chapter 11

The Facts about Alcohol and Your Health

Findings about the relationship between alcohol and health appear to have been swerving all over the scientific road. In the last year alone, one study suggested that the lowest death rates are found among men who have only two to four drinks a week, while another found that three to five drinks a day are associated with the greatest longevity—for men and women. It's enough to drive a person to, well, drink.

Such conflicting results say nothing of the myriad other areas of confusion when it comes to drinking and health: Do the benefits accrue only if you drink wine and, more specifically, red wine? Will grapes or grape juice confer similar protective effects? Should women at high risk for breast disease abstain? And what about pregnancy and breast-feeding? Hasn't the prohibition against alcohol for women about to give birth or nursing their babies eased up some? Here is a look at some of the common misperceptions about alcohol and health and the facts behind them.

Myth: The Best Alcoholic Beverage for Protecting against Heart Disease Is Red Wine

The popular notion that red rather than white wine, beer, or mixed drinks is the "magic" potion has never been confirmed, even though at least one company has started selling French Parad'ox red wine

Reprinted with permission, *Tufts University Health & Nutrition Letter*, August 1995, tel: 1-800-274-7581.

pills that promise "all the benefits of red wine without alcohol." To the contrary, the bulk of the evidence indicates that any alcoholic beverage protects against heart disease.

Granted, researchers have singled out certain substances present only in red wine that may help ward off coronary ills. Called flavonoids, which include a subclass of compounds known as phenols, these substances come from grape skins. And they appear to act as antioxidants that keep "bad" LDL-cholesterol from forming artery-blocking plaques. Some preliminary evidence also indicates they might have an anti-clotting effect on the blood, which could protect against heart attacks.

But even if the substances in red wine do prove to confer a little extra protection against heart disease, the added benefit will turn out to be very small, says Harvard University's Eric Rimm, MD, one of the leading researchers looking into the connection between alcohol and health. That's because the ingredient in alcoholic beverages that has the most salutary effect by far, he explains, is the alcohol itself. Some 40 studies have consistently linked the consumption of all kinds of alcohol to a reduced risk of heart disease.

In a look at almost 8,000 men participating in the Honolulu Heart Study, for instance, beer drinkers were at significantly less risk of developing heart disease than teetotalers. And in a 10-year look at almost 130,000 people in California, those who did not drink red wine edged out the red wine preferrers in warding off cardiovascular death. Red wine also wasn't the "winner" in a Harvard study involving 44,000 middle-aged men; no matter what they drank, moderate drinkers fared better than abstainers. In fact, in this case, hard liquor such as whiskey appeared to have the strongest protective effect.

That red wine isn't the "drink of choice" when it comes to staving off heart disease makes sense when you consider that the substances which set it apart—antioxidants—are present in low concentrations, much lower than, say, the concentration of antioxidants that a balanced diet high in fruits and vegetables would bring. In fact, you'd have to drink dangerously large amounts of red wine to get the amount of antioxidant protection contributed by several daily servings of produce.

Myth: Alcohol Protects against Heart Disease by Thinning the Blood

Alcohol does appear to help render cells in the blood called platelets less "sticky" and therefore less likely to aggregate and form a clot

The Facts about Alcohol and Your Health

that could block the flow of blood to the heart. But the largest proportion of alcohol's benefit appears to be that it raises HDL-cholesterol, the "good" kind that clears cholesterol from the blood rather than causes the build-up of "debris" along the artery walls.

The totality of evidence suggests that drinking can raise HDL-cholesterol levels from 10 to 20 percent or, say, 4 to 8 milligrams (per deciliter of blood) for someone whose HDL is 40. (An HDL-cholesterol level below 35 is considered low; an HDL of 55 or more is particularly advantageous.)

While alcohol boosts HDL-cholesterol levels, exercising and losing excess weight raise them even more.

Regular exercise along with taking off extra pounds does indeed raise HDL-cholesterol, but in many cases a couple of drinks a day can raise it at least as high. According to Margo Denke, MD, a heart disease specialist at the University of Texas Southwestern Medical Center, if you start out with low HDL-cholesterol and start an exercise program of moderate intensity, you might only raise HDL-cholesterol three to four points. You could expect the same results from losing five to 10 excess pounds.

Of course, engaging in physical activity on a regular basis does a lot of life-protecting things that drinking doesn't: making the heart beat more efficiently, reducing the risk of diabetes, decreasing blood pressure, and increasing bone density. Taking off extra pounds also decreases blood pressure and staves off diabetes as well as takes stress off the joints, puts less pressure on the heart muscle, lowers the chances of ending up with respiratory and orthopedic disorders, and makes it easier to get around.

Myth: Because Alcohol Raises the Risk for Breast Cancer, the Hazards of Drinking Outweigh the Benefits for Women

It's true that alcohol seems to raise the risk of breast cancer, apparently by raising a woman's levels of the hormone estrogen, which promotes the development of certain types of breast tumors. Consider that in a Harvard study of almost 90,000 middle-aged women three to nine drinks a week reduced the risk of heart disease by 40 percent but raised the risk of breast cancer by 30 percent.

That might make it seem like a wash but, contrary to popular belief, only 4 percent of women die of breast cancer, whereas 40 percent of women die of heart disease. In other words, moderate drinking would extend more lives than it would end prematurely.

Many professionals advise women to consider their personal situations and discuss their health histories with their doctors. For example, a woman might want to abstain or at least drink on a very infrequent basis if she has one or more risk factors for breast cancer: A mother or sister who has developed the disease, onset of menstruation before age 12, first pregnancy after 30, never having children, menopause later than 55.

On the other hand, if a woman does not have any particular risk factors for breast cancer yet has developed some heart disease risks—high blood pressure, diabetes, or high blood cholesterol—she might choose not to stop drinking moderately if that is already one of her habits.

Myth: Moderate Drinking Means a Maximum of Two Drinks a Day

The two drinks a day recommendation—often made in reference to men—is not engraved in stone. And it certainly is not appropriate for women, older people, and those taking prescription drugs and over-the-counter medications that do not mix with alcohol. Women are not supposed to have more than one drink daily, according to the U.S. Dietary Guidelines for Americans, because they are smaller than men and therefore don't hold their liquor as well. In addition, women have proportionately more fat and less water than men, so alcohol does not get diluted as well in their bodies. Then, too, women have less of an enzyme called alcohol dehydrogenase that breaks down alcohol before it reaches the bloodstream, so it is more likely to go to their heads.

Even one drink a day may be more than optimal for women. A recently released study of 85,000 middle-aged women spanning 12 years found the greatest longevity was associated not with a daily glass of wine, beer, or mixed drink but with one to three drinks a week. A drink a day lowered mortality risk too, but not as much.

As concerns older people, a reasonable definition of moderate drinking is also no more than one drink a day, according to researchers at the Centers for Disease Control and Prevention. While older drinkers metabolize alcohol as efficiently as younger ones, an identical dose of alcohol produces a higher blood alcohol concentration in an older drinker because total body water content decreases with age.

Of course, many older people, as well as a significant proportion of middle-aged men and women, take medications that don't interact well with alcohol. Heart drugs like Nitrostat, for instance, can combine with alcohol to make blood pressure drop precipitously. Drinking also increases the risk of gastrointestinal bleeding in people who

The Facts about Alcohol and Your Health

regularly take aspirin, like some arthritis sufferers. And medications like anticonvulsants have a sedative effect that might work with alcohol to heighten a sleepy or fatigued effect and therefore make somebody more likely to, say, fall asleep at the wheel. Anyone who takes a particular drug on a regular basis should speak to a physician about its interaction with alcohol before mixing the two at any level.

Finally, it is not crystal clear that even young and middle-aged men who don't take medication should feel sanguine about a two drinks a day habit. Last fall an 11-year Harvard study of 22,000 men found those who had the lowest rate of death from all causes drank only two to four drinks a week, or something on the order of a drink every two to three days. Specifically, their death rate was about 22 percent lower than men who didn't drink at all.

Harvard's Dr. Rimm notes that this is just one study and that, on average, two drinks a day remains a reasonable limit for most men. But men, like women, need to consider certain personal factors. "Clearly," he states, "if you're six feet two inches and weigh well over 200 pounds, two drinks a day is going to be okay. But if you're a small man with a slight frame, you might be better off at a maximum of one."

Beyond two drinks a day, alcohol has direct adverse effects on the heart.

Even at as many as four drinks a day, a man is less likely to die of heart disease than a nondrinker. But by drinking more than two alcoholic beverages daily, his risk of death from other illnesses appears to go up sharply. Specifically, he has a greater chance of dying from several different types of cancer, including cancer of the esophagus and stomach, and perhaps cancer of the colon and rectum as well. He might also be more likely to die of a stroke. Cirrhosis of the liver, falls, and automobile accidents also increase.

To be sure, a recently released study from Denmark suggests that men and women who have as many as three to five daily glasses of wine are less likely to die as soon as people who drink less. But most researchers in the field are quick to point out that those findings are an anomaly that has yet to be explained and that the totality of evidence suggests very strongly that for anyone, more than two drinks a day (one for women and older people) is a dangerous habit.

Myth: Because the French Are Regular Consumers of Alcohol, They Live Longer than Americans

The French do consume much more alcohol than Americans. Indeed, they drink eight to 10 times as much wine. But a recent study looking at drinking patterns and death rates in 21 developed nations showed that the protective effects of alcohol enjoyed by the French are, in effect, wiped out by alcohol abuse that leads to early death from cirrhosis of the liver, accidents, suicides, and other problems.

Interestingly, alcohol consumption in France has gone down dramatically over the last few decades—from 19 quarts per person a year in 1965 to 14 quarts in 1988. And so have coronary death rates—from 95 people per 100,000 in 1965 to 71 people per 100,000 in 1988. Deaths from cirrhosis of the liver have practically been cut in half during that same period.

Myth: Drinking Small Amounts of Wine during Pregnancy and Breast-Feeding Is Now Considered Harmless

A 1994 book entitled *To Your Health: Two Physicians Explore the Health Benefits of Wine* does say that light drinking (which the authors do not define for pregnant women) is safe because it will not cause fetal alcohol syndrome and its attendant problems: malformation of the face, central nervous system deficiencies, and long-term mental retardation. But research suggests that drinking even less than one drink a day can still result in decreased weight, height, and head size as well as reduced IQ scores. Both the Surgeon General and the American College of Obstetricians advise that no amount of alcohol is safe for the baby during pregnancy.

As for drinking while breast-feeding, an old wives' tale says that a glass of wine or beer before breast-feeding relaxes the mother and thereby allows her to produce more milk for her baby. But a study at the Monell Chemical Senses Center in Philadelphia found that breast-fed infants end up with about 20 percent less milk after their mothers have a drink than when they abstain.

It Goes to More Than Your Head

Researchers agree almost universally that no one should take up drinking for the express purpose of staving off heart disease. The potential for alcohol abuse is too strong, and there are much safer and generally more healthful ways to protect the cardiovascular system: following a diet low in fat, particularly saturated fat; eating more vegetables and fruits; exercising more; and losing excess weight.

The calories in alcoholic beverages need to be considered too. Most wines, beer, or other alcoholic drinks contain at least 100 calories each,

The Facts about Alcohol and Your Health

which at a drink a day could easily add more than 10 pounds in less than a year's time.

If your drink of choice is a cocktail such as a martini, gin and tonic, or screwdriver, one drink will come closer to 200 calories. It's the same for many of the beers brewed at one of the many microbreweries now popping up around the country. Microbrewed beers like stouts and porters don't necessarily contain more alcohol than regular beer, but they do contain more carbohydrates. Take a look at Table 11.1 to see how many calories are in your favorite alcoholic beverage.

Note that each choice contains in the neighborhood of one half ounce of alcohol—the definition of one drink. But serving sizes and percentages of alcohol by volume differ because that half ounce is more diluted in some drinks than in others.

Table 11.1. Calories in Alcoholic Beverages

Beverage (% alcohol by volume)	Serving size(oz)	Calories
wine (11.5%)	5	105
sherry (19%)	3	125
beer (4.5%)	12	150
stout or porter on tap (about 3%)	12	200
gin, vodka, rum, whiskey (rye, Scotch), 80 proof (40%)	1.5	100-10
cordials, liqueurs, 25-100 proof (12.5-50%)	1	50-100
martini (38%, 3/4 oz alcohol)	2.5	156
manhattan (37%)	2	128
bloody mary (12%)	5	116
Tom Collins (9%)	7.5	121
daiquiri (28%)	2	111
gin & tonic (9%)	7.5	171
pina colada (12%)	4.5	262
screwdriver (8%)	7	174
tequila sunrise (14%)	5.5	189
whiskey sour prepared from bottled mix (17%)	3.5	160

Chapter 12

Common Diagnostic Tests

Blood Tests

The most common blood tests related to heart disease measure blood cholesterol, triglyceride and HDL cholesterol levels, cardiac enzymes, oxygen content and prothrombin time, and check for thyroid disorders.

- **Cholesterol:** Measurement of total cholesterol, HDL cholesterol and, triglycerides allows a calculation of LDL cholesterol, and the ratio of LDL cholesterol to HDL cholesterol. Blood levels of triglycerides vary according to recent food intake. To get a true reading, be sure to fast for 12 hours before the blood is drawn.

- **Cardiac enzymes:** Enzymes found in the heart may leak into blood from damaged heart cells after a heart attack. If you experience chest pain, your doctor may test your blood for the enzymes creatine kinase (CK) and lactate dehydrogenase (LDH).

- **Oxygen content:** Measurement of blood oxygen helps to determine whether your overall circulation is sufficient, whether the lungs are providing enough oxygen to the bloodstream, and

---

This chapter includes "Blood Tests," from Johns Hopkins InteliHealth (www.intelihealth.com), © 1997 The Johns Hopkins University, reprinted with permission of InteliHealth; and "Cardiac X-rays," "Heart Scan," "Heart Scan with Endoscopy," Electrocardiography," "Stress Test," "Holter Monitoring," and "Cardiac Blood Pool Scan," used with permission from *Everything You Need to Know about Medical Tests*, 1996. © Springhouse Corp.

whether there is evidence of poor blood flow from the heart to the lungs. Oxygen is measured in blood drawn from an artery whereas standard blood tests use blood from a vein, usually drawn at the bend of the elbow.

- **Prothrombin time (clotting time):** Medications that slow blood clotting are anticoagulants, warfarin (Coumadin), for example, or antiplatelet drugs, such as plain old everyday aspirin. Although they are referred to as "blood thinners," they don't actually "thin" the blood; instead anticoagulants alter proteins in the blood that are responsible for clotting, while antiplatelet drugs prevent platelets from clumping and forming clots. Because people respond differently to anticoagulants, blood tests that measure prothrombin time are used to determine whether the drug dose is correct—effective, yet safe (too high a dose can cause bleeding). Prothrombin time is measured in people taking an anticoagulant, not in those taking aspirin.

- **Thyroid:** Doctors often check for thyroid disease because an abnormally functioning thyroid gland can lead to a racing heartbeat. One of the most common thyroid disorders is known as Grave's disease. The disorder results from an overactive thyroid gland that produces excessive amounts of thyroid hormones.

Cardiac X-rays

These X-rays are among the most frequently used tests for evaluating heart disease and its effects on the blood vessels of the lungs. They show images of the thorax, mediastinum, heart, and lungs. In a routine evaluation, two different views are taken.

Why is this test done?

Cardiac X-rays may be performed for the following reasons:

- To help detect heart disease and abnormalities that change the size, shape, or appearance of the heart and lungs
- To check for the correct position of pulmonary artery and cardiac catheters and of pacemaker wires

What should you know before the test?

- You'll learn about the test, including who will perform it and where. The test exposes you to little radiation and is harmless.

Common Diagnostic Tests

- You'll remove jewelry, other metal objects, and clothing above your waist and put on a hospital gown.

What happens during the test?

The procedure depends on how the X-rays are taken.

- Front and back views
  - You stand up about 6 feet (2 meters) from the X-ray machine with your back to the machine and your chin resting on top of the film cassette holder.
  - The holder is adjusted to slightly extend your neck. You then place your hands on your hips, with your shoulders touching the holder, and center your chest against it.
  - You take a deep breath and hold it while the X-ray film is exposed.
- Left side view
  - You extend your arms over your head and put your left side flush against the cassette.
  - You then take a deep breath and hold it while the X-ray film is exposed.

Does the test have risks?

Cardiac X-rays usually aren't done during the first 3 months of pregnancy. However, when they're absolutely necessary, a lead shield or apron should cover the mother's stomach and pelvic area during the X-ray exposure.

What are the normal results?

The heart and lungs should have a normal size, shape, and condition on the X-rays.

What do abnormal results mean?

Cardiac X-rays must be evaluated in light of a person's medical history, physical exam, and the results of previous X-rays and electrocardiograms. An abnormal silhouette of the heart usually indicates enlargement of the left or right ventricle or the left atrium. The test can also show the first signs of congestion in the lungs' blood vessels.

Heart Scan

Called an echocardiogram by doctors, this test evaluates the size, shape, and motion of various structures within the heart. It's a noninvasive test, which means that nothing enters your body during the procedure.

In an echocardiogram, a microphone-like transducer directs extremely high-pitched sound waves (which can't be heard by the human ear) toward the heart, which reflects these waves, producing echoes. The echoes are converted to images that are displayed on a monitor and recorded on a strip chart or videotape.

The doctor may use an echocardiogram when evaluating people with chest pain, enlarged heart silhouettes on X-rays, suspicious changes on electrocardiograms, and abnormal heart sounds.

Why is this test done?

An echocardiogram may be performed for the following reasons:

- To help the doctor diagnose and evaluate abnormalities of the heart's valves
- To measure the size of the heart's chambers
- To evaluate chambers and valves in congenital heart disorders
- To help diagnose hypertrophic and related cardiomyopathies
- To detect tumors in the atria
- To evaluate cardiac function or wall motion after a heart attack
- To detect pericardial effusion, a disorder marked by excessive fluid in the sac surrounding the heart

What should you know before the test?

- You won't need to change your diet before the test.
- The test usually takes 15 to 30 minutes, and it's safe and painless.

What happens during the test?

- The room may be darkened slightly to help the examiner see the oscilloscope screen. Other procedures, such as electrocardiography, may be performed at the same time.

Common Diagnostic Tests

- You lie on an examining table for the test.
- Conductive jelly is applied to your chest and a transducer is placed on it.
- The transducer is systematically angled to direct ultrasonic waves at specific parts of your heart.
- Significant findings are recorded on a strip chart recorder or on a videotape recorder.
- To record heart function under various conditions, you may be asked to inhale and exhale slowly or to hold your breath.
- You may be asked to inhale a gas with a slightly sweet odor (amyl nitrite) while changes in your heart function are recorded. The gas can cause dizziness, flushing, and an abnormally rapid heartbeat, but these symptoms quickly subside.

What happens after the test?

- The conductive jelly is removed from your skin.

What are the normal results?

An echocardiogram can show the doctor the normal motion patterns and the structures of the four heart valves.

What do abnormal results mean?

Abnormalities in heart valves, such as mitral stenosis, readily appear on the echocardiogram. The test may also indicate that one of the heart's chambers is especially large, possibly indicating congestive heart failure. Other chamber or valve abnormalities may indicate a congenital heart disorder. The doctor can use these and other signs to chose more definitive tests.

The echocardiogram is especially sensitive in detecting pericardial effusion. Normally, the heart linings are continuous membranes, and thus produce a single or near-single echo. When fluid accumulates between these membranes, it causes an abnormal echo-free space to appear.

Heart Scan with Endoscopy

This test allows the doctor to see the heart's structure and function without opening the body. It combines ultrasound with endoscopy to provide a better view of your heart's structures. The medical name for this test is transesophageal echocardiography.

During the test, a small, microphone-like transducer is attached to the end of an endoscope and inserted into your esophagus, allowing images to be taken from the back of the heart. This causes less interference from bones and other structures near the heart and produces high-quality images of the thoracic aorta.

Why is this test done?

The test may be performed to evaluate the following conditions:

- thoracic and aortic disorders, such as dissection and aneurysm
- conditions that affect the heart's valves, especially in the mitral valve and in people with prosthetic devices
- endocarditis
- congenital heart disease
- intracardiac clots
- cardiac tumors
- valve repairs

What should you know before the test?

- You'll need to fast for 6 hours before the test.
- The doctor or nurse will ask if you have any conditions that might interfere with the test, such as esophageal obstruction, gastrointestinal bleeding, previous radiation therapy, severe cervical arthritis, or allergies.
- If you're having the procedure as an outpatient, arrange to have someone take you home.

What happens during the test?

- Your throat is sprayed with a topical anesthetic. You may gag when the endoscope is inserted.
- An intravenous line is inserted to sedate you before the procedure; you may feel some discomfort from the needle puncture and the pressure of the tourniquet.

Common Diagnostic Tests

- You're made as comfortable as possible during the procedure and your blood pressure and heart rate are monitored continuously.
- After the endoscope is put down your throat, ultrasound images are recorded. These images are reviewed by the doctor after the procedure.

What happens after the test?

- You'll remain in bed until the sedative wears off.
- The nurse will encourage you to cough after the procedure, either while lying on your side or sitting upright.
- You can have food or water after your gag response returns.

What are the normal results?

The test should reveal no cardiac problems.

What do abnormal results mean?

The test can reveal thoracic and aortic disorders, endocarditis, congenital heart disease, intracardiac clots, or tumors, or it can be used to evaluate valvular disease or repairs. Findings may indicate aortic dissection or an aneurysm, mitral valve disease, or congenital defects such as patent ductus arteriosus.

Electrocardiography

An electrocardiogram, commonly known as an EKG, is the most common test of the heart's condition. It's used to graphically record the electrical current generated by the beating heart. This current radiates from the heart in all directions and, on reaching the skin, is measured by electrodes. These electrodes are connected to an amplifier and strip chart recorder, which prints tracings. The doctor interprets the tracings to obtain information about the heart's functioning.

Why is this test done?

An electrocardiogram may be performed for the following reasons:

- To help identify irregular heartbeats, an enlarged or inflamed heart, heart damage, and the site and extent of a heart attack

- To check on recovery from a heart attack
- To evaluate the effectiveness of drugs for heart problems
- To check the performance of a cardiac pacemaker

What should you know before the test?

- You'll learn about the test, including who will perform it, where it will take place, and its expected duration (5 to 10 minutes). During the test, electrodes will be attached to your arms, legs, and chest. The procedure is painless and you should relax, lie still, and breathe normally.
- Don't talk during the test because the sound of your voice may distort the electrocardiogram tracing.
- Tell the doctor or nurse if you're taking any medications.

What happens during the test?

- You lie on your back, and a nurse attaches electrodes to your chest ankles, and wrists.
- The nurse connects leadwires after all electrodes are in place and may secure the limb electrodes with rubber straps, but won't tighten them too much.
- The nurse presses the START button and the machine records and prints the electrocardiogram.
- When the machine finishes, the nurse removes the electrodes.

What are the normal results?

An electrocardiogram should show no disturbances in the heart's function.

What do abnormal results mean?

- An electrocardiogram may show evidence of a heart attack, enlargement of the right or left ventricle, irregular heartbeats, inflammation of the heart, and other problems. Sometimes, an electrocardiogram may only show problems during exercise or an episode of chest pain.

Stress Test

Referred to as an exercise electrocardiogram or an exercise EKG by doctors, this test evaluates the heart's response to physical stress. It provides important information that can't be obtained from a resting electrocardiogram.

In this test, an electrocardiogram and blood pressure readings are taken while a person walks on a treadmill or pedals a stationary bicycle. In the multistage treadmill test, the speed and incline of the treadmill increase at predetermined intervals. In the bicycle test, the resistance in pedaling increases gradually as a person tries to maintain a specific speed.

Unless complications develop, the test goes on until a person reaches the target heart rate (set by the doctor) or feels chest pain or fatigue. A person who's had a recent heart attack or bypass surgery may walk the treadmill at a slow pace to determine his or her activity tolerance before being discharged from the hospital.

Why is this test done?

A stress test may be performed for the following reasons:

- To help diagnose the cause of chest pain
- To determine the heart's condition after surgery or a heart attack
- To check for blockages in the heart's arteries, particularly in men over age 35
- To help set limits for an exercise program
- To identify irregular heartbeats that develop during physical exercise
- To evaluate the effectiveness of drugs given for chest pain or irregular heartbeats

What should you know before the test?

- You'll learn who will perform the test, where it will take place, and its expected duration. Electrodes will be attached to several areas on your chest and, possibly, your back. You won't feel any current from the electrodes; however, they may itch slightly.

- Expect that the test will make you tired, sweaty, and out of breath, but it poses few risks. The doctor may, in fact, stop the test if you feel tired or get chest pains.
- Don't eat, smoke, or drink alcohol or caffeinated beverages for 3 hours before the test. Continue to take any prescribed medications unless your doctor tells you otherwise.
- Wear comfortable socks and sneakers and loose, lightweight shorts or slacks. Men usually don't wear a shirt during the test, and women generally wear a bra and a lightweight short-sleeved blouse or a hospital gown with a front closure.
- Tell the doctor or nurse how you feel during the test.
- You'll be asked to sign a form that gives your permission to do the test. Read the form carefully and ask questions if any portion of it isn't clear.

What happens during the test?

- The electrode sites are cleaned with an alcohol swab, and excess skin oils are removed with a gauze pad or fine sandpaper.
- Electrodes are placed on your chest. The leadwire cable is placed over your shoulder and the leadwire box is placed on your chest. The cable is secured by pinning it to your clothing or taping it to your shoulder or back. Then the leadwires are connected to the chest electrodes.
- The monitor is started, and a tracing is obtained. The doctor checks this tracing, takes your blood pressure, and listens to your heart.
- In a treadmill test, the treadmill is turned on to a slow speed, and you're shown how to step onto it and how to use the support railings to maintain your balance. Then the treadmill is turned off. Next, you step onto the treadmill, and it's turned on to slow speed until you get used to walking on it.
- For a bicycle test, sit on the bicycle while the seat and handlebars are adjusted to comfortable positions. Don't grip the handlebars tightly; just use them for maintaining your balance. Pedal until you reach the desired speed, as shown on the speedometer.
- During both tests, the doctor checks the monitor for changes in the heart's rhythm. The doctor also checks blood pressure at the

Common Diagnostic Tests

end of each test level. Tell the doctor if you feel dizzy, light-headed, short of breath, or unusually tired. If your symptoms become severe, the doctor will halt the test.
- Usually, testing stops when you reach the target heart rate. As the treadmill speed slows, you may be instructed to continue walking for several minutes to prevent nausea or dizziness. When the treadmill is turned off, you are helped to a chair, and your blood pressure and electrocardiogram are monitored for 10 to 15 minutes.

What happens after the test?
- You may resume your usual diet.
- If any drugs were discontinued before the test, you may resume taking them.

Does the test have risks?
- Because a stress test places considerable demands on the heart, it's not usually performed if a person has an aneurysm, uncontrolled irregular heartbeats, an inflammation of the heart, severe anemia, uncontrolled high blood pressure, unstable angina, or congestive heart failure.
- You may become exhausted from the test, experience chest pain or irregular heartbeats, or have significant changes in your blood pressure. The doctor will stop the test if any of these conditions develops.

What are the normal results?

In a normal exercise electrocardiogram, a person's heart rate rises in direct proportion to the workload and increased need for oxygen. Blood pressure also rises as workload increases. A normal person attains the endurance levels appropriate for his or her age.

What do abnormal results mean?

The test can detect the damage caused by a heart attack. Specific changes in electrocardiogram waveforms may indicate disease in the left coronary artery or in multiple blood vessels in the heart.

The usefulness of the test for predicting coronary artery disease varies. Much depends on the person's medical history. However, inaccurate test results are common. To detect coronary artery disease accurately, a thallium scan and stress test, exercise multiple-gated acquisition scan, or an angiogram may be necessary.

Holter Monitoring

This test continuously records the heart's electrical activity as a person goes about a normal routine. In effect, Holter monitoring is an around-the-clock electrocardiogram.

During the test period, which usually lasts for 24 hours but can extend up to 7 days, a person wears a small reel-to-reel or cassette tape recorder that's connected to electrodes placed on the chest. The person also keeps a diary of his or her activities and any associated symptoms. At the end of the recording period, the tape is analyzed by a computer that correlates heart abnormalities, such as irregular beats, with the activities in the diary.

Why is this test done?

Holter monitoring may be performed for the following reasons:

- To detect irregular heartbeats missed by a stress test or resting electrocardiogram
- To evaluate chest pain
- To check the heart's condition after a heart attack or insertion of a pacemaker
- To evaluate the effectiveness of drugs given for irregular heartbeats

What should you know before the test?

- You'll learn that you'll wear a small tape recorder for 24 hours (or for 5 to 7 days if a self-activated monitor is being used). The nurse will show you how to position the recorder when you lie down.
- The nurse or doctor will demonstrate the proper use of specific equipment, including how to mark the tape (if applicable) at the onset of symptoms.
- If a self-activated monitor is being used, you'll be shown how to press the event button to activate the monitor if you experience any unusual sensations. Don't tamper with the monitor or disconnect the leadwires or electrodes.

Common Diagnostic Tests

- If you won't be returning to the office or hospital right after the test, the nurse or doctor will show you how to remove and store the equipment.

What happens during the test?

- The nurse or doctor cleans the electrode sites, applies the electrodes to your skin, attaches the leadwires to the electrodes, and shows you how to wear the monitor on a belt or over your shoulder.
- Continue your routine activities during the test period.
- Write in a diary your usual activities (such as walking, climbing stairs, urinating, sleeping, and sexual activity) and their time. Also write down any emotional upsets, physical symptoms (dizziness, palpitations, fatigue, chest pain, and fainting), and use of medication.
- Wear loose-fitting clothing with front-buttoning tops during the test.
- Avoid magnets, metal detectors, high-voltage areas, and electric blankets during the test.
- Check the recorder to make sure it's working properly. If the monitor light flashes, one of the electrodes may be loose and you should depress the center of each one. Notify the nurse if one comes off.

What happens after the test?

The nurse will remove all chest electrodes and clean the area.

What are the normal results?

Electrocardiogram readings are compared with the person's diary. These readings reveal changes in heart rate that normally occur during various activities. The electrocardiogram should show no significant irregular heartbeats.

What do abnormal results mean?

The test can detect many different types of irregular heartbeats. During recovery from a heart attack, this test can help determine the prognosis and the effectiveness of drug therapy.

Although Holter monitoring matches symptoms and electrocardiogram changes, it doesn't always identify the symptoms' causes. If initial monitoring proves inconclusive, the test may be repeated.

Cardiac Blood Pool Scan

This test is used to check the function of the ventricles, the heart's two lower chambers. (The two upper chambers are called the atria.) To perform this test, the doctor first gives an injection of red blood cells or a protein (albumin) that's tagged with a mildly radioactive substance called technetium. A scintillation camera records radioactivity as the technetium passes through the left ventricle.

Gated cardiac blood pool imaging, performed after a first-pass scan or as a separate test, has several forms. The basic principle is that multiple images are taken to show the heart in motion. This helps the doctor find problem areas in the ventricle.

Another variant of the cardiac blood pool scan, called a MUGA scan, may be done. MUGA stands for a multiple-gated acquisition scan. In this test, a special camera records sequential images of the heart wall that can be studied like motion picture films. These images capture events in the heart's pumping cycle: the contraction of the heart, followed by its relaxation.

Why is this test done?

A cardiac blood pool scan may be performed for the following reasons:

- To check the function of the left ventricle, the chief pumping chamber of the heart
- To detect aneurysms of the left ventricle and other motion abnormalities of the heart wall

What should you know before the test?

- You'll learn about the test, including who will perform it, where it will take place, and its expected duration. During the test, the doctor will inject the test solution into a vein in your forearm. Then a detector positioned above your chest will record the circulation of this solution through the heart. The solution, although slightly radioactive, poses no radiation hazard and rarely produces side effects.

Common Diagnostic Tests

- You'll be directed to remain silent and motionless during the test, unless otherwise instructed.
- You'll be asked to sign a consent form. Carefully read the form and ask questions if any portion of it isn't clear.

What happens during the test?

- At the start of the test, a nurse attaches electrodes to your body so that an electrocardiogram can be performed during the test.
- You lie beneath the detector of a scintillation camera, and the doctor injects the solution.
- For the next minute, the camera records the first pass of the solution through the heart so that heart valves can be located.
- Then the camera records the end of the contraction and relaxation stages of the heartbeat. In all, it records 500 to 1,000 cardiac cycles on X-ray or Polaroid film. An electrocardiograph is used to help time the taking of pictures.
- You may be asked to change your position during the test. You may also be asked to take the drug nitroglycerin or to exercise briefly.

Does the test have risks?

The test shouldn't be performed on a pregnant woman.

What are the normal results?

Normally, the left ventricle contracts symmetrically, and the technetium appears evenly distributed in the scans. Higher counts of radioactivity occur during the heart's contraction because there's more blood in the ventricle. Lower counts occur during its relaxation as the blood is ejected.

What do abnormal results mean?

The test can be used to detect coronary artery disease, which causes asymmetrical distribution of blood to the heart. The test also can detect cardiomyopathies and shunting of blood within the heart.

Part Three

Preventing Heart Disease

Chapter 13

How to Be Heart Healthy

The heart can be compared to an automobile's engine. Both are power units that keep bodies moving. The human heart is responsible for circulating 10½ pints of blood throughout our bodies. When everything is in working order, the heart efficiently supplies every cell with oxygen and nutrients and washes away wastes. But when things go wrong and the flow of blood is interrupted or the heart beats irregularly, life itself is endangered. Like the engine, how you treat your heart, to a large extent, will determine how long and well it will continue to work for you.

"A healthier heart is within everyone's reach," says Denton A. Cooley, M.D., founder, president, and surgeon-in-chief of the Texas Heart Institute. "Each of us, regardless of our age or physical shape, can reduce our risk of heart disease."

Even though there has been an extensive educational effort to make people aware of the causes of heart disease and the measures necessary to prevent it, heart disease remains the leading cause of death in America for both men and women, claiming a life every 33 seconds. Each day 2,600 people die of the disease. In fact, heart disease is responsible for more deaths in America than cancer, AIDS, and accidents combined. Heart disease is any disease that affects the heart or blood vessels. New diagnostic and treatment methods have reduced the number of deaths due to heart disease; yet, they have not affected its prevalence.

"How to Be Heart Healthy," © 1998 Texas Heart Institute, reprinted with permission; and "The Texas Heart Institute Heart-Health Test," © 1997 Texas Heart Institute; reprinted with permission.

"Many people take better care of their cars than their bodies," says Dr. Cooley. "They are careful to change the oil, have regular tune-ups, and use the proper gasoline. However, when it comes to their bodies, they fuel them with high-fat and high-salt meals, smoke, and don't exercise routinely. Medical advances can't eradicate heart disease. Good health depends largely on people taking positive action."

Certain personal habits, as well as physical characteristics, increase your risk for acquiring heart disease. You cannot control risk factors such as gender, age, and genetics, but you need to be aware of how they affect your heart health. Throughout early to middle adulthood, men have a much higher risk for development of heart disease, while women's risk remains fairly low. But between the ages 65 and 84, the risk for heart disease becomes about equal for both sexes. By the time a woman reaches 85, she is twice as likely as a man to have heart disease.

"Women usually develop heart disease about a decade later than men," says Dr. Cooley. "Men tend to show signs of heart disease in their 40's and 50's. As women age, their risk for heart disease markedly increases. This is probably due to the decreasing estrogen levels during and after menopause."

Medical studies indicate that the female hormone estrogen, which regulates the menstrual cycle, protects young women against heart attacks by increasing the high-density lipoprotein (HDL) cholesterol levels in the blood. HDL cholesterol aids in preventing plaque from collecting in the arteries. Plaque is composed of low-density lipoprotein (LDL) cholesterol, fats, and other debris in the blood. Plaque buildup narrows the arteries, restricting the flow of oxygen-rich blood. If the heart is denied blood for approximately 30 minutes, a heart attack occurs—death of a portion of heart tissue. If plaque clogs an artery to the brain and blood flow is halted, it causes a stroke or death of brain tissue.

"Heart disease poses the biggest threat to the average woman's life," says Dr. Cooley. "Postmenopausal women may be able to reduce the risk of cardiovascular disease by taking estrogen or hormone replacement therapy."

As you age the risk for heart disease increases. Your arteries become stiff and less flexible, heart walls may thicken, and the heart muscles may not relax as fully as they did when you were younger. As a result, your heart loses some of its ability to pump blood to muscles, increasing your likelihood of acquiring cardiovascular disease.

One serious threat to individuals as they age is coronary artery disease (CAD), narrowing of the arteries supplying the heart with blood. CAD is a progressive disease that develops over the years as plaque collects in the arteries, restricting the flow of blood to the heart. As plaque limits the flow, you may experience angina or chest pain. If the plaque completely blocks the artery, a heart attack occurs. CAD and other health problems associated with age can be minimized through a heart-healthy diet, regular exercise, and heart-healthy habits, which will be discussed.

Genetics is another predictor of heart disease. The occurrence of heart disease in a direct blood relative (i.e., grandparent, parent, or sibling) before the age of 55 increases your risk of developing heart disease. A family history simply means that you are more likely to develop heart disease than another person your same age and gender who does not have a family history of heart disease. It does not mean that you will definitely acquire heart disease. Researchers are still trying to determine the role of our genes versus our environment. Two risk factors, high blood pressure and high cholesterol, can be inherited, which might explain why some families have a tendency toward heart disease. Also, our families shape many of our attitudes toward lifestyle habits that affect our heart health. Our families influence our views toward diet, exercise, and tobacco usage.

"Although you cannot control risk factors such as gender, age, and genetics, there are many lifestyle risk factors you can alter to prevent or postpone heart disease," says Dr. Cooley. "Medical studies indicate that following a diet low in fat, salt, and cholesterol; refraining from the use of all types of tobacco; exercising at least three times a week; maintaining your ideal weight; and decreasing your blood pressure can reduce your odds of acquiring heart disease."

Smoking is a significant risk factor, especially for women, because it reduces the protective effect of the female hormone estrogen, which aids in the prevention of artery-clogging plaque buildup. Additionally, smoking cigarettes or cigars deprives the heart of oxygen, encourages the blood to clot, promotes irregular heartbeats, and injures the lining of the arteries.

"Smokers have two to ten times the risk for heart attacks," states Dr. Cooley. "By quitting smoking, you can significantly reduce your risk for heart disease. Within 20 minutes of putting down the cigarette, your blood pressure, pulse rate, and body temperature return to normal. The benefits of not smoking increase with time. Studies have shown that after 10 to 14 years, ex-smokers may reduce their risk for heart disease to that of nonsmokers."

Smoking poses even more of a problem for women taking oral contraceptives. Studies have shown that smokers who take oral contraceptives are 39 times more likely to have a heart attack and 22 times

Heart Diseases and Disorders Sourcebook, Second Edition

more likely to have a stroke than women who neither smoke nor take oral contraceptives.

Another significant risk factor for both men and women is weight. Weighing even slightly more than ideal for your height increases your risk for heart disease. The more overweight you are, the greater the risk factor. Where the weight is accumulated is also of extreme importance for both sexes. People who are apple-shaped (gain fat around their middle) are at a much higher risk than those who are pear-shaped (gain fat around the hips).

Exceeding your ideal weight by 30 percent significantly increases your risk for development of heart disease, as well as for high blood cholesterol, high blood pressure, and diabetes—three other risk factors for heart disease. Also, carrying too much weight can harm the circulatory system. A heart-healthy diet and regular physical exercise are the best weapons for weight loss.

Diets high in cholesterol and saturated fat are often the cause for high blood cholesterol, a risk factor for heart disease. A high level of LDL (bad) cholesterol in the blood leads to deposits of plaque in the arteries, narrowing the arteries and reducing the supply of blood to the heart. Extensive plaque buildup is called atherosclerosis or hardening of the arteries because it causes the artery walls to thicken and lose flexibility. It is linked to heart attacks and strokes. Studies indicate that one's total cholesterol should not exceed 200 mg/dL. When cholesterol levels reach 300 mg/dL, the risk for heart disease increases three to five times. Cholesterol levels can be lowered by quitting smoking, drinking alcohol only in moderation (if at all), exercising, and eating a heart-healthy diet.

Another major risk factor is high blood pressure or hypertension. Hypertension is often called the silent killer because it can kill people before it is ever discovered. It forces the heart to pump harder to keep blood moving throughout the body. The heart muscle becomes enlarged and the overworked system performs poorly, delivering less oxygen to other vital organs. If untreated, high blood pressure can lead to a heart attack, stroke, and kidney disease. Blood pressure is a measurement of the force of the blood against the walls of the arteries at the time the heart contracts (the top number or systolic pressure) and a measurement of the heart at rest between beats (the lower number or diastolic pressure). A normal blood pressure reading for an adult at rest is a systolic pressure of 120 to 130 and a diastolic pressure of 80 to 90. However, your blood pressure will vary with your age and activity. No symptoms accompany high blood pressure; thus, it is important to have yearly checkups. The disease can

How to Be Heart Healthy

be controlled by maintaining a heart-healthy lifestyle—no tobacco, a heart-healthy diet, exercise, stress management, and regular physical check-ups.

Diabetes, or high blood sugar, is another risk factor for heart disease. Diabetes is a disease in which the body loses its ability to produce or properly use insulin, which is needed to convert sugar and starch into energy. People who are overweight or have a family history of diabetes face an increased risk of acquiring the disease. Often, the symptoms for diabetes go unnoticed. If the disease is untreated, it can cause serious damage to the heart, eyes, kidneys, and nerves. It also has a tendency to mask the symptoms of heart disease. Diabetics have a threefold probability of acquiring heart disease. Although there is no cure for diabetes, diabetics may prevent or delay heart problems by reducing other risk factors.

"High blood cholesterol, high blood pressure, diabetes, and weight can all be controlled and, in many cases, prevented by a diet low in fat, salt and cholesterol, by regular exercise, and if necessary, by medication," says Dr. Cooley.

Exercise or the lack of it plays a significant role in our health. Research has shown that we need to exercise aerobically (i.e., brisk walking, jogging, cycling, etc.) at least three times a week for 30 minutes to condition our hearts. Also, medical studies indicate that short bouts of exercise equaling 30 minutes are just as beneficial as a continuous 30-minute workout for becoming heart-healthy. Exercise improves our circulation, helps in managing stress, controls our weight, increases HDL (good) cholesterol levels, creates more energy, and helps in lowering blood pressure.

"One of the best things we can do for ourselves is to fuel our body with low fat food and exercise regularly," states Dr. Cooley. "Exercise burns off calories, reduces the appetite, lowers blood pressure, reduces stress levels, and raises HDL cholesterol levels (good cholesterol). It has the added benefit of making us look better and feel more vigorous. It's almost too simple. The foods we eat and our activity level directly influence our heart health. By beginning a weight loss and exercise program, we may postpone or prevent heart disease."

You may be pleasantly surprised to find that by making only a few sensible changes in your diet, you can enjoy the benefits of a heart-smart diet. Heart-healthy habits include limiting your intake of salt to no more than a teaspoon (6 grams) or 2,400 milligrams of sodium a day. If you have high blood pressure, your physician may suggest an even lower level of salt intake. Many snack and convenience foods contain our daily requirement of salt and a large amount of fat.

Your diet should consist primarily of fruits, vegetables, grain products, lean meats, and fish. Try to decrease your level of fat (especially saturated fat) and cholesterol (i.e., fatty red meats, whole milk, whole milk cheeses, eggs, cream-based dishes, and rich desserts). Only 30 percent of your calories should come from fat. You can cut fat and cholesterol by replacing fried foods with roasted, baked, grilled, steamed, and broiled foods. Buy only lean cuts of meat and pare away visible fat prior to cooking. Remove the skin of chicken and turkey prior to cooking—the skin doubles the fat. Also, limit your intake of nuts and seeds, which are high in fat and calories. Replace butter and lard with oils high in monounsaturated fats (i.e., olive, canola, and peanut oil). These oils are not harmful and might be beneficial to your heart health. Your cholesterol consumption should be no more than about 300 milligrams. One egg has approximately 213 milligrams. Eat in small quantities bacon, sausage, hot dogs, bologna, salami, and processed meats, which are high in fat, cholesterol, and salt.

"You can reduce your blood cholesterol level by five to ten percent by eating a heart-healthy diet—consuming more dietary fiber (fruits, vegetables and grains) and less fat (butter) and cholesterol (dairy products and meats)," states Dr. Cooley. "By eating foods high in fiber, people tend to feel full and eat less high-calorie, high-fat, and high-cholesterol foods."

Also, alcohol consumption affects your heart. Medical research indicates that having one ounce of alcohol per day protects against heart disease and heart attacks. One ounce of alcohol is defined as the amount in one 8-ounce glass of wine, two 12-ounce glasses of beer, or one cocktail made with 2-ounces of 100-proof liquor. This moderate amount of alcohol raises the level of HDL (good) cholesterol levels, which helps to move more of the LDL (bad) cholesterol out of the body. Whereas drinking this modest amount of alcohol is helpful to the heart, excessive amounts of alcohol can seriously damage the heart and liver. Overindulging can result in high blood pressure, strokes, irregular heartbeats, and cardiomyopathy, a serious disease which can cause heart failure. Alcohol raises the blood sugar; thus, if you are diabetic avoid alcohol. Additionally, alcohol will worsen the condition of those with high blood pressure and liver disease. Also, pregnant women should limit or avoid alcohol because it can gravely damage the fetus. If you drink, medical experts advise having no more than one to two drinks a day. As with most things, moderation is important, states Dr. Cooley.

Managing stress is important to everyone's well-being, but it is a special concern for those with heart disease. Stress is our mental, physical, and emotional reaction to perceived threats, irritants, and challenges in our lives. It is highly individualized. What one person finds stressful, another finds exhilarating. For instance, some may enjoy driving at high speeds on the freeway, whereas just the thought of driving on the freeway produces symptoms of stress in others.

Those with heart disease often complain of heart pain during emotionally stressful situations. Heart attacks are also more likely during times of stress. When we feel stressed, our hearts race and blood pressure rises, increasing the demand by the heart for oxygen, which can cause chest pain. Also, our arteries can become injured by the combination of excess hormones and blood circulation required during the stress response. As the arterial walls begin to heal, they thicken, making them prone to plaque buildup, which narrows the artery. Additionally, when we are stressed, our blood is more likely to clot and block a narrow artery, causing a heart attack. Researchers, at this time, are not saying that stress causes heart disease, but they do believe it aggravates heart conditions.

Managing stress can improve your life, no matter how healthy you are, says Dr. Cooley. In order to manage stress, you must first be able to identify when you are feeling stressed. Common symptoms of stress include a racing heart, sudden sweating, sudden anger, an upset stomach, headaches, anxiety, tensing-up of muscles, binge eating and drinking, to name a few. Once you recognize that you are under stress, try to pinpoint the cause of it. One helpful way to identify the cause is to write down when you are stressed to find the pattern. Think about ways you could avoid these situations from recurring. You cannot change all the situations that cause you stress but you can change your response to those situations. There are a number ways to reduce the effects of stress on your mind and body. Exercising, crying, taking warm baths, and breathing deeply are just a few ways to minimize stress. Find a method that works for you.

"No one believes that they will have heart disease," says Dr. Cooley, "but many will unless they take steps to change unhealthy habits. The good news is that many heart diseases can be treated or prevented through innovative medicines, technology, and surgery."

If you are experiencing shortness of breath, fatigue, dizziness, fainting, palpitations, swelling of tissue, skin discoloration, or chest pain see your physician immediately. These are common symptoms of heart disease. Early diagnosis and treatment are important in preventing further damage.

"Most of us consider ourselves healthy, as long as we are not experiencing symptoms of illness; however, sometimes the first noticeable symptom of heart disease is a heart attack," says Dr. Cooley. "Once you begin to notice symptoms of heart disease, damage has already occurred. Thus, it is important to be aware of your risk for heart disease and take the necessary steps to reduce your risk."

"The secret to longevity and good health is prevention," says Dr. Cooley. "Make the lifestyle changes necessary to promote good health in the future. By simply controlling one or more of your heart-health risk factors, you can add months and possibly years to your life. You will likely feel more vigorous, too."

To find out more about your personal risk factors, take The Texas Heart Institute Heart-Health Test, shown below.

The Texas Heart Institute Heart-Health Test

The physicians at the Texas Heart Institute have identified nine factors which affect your heart and when added together will give an accurate assessment of the health of your heart. These factors are your personal health history, activity level, weight, use of tobacco, blood pressure, total cholesterol, diabetes, gender, and age. Although other factors such as alcohol use, diet, family history, and stress also affect your heart, the nine identified factors provide the most reliable measurement based on current data. Texas Heart Institute physicians developed this test, excerpted from Texas Heart Institute Heart Owner's Handbook, to provide a quick rating of your heart health. Through this test, you will become aware of your risk for heart disease and how you can improve your heart's health.

To discover how healthy your heart is, please answer the following questions and add the total points for your score.

Personal Health History

1. I have a diagnosed heart or blood vessel disease.

    Yes: 4
    No: 0

Exercise

2. I perform aerobic exercise (i.e., walking, swimming, dancing) for a total of 30 minutes four or more times a week.

    Yes: 0
    No: 4

Weight

3. Using the weight table [you may refer to the weight table posted on the Texas Heart Institute's web site at www.tmc.edu/thi/weightlb.html or you can use the table provided in Chapter 14—Identifying Risk Factors for Heart Disease], find your healthy weight range. Using an appropriate table for your gender, look up your height (without shoes) and body frame size to find your healthy weight range (ranges include 3 pounds of clothing for women, 5 pounds for men). To determine your body frame size, place your left thumb and middle finger around your right wrist and squeeze tightly. If your thumb and finger overlap, you have a small frame; if they touch, you have a medium frame; and if they do not touch, you have a large frame. My weight is:

>20 pounds or more above my healthy range: 3
>10 to 20 pounds above my healthy range: 2
>5 to 10 pounds above my healthy range: 1
>Within 5 pounds of my healthy range: 0

Smoking and Tobacco

4. I smoke cigarettes

>every day: 4
>I used to smoke, but I quit less than 3 years ago: 3
>I don't smoke but I live or work with people who do: 2
>I used to smoke, but I quit more than 3 years ago: 1
>I don't smoke: 0

Blood Pressure (for adults 18 or older)

5. My blood pressure is

>Above 160/90: 4
>Between 140/90 and 160/90: 2
>Below 140/90: 0

Total Cholesterol

6. My cholesterol is

>Above 240 mg/dL: 3
>200 to 240 mg/dL: 2
>I don't know what it is: 1
>200 mg/dL or below: 0

Heart Diseases and Disorders Sourcebook, Second Edition

Diabetes

7. I have high blood sugar or diabetes
   Yes: 4
   No: 0

Gender

8. I am

   male: 4

   I am female, have gone through menopause,
   and am not taking hormone replacement therapy: 3

   I am female, have gone through menopause,
   and am taking hormone replacement therapy: 2

   I am female and have not gone through menopause: 0

Age

9a. I am male and

   over 60: 4
   45 to 60: 3
   30 to 44: 2
   Under 30: 0

9b. I am female and

   Over 60: 3
   45 to 60: 2
   30 to 44: 1
   Under 30: 0

ADD YOUR TOTAL OF POINTS _____

0-12 You are at low risk. Congratulations! Your current lifestyle should keep you healthy for many years.

13-24 You are at medium risk for heart disease. You should modify your lifestyle to reduce your risk of heart disease. If you have not yet discussed your heart risks with your doctor, make an appointment for a complete checkup.

25-34 You are at high risk for heart disease. If you are not already being treated for heart disease, see your doctor immediately. It is important that you begin to reduce your risk as soon as possible. If you already have a heart problem, you can do much to prevent your condition from becoming worse.

Also, if you are experiencing shortness of breath, fatigue, dizziness, fainting, palpitations, swelling of tissue, skin discoloration, or chest pain see your physician immediately. These are common symptoms of heart disease. Early diagnosis and treatment are important in preventing further damage.

"The secret to longevity and good health is prevention," says Dr. Cooley. "Make the lifestyle changes necessary to promote good health in the future."

The Texas Heart Institute at St. Luke's Episcopal Hospital was founded by world renowned cardiovascular surgeon Dr. Denton A. Cooley in 1962 for the study and treatment of diseases of the heart and blood vessels. More than 90,000 open heart operations and 160,000 diagnostic cardiac catheterizations procedures have been performed at the Institute—experience no other facility can match. The Institute's physicians also rank as world leaders in nonsurgical treatment methods. The Texas Heart Institute is consistently counted among the top ten cardiology centers in the United States in U.S. News and World Report's annual guide to "America's Best Hospitals."

If you need information about keeping your heart healthy, e-mail the Heart Information Service or call 1-800-292-2221. (Outside the U.S., call 713/794-6536.) URL: http://www.tmc.edu/thi/heartest.html (Modified 6/17/98)

Chapter 14

Identifying Risk Factors for Heart Disease

Risk Factors and Prevention

Certain risk factors increase your chances of developing cardiovascular disease—especially coronary artery disease, the most common type. Blockages in coronary arteries can lead to angina, heart attack, and death. Some of these factors cannot be controlled, such as heredity, age, and gender. But most risk factors for heart disease can be controlled—often with measures as simple as maintaining a healthy lifestyle, including proper diet and participating in a regular fitness program.

- *Heredity*: When genes are to blame
- *Age*: The older you get, the higher your risk
- *Gender*: Sex influences potential problems
- *High Blood Pressure*: Lower your risk of the "silent killer"
- *Smoking*: The leading cause of preventable death
- *High Cholesterol*: The buildup of plaque that can bring you down
- *Obesity*: Lose pounds to lower risk
- *Diabetes*: A 5-fold risk in heart disease
- *Stress*: Manage your moods to prevent heart disease
- *Sedentary Lifestyle*: Get moving to reduce risk

© 1997 Johns Hopkins InteliHealth (www.intelihealth.com); reprinted with permission of InteliHealth.

Heredity

Your risk of developing coronary artery disease is higher if you have a close relative (mother, father, brother or sister) who developed the disease before age 55. This increased risk holds true even if you have eliminated risks that weren't as well known a generation ago, such as smoking or high blood cholesterol. The greatest inherited risk of heart disease is a genetic predisposition to have dangerously high cholesterol levels, a condition known as familial hypercholesterolemia that is marked by blood cholesterol levels above 300 mg/dl. Other genetic factors passed on from parents to children may promote the development of moderately high cholesterol or triglyceride levels, low HDL cholesterol levels, high blood pressure, diabetes, or obesity.

Although you can't alter your genetic background, you can do your best to control those risk factors under your control—high cholesterol levels, stress, smoking, obesity, and a sedentary lifestyle.

Race also plays a role in the development of cardiovascular disease, mainly for high blood pressure. Compared with whites, African Americans develop high blood pressure at an earlier age. And no matter their age, the disease is more severe in blacks than in whites. Because high blood pressure increases the risk of other cardiovascular diseases, blacks are 1.8 times more likely to have a nonfatal stroke, 1.3 times more likely to have a fatal stroke, and 1.5 times more likely to die from heart disease than are whites. Although many theories have been proposed to explain these inequalities in the risk of developing and dying from heart disease, to date, researchers have had difficulty determining the exact reasons. One theory is that blacks may suffer from a lack of access to health care. And high blood pressure is thought to be more common in blacks because of racial differences in the way sodium is excreted by the body; some researchers believe that blacks retain more sodium than whites, a factor that can work to increase blood pressure.

Genes may play a role in another way, too: Evidence is mounting that high levels of an amino acid called homocysteine may also play a role in clogging the arteries that feed the heart and the brain. In Harvard's ongoing Physicians' Health Study, men with high homocysteine levels had three times the risk of heart attack compared to men with lower levels—even when other risk factors were taken into account. Although more research is needed, other major studies have found that people who had heart attacks or strokes had higher homocysteine levels than control groups of healthy people. Some people inherit extremely high levels of homocysteine and may die of complications of

Identifying Risk Factors for Heart Disease

arteriosclerosis at an early age. A diet high in folic acid has been found to lower blood homocysteine levels. Orange juice, lentils, spinach and vitamin-fortified cereals are all good sources of folic acid.

Age

Cardiovascular disease becomes more common as you age. About 10,000 women and 18,000 men under age 45 die of cardiovascular disease each year. But between the ages of 45 and 64, that figure climbs to about 40,000 women and 85,000 men. From ages 65 and 84, it soars to about 240,000 women and 260,000 men. That is why it becomes increasingly important as you age to pay careful attention to diet, fitness, and other factors that can prevent or reduce the risk of heart disease.

Years or decades of a poor diet take their toll as you age and fatty plaques that have collected along artery walls slow or impede blood flow. Older people also are less likely to exercise regularly, and more likely to have developed other cardiovascular risk factors such as high blood pressure and diabetes. The effects of age also are felt directly by the blood vessels and the heart. As blood vessels age, they become less flexible and thus make it harder for blood to move through them. The heart itself expands with age. As any muscle, the heart grows the more it is worked. After a lifetime of pumping, the heart may become enlarged. An enlarged heart is less able to pump blood efficiently than a firm smaller heart.

Gender

It's hard to separate the role of gender from other risk factors in the development of coronary artery disease. Men are more likely to have coronary artery disease than women until women reach menopause. The hormone estrogen protects women from heart disease until they reach menopause. But after menopause, women catch up with men and have nearly the same rate of heart attacks.

For many years, heart disease was thought to be primarily a male concern, though recently doctors have come to realize that this is not true—heart disease is an equal opportunity destroyer. About 44 percent of women die within a year of heart attack, compared to only 27 percent of men, according to the American Heart Association. During the first four years following a heart attack, about 20 percent of women will suffer another heart attack, compared to 16 percent of men.

The reasons are unclear, but doctors do know that about one of every four women over age 20 will develop high blood pressure, and that women who have never had the condition may develop it during pregnancy. After menopause, about half of all women over age 55 develop high blood pressure; by age 75, women are about 15 percent more likely to have the condition than men. Also, the average cholesterol level in women rises from 199 mg/dl before age 55 to an average of 237 mg/dl after menopause. The combination of these factors may help explain why older women are at increased risk of heart disease.

The female hormone estrogen is one protector against heart disease. Estrogen boosts levels of protective HDL cholesterol, which helps to carry cholesterol out of the body. As levels of the hormone decline at menopause, a woman's risk of heart disease increases. About 3,000 women between the ages of 29 and 44 have a heart attack each year; that figure climbs to 136,000 among women aged 45 to 64, and skyrockets to 374,000 among women over age 65, according to the Framingham Heart Study.

The good news: Estrogen replacement therapy seems to reduce a women's risk of heart disease (as well as osteoporosis, the bone-thinning disease). But since estrogen may increase your risk of uterine cancer and possibly breast cancer, the decision to use hormonal therapy should be made after discussing your personal risk factors with your doctor.

High Blood Pressure

Blood doesn't flow in a steady stream, but moves through the circulatory system in spurts determined by your heart's beats. With each beat, about two ounces of freshly oxygenated blood is forced out of the left ventricle (the main pumping chamber) into the aorta and into the body's 60,000 miles of blood vessels. The tension or force that is placed on the inside walls of arteries to keep blood flowing is known as "blood pressure."

Your blood pressure is constantly changing, depending on how hard the heart is working. During exercise, for instance, the heart can pump up to three times as fast as during periods of rest. Between heartbeats the heart muscle rests momentarily and gets ready for the next beat. Blood pressure is measured by two numbers, such as 110 over 70 or 110/70. The higher number—called the systolic pressure—is the highest pressure in your arteries when your heart contracts to exert maximum force on the walls of blood vessels during a heartbeat.

Identifying Risk Factors for Heart Disease

The lower number—called the diastolic pressure—is the lowest pressure in your arteries when your heart relaxes momentarily between beats and fills with blood.

How It's Measured

Blood pressure is measured in millimeters of mercury (mm Hg). This unit refers to how high the pressure inside your arteries can raise a column of mercury. A typical normal blood pressure is considered to be 120/70 mm Hg, and high blood pressure is generally categorized as consistent readings of 140/90 mm Hg or higher; severe high blood pressure constitutes a reading of 200/115 mm Hg. A doctor shouldn't make a diagnosis of high blood pressure based on a single reading. Normal blood pressure refers to your pressure when you're resting, but your blood pressure varies with exercise, strong emotion, and stress. What's more, blood pressure increases gradually with age as the artery walls become less elastic.

Blood pressure is usually measured with a sphygmomanometer, a device that consists of an inflatable rubber cuff, an air pump, and a column of mercury or a dial or digital readout reflecting pressure in the air column. The cuff is wrapped around the upper arm and tightened until blood flow through the large artery in the arm is stopped. As air is pumped into the cuff, it pushes up a column of mercury or air. The doctor or nurse places a stethoscope over the artery and listens first for the cessation of blood flow, then as the cuff is loosened, the first thumping sound of blood flow resuming in the vessels. The height of the mercury or air indicates the systolic pressure. The pressure when the thumping sound stops is the diastolic pressure. While doctors had thought that the presence of hypertension required both an elevated systolic (first number) and diastolic (second number), they now believe that you have high blood pressure if either your systolic pressure exceeds 140 or your diastolic is greater than 90.

High blood pressure is not a condition to take lightly, because it can damage components of the circulatory system—including the blood vessels of the heart, brain, eyes, and kidneys. And the longer it goes undiagnosed and untreated, the worse the outlook, because it forces your heart to work harder than normal. Blood pressure is like a weight or load that the heart muscle must lift, and like any muscle, your heart gets larger with heavy work. Eventually, the muscle can no longer adapt to the excessive work load, and the heart's pumping efficiency decreases. If this occurs, the heart muscle may weaken and heart failure may develop. High blood pressure also accelerates the development of atherosclerosis in your arteries as you age, increasing the chances of a stroke or heart attack. And by putting increased pressure on your artery walls, high blood pressure also can lead to an aneurysm, a bulge in a weakened artery.

Because high blood pressure is a risk factor for so many forms of heart disease, it's important to get it under control. Many studies have demonstrated a direct relationship between high blood pressure and stroke, coronary artery disease, heart failure, and kidney failure. Compared with people whose high blood pressure is under control, those with uncontrolled high blood pressure are about 3 times more likely to have coronary artery disease, about 6 times more likely to have congestive heart failure, and about 7 times more likely to have a stroke.

Know Your Numbers

Systolic *(first number)*

- *Less than 130 mm Hg*: normal blood pressure; recheck within two years
- *130 to 139 mm Hg*: high normal; recheck within one year
- *140 to 150 mm Hg*: mild high blood pressure; recheck within two months
- *160 to 179 mm Hg*: moderate high blood pressure; see your doctor within one month
- *180 to 209 mm Hg*: severe high blood pressure; see your doctor within one week
- *210 mm Hg or higher*: very severe high blood pressure; see your doctor immediately

Diastolic *(second number)*

- *Less than 85 mm Hg*: normal blood pressure; recheck within 2 years
- *85 to 89 mm Hg*: high-normal blood pressure; recheck within 1 year
- *90 to 99 mm Hg*: mild high blood pressure; recheck within 2 months
- *100 to 109 mm Hg*: moderate high blood pressure; see your doctor within 1 month

Identifying Risk Factors for Heart Disease

- *110 to 119 mm Hg*: severe high blood pressure; see your doctor within 1 week

- *120 mm Hg or higher*: very severe high blood pressure; see your doctor immediately

Treatment

A kidney disorder, adrenal gland or pituitary tumor, defects or constriction of the aorta, or thyroid disease are sometimes the underlying cause of high blood pressure; but in more than 90 percent of cases, no specific cause can be found. If you have high blood pressure, it's very important to work with your doctor to get your blood pressure down to safe levels. Treatment may include lifestyle changes (losing weight may be all that's necessary), drug therapy or some combination of both. In fact, one recent study called the Dietary Approaches to Stop Hypertension Trial (DASH) found that a diet high in fruits, vegetables, and low-fat dairy products may be enough on its own to reduce blood pressure in some people.

In the DASH trial, people with high blood pressure, (averaging 160/95) were split into two groups, each following a slightly different diet. One was the typical American diet—consisting of 3.5 pieces of fruit and vegetables a day, one-half serving of low-fat dairy products, and 3.5 servings of fish, poultry, or meat. The second diet consisted of nine pieces of fruit or vegetables, 3.5 servings of low-fat dairy products and only about two servings of fish, poultry or meat. The study found that people who followed the second diet lowered their blood pressure to an average of 150/90, while blood pressure did not change in those following the typical American diet.

Besides eating right, here's what experts generally recommend for controlling high blood pressure:

- **Don't smoke.** Smoking promotes artherosclerosis and contributes to high blood pressure.

- **Lose weight** (if necessary). Weight loss lowers blood pressure, eases the burden on your heart and may prevent diabetes and its complications.

- **Reduce salt intake to about 2,500 mg a day.** Cutting down on salt (actually the sodium it contains) may lower your blood pressure, as about two-thirds of Americans are sensitive to salt. Since it's hard to know whether your blood pressure is affected by salt, it pays to cut back if you have hypertension or are at risk for it. Excess sodium encourages the body to retain fluid. This excess fluid puts undo strain on the heart by increasing the volume of blood, leaving the heart with more to pump. Excess fluid in the body's tissues is a problem for people with congestive heart failure. It may also interfere with certain fluid-reducing medications, such as diuretics.

- **Increase fiber in your diet**, especially soluble fiber (found in oat bran, beans, pears and apples, for example). Soluble fiber binds with bile acids in the intestine so that they are excreted instead of being absorbed into the bloodstream. The result, increased formation of bile acids from cholesterol, can lower blood cholesterol levels.

- **Limit alcohol** to no more than one ounce a day. That's about the amount of alcohol in one mixed drink, a glass of wine, or a bottle of beer. Larger amounts of alcohol can raise blood pressure.

- **Increase physical activity** to at least three times per week, for about 30 minutes per session. Exercises best for controlling blood pressure are aerobic activities like walking, running, swimming, bicycling, or others that boost your heart rate and keep it high for an extended period of time.

- **Practice a regular form of relaxation therapy**, such as meditation, yoga, or biofeedback. That's because blood pressure tends to increase during periods of uncontrolled stress.

Medications

There are many drugs that can control blood pressure effectively with different modes of action and different side effects. These medications are divided into six categories: diuretics, vasodilators, alpha-blockers, beta-blockers, ACE inhibitors, and calcium channel blockers. Within each category are a number of different drugs. Because of their variety, as well as their variable actions (age, race, and severity of hypertension make a difference) and side effects, national consensus guidelines have been developed as a standardized approach to treating hypertension.

- The first step is to try to lower your blood pressure with lifestyle changes. If this effort doesn't reduce pressure sufficiently or if the level of blood pressure is very high, drugs are added.

Identifying Risk Factors for Heart Disease

- Your doctor may first prescribe a diuretic or beta-blocker.
- If these drugs aren't effective, your doctor has three treatment options: increase the dose, substitute another drug, or add a second drug from a different class of antihypertensives. If your blood pressure still is not controlled, a third drug may be added.

It may take trying a number of different drug combinations before you and your doctor find the drug or drugs that work best for you. Don't get discouraged during this phase. It's important for you to follow your doctor's advice, return as advised to check your blood pressure and tell your doctor how you are adjusting to the medications. Working together, you'll find the best way to reduce your blood pressure and your risk of heart disease or a stroke.

- **Drug Category:** Diuretics
- **How They Work:** By helping the kidneys remove sodium and extra water
- **Some Common Agents:** Chlorthalidone, Chlorthiazide, Hydrochlorthiazide

- **Drug Category:** ACE inhibitors
- **How They Work:** By dilating arteries and decreasing the resistance of the blood pumped from the heart
- **Some Common Agents:** Captopril, Enalapril, Lisinopril

- **Drug Category:** Angiotensin Receptor Blockers
- **How They Work:** Like ACE inhibitors, by dilating arteries and decreasing the resistance to blood flow
- **Some Common Agents:** Losartan, Valsartan

- **Drug Category:** Vasodilators
- **How They Work:** By relaxing the muscles in the walls of the blood vessels
- **Some Common Agents:** Hydralazine, Minoxidil

- **Drug Category:** Calcium Channel Blockers
- **How They Work:** By slowing the flow of calcium into blood vessels, which in turn relaxes the vessels
- **Some Common Agents:** Diltiazem, Verapamil, Nifedipine

- **Drug Category:** Alpha-blockers
- **How They Work:** By relaxing the nerves that are central to regulating blood pressure
- **Some Common Agents:** Terazosin, Doxazosin

- **Drug Category:** Beta-blockers
- **How They Work:** By blocking receptors in the brain that are increasing blood pressure
- **Some Common Agents:** Metoprolol, Propranolol, Atenolol

Smoking

Smoking is the leading cause of preventable illness and death in the United States where more than 400,000 deaths every year are attributed to smoking. At least one in three of these deaths is related to cardiovascular disease.

The reason: Tobacco smoke contains about 4,000 substances, many of them known to cause adverse health effects. The dangers of three of them, nicotine, tar, and carbon monoxide are particularly important.

- Nicotine is the substance that causes addiction to tobacco. It stimulates the release of epinephrine—adrenaline—into the smoker's bloodstream, forcing the heart to work harder (and offering a possible explanation for why smokers have raised blood pressure). By constricting blood vessels, including the coronary arteries, nicotine compromises the heart's own blood supply.

- Tar in tobacco produces chronic irritation of the respiratory system and is a major cause of lung cancer.

- Carbon monoxide passes from the lungs into the bloodstream, where it combines with hemoglobin and reduces the amount of oxygen that can be carried in your red blood cells. It also damages blood vessel linings, contributing to atherosclerosis. In the long term, persistently high levels of carbon monoxide in the blood lead to hardening of the arteries, which increases the risk of a heart attack.

- Smoking also contributes to hardening of the arteries and to atherosclerosis by lowering HDL cholesterol levels. Triglyceride (fat) levels may also be higher in smokers. And smoking also raises blood levels of fibrinogen, a substance involved in clotting,

Identifying Risk Factors for Heart Disease

thereby increasing the likelihood of a blood clot forming in an already narrowed heart artery.

The main cardiovascular risk from smoking is that it promotes atherosclerosis in blood vessels. The mechanism for this effect isn't certain, but several potential links have been identified. Smoking reduces the proportion of HDL (good) cholesterol to LDL (bad) cholesterol in the blood and increases the tendency for blood to clot inside blood vessels and obstruct blood flow. Components of tobacco smoke, particularly carbon monoxide, may also directly damage the internal lining of the blood vessels.

Inhaling cigarette smoke—even through second-hand smoke, which causes an estimated 35,000 to 40,000 deaths from cardiovascular disease each year—also has a temporary but harmful effect on your heart and blood vessels that may lead to serious consequences, such as a heart attack. That's because the nicotine in smoke raises your blood pressure and increases heart rate. Carbon monoxide, the same gas in car exhaust that's lethal in closed spaces, gets into your blood and reduces the amount of oxygen your blood can carry to your heart and the rest of your body. These effects of smoking may lead to ischemia (a lack of blood flow and oxygen to the heart muscle) and cause chest pain (angina) or a heart attack. Besides these effects on the heart and its arteries, smoking is the main cause of chronic lung diseases such as chronic bronchitis, emphysema and, of course, lung cancer.

You Can *Stop Smoking*

If you smoke, it's never too late to get the benefits of stopping—as demonstrated by the fact that millions of American smokers have managed to kick the habit. The good news is that the day after you quit, your heart already starts to recover. Your risk of heart disease will drop dramatically within the first two years after kicking the habit. According to the American Lung Association, a two-pack a day smoker is at double the risk of heart disease compared with non-smokers; Once you quit, however, that risk is only about 30 percent higher than non-smokers.

So how do you do it? You can try smoking fewer cigarettes, but you're likely to end up smoking just as many as you used to. And switching to "low-tar, low-nicotine" cigarettes usually does little good: Because nicotine is so addictive, most smokers who switch brands automatically compensate by puffing on each cigarette harder and more often. Just because a cigarette is listed as low-tar or low-nicotine, doesn't mean the smoker is inhaling less nicotine. By inhaling more deeply smokers can get as much nicotine (and tar) out of a low-nicotine cigarette as from a regular one. The only safe choice is to quit completely. And here's how:

Try the Write Stuff. Write down your most important personal reason to quit. Is it to regain control of your life and health? To set a good example for your children? To protect your family from the dangers of secondhand smoke? Personal motivation is a key predictor of success in quitting smoking, and keeping a personal "record" of that motivation helps many smokers quit. It also helps to write a letter to loved ones stating the reasons why smoking is so important that you choose to die early rather than be with them. This type of letter is especially powerful, because it helps make you feel selfish and foolish for continuing a habit that will surely harm you (and them), and offers some people the motivation to finally quit.

Take It Slowly. Most smokers fail at their first attempt to quit, and nearly all smokers experience some degree of nicotine withdrawal. So give yourself a month to overcome these symptoms. The quitting process should be taken one day at a time to ensure long-term success. Some people pay themselves for each day they go smokeless—just take the money you'd normally spend on cigarettes or cigars and put it in a jar. At the end of each week or month, buy yourself some "reward" item.

Avoid the Triggers. To be successful at quitting, you have to avoid or even leave situations that trigger the urge to light up. That includes social gatherings where smoking is permitted, restaurants, and maybe even your morning coffee. In fact, many smoking cessation experts recommend that you cut back on both caffeine and alcohol while you're trying to quit; both are triggers for smoking. If you like to smoke after a meal, go for a walk instead. If you smoke while watching TV, munch on celery. Keep a diary of when you smoke. The diary can help determine your triggers, so you can avoid or modify them.

Get with a Program. Deciding to "tough it out" on your own may not work well over the long-term. Women in particular seem to benefit from group support while trying to quit; but even if you go it alone, following a regimen from a smoking cessation program offers you a better chance at success. You can find these programs in your local Yellow Pages, but can also get information from these national agencies:

Identifying Risk Factors for Heart Disease

- Agency for Health Care Policy and Research at 800-358-9295
- American Cancer Society at 800-ACS-2345
- American Heart Association at 800-AHA-USA1
- American Lung Association at 800-LUNG-USA
- Centers for Disease Control and Prevention (CDC), Office on Smoking and Health at 800-CDC-1311
- National Cancer Institute (NCI) at 800-4-CANCER

Don't Worry about Your Waistline. Fear of gaining weight is one of the most commonly cited reasons smokers—especially women—give when explaining why they don't want to quit. But it needn't be. About one in three smokers gain weight when they quit, but 90 percent of them actually lose that weight within a year or two. Meanwhile, two in three either lose weight (usually by starting an exercise program) or stay at the same weight.

Ex-smokers may gain weight for two reasons: their metabolism slows from the lack of nicotine and they may compensate for the lack of cigarettes by snacking on candy and junk food. But if you need "finger food," choosing low-fat snacks such as carrot sticks and fruit can help. Meanwhile, the American Heart Association has helpful guidelines for avoiding weight gain. To request a free copy, call the American Heart Association at 800-AHA-USA1, or visit their site on the World Wide Web at www.americanheart.org.

Get Help with a Nicotine Replacement Therapy. Using a nicotine patch or gum has been shown to increase your chances of successfully kicking the smoking habit; one recent study showed that 21 percent of smokers successfully quit with the aid of patches, compared to only 9 percent of a placebo group. Both patches and gum provide the body with a steady stream of nicotine, to help reduce the withdrawal symptoms caused by not smoking.

The patches now available over-the-counter are placed on your shoulder or back each morning and worn for about eight weeks; most smokers start with full-strength patches containing 15 to 22 mg of nicotine and then switch to "weaker" patches containing 5 to 14 mg of nicotine. Some people develop slight skin irritations at the patch site, but this is usually easily treated and moving the patch to another part of the body usually helps.

Nicotine gums, also available over-the-counter, must be chewed slowly for about 30 minutes for best results—usually one piece every hour or two for up to three months. Side effects include mild hiccups, jaw aches or stomach ache. Many smokers start with a 2 mg dose, but heavy smokers—those who smoke more than one pack a day—may opt for the 4 mg dose.

Try the Alternative Route. While proponents of alternative methods of smoking cessation like acupuncture and hypnosis claim they can help reduce your cravings for nicotine, no studies have shown that they actually help smokers kick the habit. Still, many people have tried these and other alternative methods with success. With acupuncture, fine needles are inserted in and around your ear lobes and the acupuncture technician then may tape a small button on your ear lobe which you are advised to press or massage when the urge to smoke overcomes you. Hypnosis for smoking cessation may work by a process called suggestion. When you visit a hypnosis specialist, you'll be put under a trance during which the hypnotist will suggest that you do not enjoy smoking, that cigarettes taste bad, or a host of other negative ideas regarding smoking. The hypnosis theory holds that you will remember these suggestions when the urge to smoke overtakes you.

High Cholesterol

In the past decade cholesterol has become a household word as a risk factor for coronary artery disease. Cholesterol is a sterol, one of several types of fats (lipids) that play an important role in your body. Your liver makes cholesterol from nutrients in food and uses it for a variety of important functions, including building cells and manufacturing hormones. You also get cholesterol from animal foods in your diet—such as meat, eggs, and dairy products. Although dietary cholesterol can raise blood cholesterol, most of the cholesterol in your blood is made by the liver; and saturated fat is the greater villain in heart disease.

Research clearly shows that too much cholesterol in your blood can cause buildup of atherosclerotic plaques, the accumulations in arteries that can block blood flow and lead to a heart attack. Cholesterol is a fat and it doesn't dissolve in water. Therefore, to circulate through your watery blood, cholesterol and triglycerides (another blood fat) are combined with proteins to form lipoproteins.

There are four types of lipoproteins, differing in the ratio of protein to triglyceride and cholesterol. The main types are the familiar low-density lipoprotein (LDL) and high-density lipoprotein (HDL).

LDL cholesterol, the so-called "bad" cholesterol, is transported to sites throughout the body where it's used to repair cell membranes

Identifying Risk Factors for Heart Disease

or to make hormones. LDL cholesterol can accumulate in the walls of your arteries, somewhat in the way hard water promotes a buildup of lime inside the plumbing of your house. Cholesterol deposits, however, are spotty, rather than evenly coated throughout the arteries.

HDL, which carries the so-called "good" cholesterol, transports cholesterol to the liver where it's altered and removed from the body. In a sense, HDL is the clean-up crew that sops up excess cholesterol from the tissues and disposes of it before it can do any damage. In fact, there is no "good" cholesterol. The lipoprotein HDL is "good" rather than the cholesterol it carries. But laboratories measure HDL cholesterol rather than HDL itself.

Recent research indicates that the ratio of LDL cholesterol to HDL cholesterol is a good measure of your risk for developing heart disease. Ideally, LDL cholesterol levels should be below 130 mg/dl, and HDL cholesterol levels should be above 45 mg/dl. A relatively low ratio of LDL cholesterol to HDL cholesterol—less than 3—is desirable. For example: Divide LDL cholesterol (130) by HDL cholesterol (45) = 2.8.

But cholesterol isn't the only lipid circulating in your blood. Triglycerides (three fatty acids attached to a glycerol molecule) is transportable fuel used by the body to produce energy. The saturated and unsaturated fats you're always reading about are found on different types of triglycerides. All fats and oils in food contain mixtures of fatty acids, although in different proportions—the familiar saturated, polyunsaturated, and monounsaturated fats. The more the fatty acid molecule is saturated (with hydrogen atoms), the less heart-healthy the fat.

Know Your Numbers

Cholesterol and triglycerides are measured in milligrams per deciliter of blood (mg/dl).

Table 14.1. Cholesterol and Triglyceride Levels

	Desirable	Borderline	Too High
Total cholesterol	<200	200-239 mg/dl	>240 mg/dl
LDL cholesterol	<130	130-159 mg/dl	>160 mg/dl
Triglycerides	<200 mg/dl		>200 mg/dl
LDL/HDL Ratio	<3	3-5	>5

	Average	Too Low
HDL cholesterol in males	45 mg/dl	<35 mg/dl
HDL cholesterol in females	55 mg/dl	<35 mg/dl

Cholesterol in Your Body

The cholesterol in your bloodstream comes from two sources: partly from your diet, but mostly from the liver and intestines. Your body manufactures all the cholesterol you need, so you don't have to consume it to maintain your health. Your blood cholesterol level is affected by your diet and your genetic makeup. Regular aerobic exercise reduces the blood level of triglycerides and increases the level of HDL cholesterol.

Your genes can affect your cholesterol levels. Because of abnormal genes inherited from their parents, some people lack certain cell receptors that are needed for removing LDL from the blood. In this condition, called familial hypercholesterolemia, people can have extremely high levels of LDL cholesterol. This results from inheriting one bad gene (heterozygote) or two bad genes (homozygote). Heterozygotes can die prematurely of coronary artery disease, usually in their 40s to 60s, while homozygotes can die in their teens or 20s.

Cholesterol is contained in animal foods—meat, fish, poultry, and whole-milk dairy products. It's not found in any plant foods such as fruits, vegetables, and legumes, or in cooking oils. But excess saturated fat in your diet can increase your cholesterol levels. Cooking oils get all of their calories from fats, but they contain primarily monounsaturated and polyunsaturated fats which do not raise cholesterol levels.

Medications

Reducing your cholesterol and other levels of blood fats should begin with lifestyle changes, such as following a low-fat diet and controlling weight, but a number of drugs can lower total and LDL cholesterol and triglyceride levels, while increasing beneficial HDL. If your cholesterol levels are high despite dietary changes, talk to your doctor about how to reduce them with these lipid-lowering medications:

- **Drug Category:** Bile acid sequestrants
- **How They Work:** By binding bile acids (which are made from cholesterol) in the intestines and removing them in the stool. More cholesterol is then used by the liver to make bile acids.
- **Some Common Agents:** Cholestyramine, Colestipol

- **Drug Category:** Gemfibrozil
- **How They Work:** By activating an enzyme that speeds the breakdown of triglycerides in the blood.
- **Some Common Agents:** Gemfibrozil (Lopid)

Identifying Risk Factors for Heart Disease

- **Drug Category:** HMG-CoA reductase inhibitors (statins)
- **How they Work:** By blocking the production of cholesterol.
- **Some Common Agents:** Lovastatin, Pravastatin, Simvastatin, Fluvastatin, Atorvastatin

- **Drug Category:** Niacin
- **How they Work:** By reducing the liver's ability to produce very low density lipoprotein, the precursor of LDL.
- **Some Common Agents:** Nicotinic acid

Obesity

One of every three Americans is overweight, and one in 10 is obese—categorized as being 20 percent or more above the normal weight for their height. Obesity is defined as an excess of body fat. Obesity is increasing in the U.S. at all ages. Being obese is more than a cosmetic problem: It increases the risk of cardiovascular health by promoting other risk factors such as high triglycerides, low HDL, high blood pressure, and diabetes. Also, if heart disease is already present, it's further aggravated by excess pounds.

There are various ways of determining whether you are obese—none of which is perfect. One of the easiest is to compare your weight with the recommended weights on the table from the federal government's "Dietary Guidelines for Americans." But no height-weight table can take into account individual variations in proportions of fat and lean tissue (since muscle weighs more than fat) or the distribution of fat in the body. For instance, a person with a great deal of muscle may be overweight according to the table but have a very low proportion of body fat, and thus not be obese and have an increased risk of heart disease.

Where your body's weight is distributed also has an important bearing on your risk for cardiovascular disease. In some obese people, most of the excess fat is deposited in the abdomen—they are called "apple-shaped"—while it settles around the hips and thighs in "pear-shaped" folks. Apple-shaped people (more commonly men) have a higher risk of heart disease than do those shaped like a pear (more commonly women). One possible reason: While other fat cells empty their fat content directly into the general blood circulation, the contents of abdominal fat cells go directly to the liver before entering the bloodstream. Abdominal obesity is associated with a resistance to insulin; in an effort to compensate for this resistance, the pancreas secretes

Heart Diseases and Disorders Sourcebook, Second Edition

excessive amounts of insulin. The resulting high blood levels of insulin set up a complex chain of reactions that eventually leads to hypertension, elevated triglycerides, low HDL levels and accelerated atherosclerosis; diabetes and coronary heart disease may follow.

One way to estimate your risk is to divide your waist circumference by your hip measurement. A ratio less than 0.80 is desirable for women, and a ratio less than 1.0 is desirable for men.

Table 14.2. How Much Should You Weigh?

Height (inches)	Weight (pounds) Ages 19-34	Ages 35 and older
60	97-128	108-138
61	101-132	111-143
62	104-137	115-148
63	107-141	119-152
64	111-146	122-157
65	114-150	126-162
66	118-155	130-167
67	121-160	134-172
68	125-164	138-178
69	129-169	142-183
70	132-174	146-188
71	136-179	151-194
72	140-184	155-199
73	144-189	159-205
74	148-195	164-210
75	152-200	168-216
76	156-205	173-222
77	160-211	177-228
78	164-216	182-234

Note: Recommended weights for women are on the lower end of the range; weights for men are on the higher end.

Identifying Risk Factors for Heart Disease

Diabetes

Diabetes is responsible for many health complications, including an increased risk of blood vessel disease and coronary artery disease. All things being equal, diabetes increases the risk of heart disease 5-fold in a woman and 2-fold in a man. In fact, about 80 percent of people with diabetes die of some form of heart disease or a stroke. Part of the reason is that diabetes raises cholesterol and triglyceride levels, and diabetics tend to be overweight.

In Type 2 (also called "non-insulin-dependent" or "adult-onset") diabetes, the body's cells become resistant to insulin and the pancreas cannot produce enough insulin to overcome the resistance. Insulin is the hormone that permits blood glucose (sugar) to move into the body's cells where it's used for energy. Insulin also reduces the amount of glucose released by the liver.

When the body fails to respond to normal insulin levels, insulin production increases. Elevated levels of insulin, however, can raise blood pressure and encourage the deposition of fat in artery walls. The result is clogged coronary arteries, plus a variety of other vascular problems, such as the leg pain of peripheral artery disease.

Weight loss can decrease the demand for insulin and exercise can help you to use excess blood glucose, preventing or slowing the onset of diabetes. If you are at risk for cardiovascular disease, it's important that your doctor check you for diabetes, as some of its symptoms—slow-healing infections, tingling or numbness in the hands and feet, blurred vision—may be subtle or absent at first.

Stress

Harnessed constructively, stress can fuel creativity and personal accomplishment. But when unmanaged and out of control, stress takes a terrible toll on your body. Research seems to suggest that your personality, the stressful events in your life and your body's physiological reaction to stress can increase your risk of heart disease. The stress/heart disease connection, however, is still a theory. Stress is difficult to study, because it's hard to measure the psychological and physical responses to stress.

But this much is clear: When an event is perceived as a threat—whether a deadline, a divorce, stalled traffic or misplaced keys—the body harks back to that ancient "fight-or-flight" response that once meant life or death. First, the stress hormones—adrenaline and cortisol (made by the adrenal glands)—flood the body, increasing the heart's need for oxygen as it prepares for vigorous action. Heart rate and blood pressure increase. Blood vessels in your skin constrict. Muscles tense and blood sugar levels increase. The tendency for blood to clot increases and the body's cells pour stored fat into the bloodstream. Add it all up and it puts additional strain on the heart and artery linings.

People who already have coronary artery disease may experience chest pain (angina) as a pounding heart and rising blood pressure increase the heart's need for oxygen. And the increased tendency for the blood to clot may predispose certain people to develop a clot in their coronary arteries, causing a heart attack.

Blowing up now and then isn't harmful. But if your emotional responses get stuck in a constant state of irritation and anger, your physical stress responses also stall in overdrive—raising blood pressure, constricting blood vessels, and pouring out a constant flood of stress hormones. Over time, as the body becomes less sensitive to cortisol and the other stress hormones, the adrenal glands respond by increasing production, even though the original trigger is no longer there.

Treatment

Although you can't control some of the events that cause stress, you can control how you manage it. The first step is to recognize the symptoms of stress, such as muscular tension, headache, insomnia, irritability, and changes in eating habits. Other warning signs include apathy, mental or physical fatigue, and frequent illness. To determine whether you may have a Type A personality, ask yourself these questions:

- Are you generally cynical or mistrustful of others? For example, do you distrust others to do their jobs properly and feel the need to check up on them?

- Do you wish bad things to happen to people you believe don't work as hard as you?

- Do you get very irritated or angry when people leave a mess in your way—leaving dishes in the kitchen sink or forgetting to mail out a report—or interfere with your daily schedule?

- Do you mistrust people who say they want to help you?

- Do you honk your horn repeatedly when the car in front doesn't move the instant the light turns green?

Identifying Risk Factors for Heart Disease

If you answer yes to any of these questions you may benefit from these stress reduction strategies:

Calm Down, Live Longer. To lower your stress levels, try a combination of techniques, designed to relieve tension, help you avoid potentially stressful situations and, above all, change the way you view events.

Duke University stress researcher Redford Williams, author of *Anger Kills*, emphasizes asking yourself whether what you're getting all worked up about is really important in the grand scheme of things. How much time will you really save even if you could make the elevator come faster or the supermarket checkout speed up? Figure it out, then drop it. If on the other hand, the situation does deserve a response (someone has cut in front of you on the bank line), it's appropriate to assert yourself. But forget about murder. It's your body that will pay.

Avoid the Stimulants. While smoking may have an immediate effect of calming your nerves, the effect is only short-term. Nicotine actually is a stimulant, revving up the nervous system. The building addiction it causes serves to leave you excited until your next fix.

Try Exercise. Regular aerobic exercise can reduce the level of stress hormones in your blood. Even a brisk walk can help lower stress hormones and dispel anger. Most experts recommend daily exercise for at least 30 minutes, but even exercising three times a week can offer benefits.

Take Time to De-Stress. Some experts recommend joining a class to learn meditation, yoga, biofeedback, or other stress-reduction techniques. But even just taking some time each day to unwind by listening to music, reading, or gardening can also help. The key is to find some activity that helps you get your mind off your worries.

Keep a Stress Diary. Write down the occasions that were stressful to you. Jot down the time of day and the circumstances that led to it, then try altering or avoiding these circumstances. Obviously, if you are stressed by your job, quitting may not be an option, but you can do things that may help. It also helps to make a list of the tasks you have to complete in a day and check them off as you go. If you find you are stressed before a meeting or whenever you are around a specific person, such as your boss, try one of the relaxation techniques described above.

Use a Quick Fix. A host of stress reduction strategies can be completed in just a few seconds:

- *Cleansing breath.* When you find yourself getting worked up over an event, stop and take a deep breath. Hold it for a few seconds and then let it out v-e-r-y s-l-o-w-l-y. As you blow out, imagine blowing all the tension from your body.

- *Relaxing postures.* Sit anywhere, even at your desk at work. Relax your shoulders so that they are comfortably rounded. Allow your arms to drop by your sides. Rest your hands, palm side up, on top of your thighs. With your knees bent, extend your legs and allow your feet, supported by your heels, to fall gently outward. Let your jaw drop. Close your eyes and breathe deeply for a minute or two.

- *Passive stretches.* It's possible to relax muscles without effort; gravity can do it all. Start with your neck and let your head fall forward to the right. Breathe in and out normally. With every breath out, allow your head to fall more. Do the same with your shoulders, arms, and back.

- *Imagery.* Find a comfortable posture and close your eyes. Imagine the most relaxed place you've ever been. It may be a lake, a mountain, a beach, or anything.

Sedentary Lifestyle

A physically active lifestyle benefits your heart in several ways: It increases your heart's ability to pump blood, promotes weight loss, and can help protect against high blood pressure and diabetes. What's more, regular exercise lowers triglyceride levels while increasing levels of "good" HDL cholesterol.

A sedentary lifestyle doesn't exercise the heart—a muscle—so it can lose its strength, flexibility, and endurance. A sedentary life is defined as being physically inactive at work and at home, and failing to participate in exercise for at least 20 continuous minutes at least three times a week. By gradually increasing the amount of exercise you do, you can improve your cardiovascular and overall fitness level in as little as eight weeks.

Cardiovascular fitness increases the efficiency of oxygen use by your body and its capacity for work. Exercise increases your heart's strength, endurance, and efficiency. A fit heart pumps 25 percent more blood per minute when at rest and over 50 percent more blood per

Identifying Risk Factors for Heart Disease

minute during physical exertion than an unfit heart. It's therefore less subject to strain when demands on it increase. A fit heart also has a lower resting heart rate—usually 60 to 70 times a minute compared to an unfit person's heart beat rate of 80 to 100 times a minute.

In general, try to set up your program so that you expend about 1,000 to 2,000 calories a week with exercise. Some examples of the number of calories burned during some exercises are given in Table 14.3.

Table 14.3. Average Number of Calories Burned in 10 Minutes, Caloric Expenditure for Your Weight

Activity	120-130 lbs	160-170 lbs	190-200 lbs
Aerobic Dance	60-105	75-140	90-165
Bicycling, Outdoors	40-145	50-195	60-230
Bicycling, Stationary	25-145	30-195	40-230
Calisthenics	40-105	50-140	60-165
Jogging, 5 mph (12 minutes/mile)	90	115	135
Jogging, 6 mph (10 minutes/mile)	105	140	170
Cross-country skiing	60-145	75-195	90-230
Swimming	50-125	65-165	75-200
Walking, 2 mph (30 minutes/mile)	30	40	45
Walking, 3 mph (20 minutes/mile)	40	50	60
Walking, 4 mph (15 minutes/mile)	55	70	85

Workouts that Work

To increase cardiovascular fitness, you need to do aerobic exercise, which refers to activities that require the continuous, rhythmic contracting of the body's large muscle groups. To supply your muscles with the steady supply of oxygen needed to meet their energy needs during an aerobic workout, the rate and depth of your breathing increases and eventually you'll perspire.

Aerobic exercise should not be so intense that your muscle cells run short of oxygen. (If you find yourself gasping for air during aerobic exercise, slow down until your breathing is steady again.) Oxygen deficiency may occur with activities such as isometric exercises like weight-lifting. These activities increase muscle tone and bulk, but they don't appear to have cardiovascular benefits. A cardiovascular fitness program has three parts: warm-up, conditioning aerobic exercise, and cool-down.

- The warm-up phase should include stretching and low-intensity endurance exercises to gradually increase your heart rate, body temperature, and blood flow to your muscles.
- Follow this with at least 20 minutes of aerobic workout.
- End with 5 to 10 minutes of low-intensity exercises, such as walking on a treadmill or stepping very gently on a stair machine. Follow those low-intensity exercises with some stretching.

Your workout should be intense enough and long enough to achieve a cardiovascular training effect. Try for about 30 minutes a day, at least three times a week on nonconsecutive days. If you haven't exercised for a long time, start with 5 minutes or less and gradually work your way up. The intensity of your exercise should be strenuous enough so that you feel you are working, but it need not be exhausting. It's best to get a doctor's approval before starting an exercise program if you are severely overweight; over age 40; have heart or lung disease, diabetes, arthritis or kidney disease; or had parents, brothers or sisters who had evidence of coronary artery disease before age 55. And stop exercising immediately if you experience:

- Chest discomfort or pressure
- A severe shortness of breath
- A burst of very rapid or slow heart rate
- An irregular heart rate
- Excessive fatigue
- Marked joint or muscle pain
- Dizziness or fainting

For most people, the hardest part about a regular exercise program is staying motivated. To help, try these strategies:

Chart Your Progress. Keeping a workout journal is a great way to see how you're improving. When you first start exercising, you may find you can ride a stationary bicycle for only 10 minutes; gradually this will increase. The record will show how far you've come and will help you set new goals.

Choose an Activity that Fits Your Personality. No single form of aerobic exercise is best. Do you like to exercise alone or in groups? If you prefer solitude, walking may be your first choice. If group activities appeal to you, enroll in an aerobic dance or water aerobics class. Do you like being outside or would you prefer to stay indoors?

Fight Boredom. Watch television or listen to music while you use indoor exercise equipment.

Chapter 15

Stop Smoking

Kicking the cigarette habit can be tough. Yet, many people like yourself have managed to break free from cigarettes. They were ready to quit and planned ahead to avoid cravings and temptations. And many people who have quit tried several times before they succeeded. You can stop smoking too! Join the growing number of people who quit. This chapter offers tips that really work. Make a plan that works for you and stick to it. Congratulations on taking this important step to a healthy life.

When you stop smoking you:

- Lower your risk of:
    - —Heart disease
    - —Stroke
    - —Cancer
    - —Lung diseases like emphysema or bronchitis
    - —Having unhealthy babies
- Improve your chances for a longer and healthier life.
- Have fresher smelling clothes, hair, and breath.
- Save the money you used to buy cigarettes.
- Stop hurting those around you. The secondhand smoke from your cigarettes can make your family and friends have more colds and asthma attacks. It can also put them at risk for heart and lung diseases.

National Heart, Lung, and Blood Institute (NHLBI), NIH Pub. No. 97-4065, September 1997.

Get Started!

Pick a quit day within 2 to 4 weeks from today. This is the most important day of your life. Set a quit date now.

Celebrate the Healthier You!

I will quit on (date) .

Before You Quit

- Tell your family, friends, coworkers, pastor, and congregation. Ask them for support and understanding.
- Write down the reasons you want to quit. Put a copy on the refrigerator where you will see it each day.
- Throw out all your cigarettes, lighters, and ash trays.
- Do not buy any more cigarettes.

Make a Plan to Stay Off Cigarettes

- Stay away from other tobacco products, such as cigars, pipes, and chewing tobacco.
- At first, avoid places that make you want to smoke. Instead, plan to spend time where smoking is not allowed, like the library, movie theaters, church, department stores, or a museum.
- Review your past attempts to quit. Think about what worked and what did not.
- Reward yourself. Quitting can be hard work. Don't think of quitting as giving something up. Rather, think of it as gaining good health. Treat yourself to something special with the money you will be saving.
- Get other smokers in your household to join you in quitting.

Dodge the Urge

Try These Healthier Substitutes for Smoking

- To keep your hands busy: Draw, write, read the paper, knit, work crossword puzzles, polish your nails.

Stop Smoking

- Frustrated? Angry? Stressed out? Upset?: Relax, take a deep breath, walk away. Talk with someone close to you, walk outside, exercise, listen to music.
- When you first get up in the morning: Brush your teeth, use mouthwash, change your routine.
- While on the phone: Chew sugarless gum or drink water through a straw.
- After meals: Brush your teeth; call a friend; or sip a cup of hot tea.
- Going to a party or restaurant?: Do not order alcohol or fatty foods. Do chew gum; drink lots of water; after dinner try flavored tea instead of coffee.

The Best Ways to Quit

Use a Combination of These Three

Use the nicotine patch or gum. The patch or the gum helps slow down the urge to smoke. This reduces the craving for nicotine when you stop smoking. Follow the package directions when you use the patch or gum. Ask your doctor for advice.

Get support and encouragement. You may want to join a quit smoking program. Seek advice from a health care provider.

Learn how to handle stress and urges to smoke. Be aware of the things that may cause you to want to smoke.

Be Aware of Temptations and Slips

The nicotine in cigarettes is addictive. The first few weeks after you stop smoking are the most difficult ones. Your body goes through nicotine withdrawal. Stay focused. Soon you will be SMOKE FREE. If you start smoking again, don't give up. Slips are a chance to learn, not to give up. It takes practice to quit. Keep trying!

Be the Person You Would Like to Be!

Celebrate your success: 1 week, 1 month, 1 year at a time.

- Keep a calendar and chart your success.

- Occasionally write down new reasons why you're glad you've quit.
- Use the money you have saved to buy something you've always wanted.

What about Gaining Weight?

Most people gain weight after quitting. While it is hard to change a lot of habits at one time, try going out for a walk after dinner. You'll avoid the urge to reach for a cigarette after you eat, and you'll get some exercise.

Chapter 16

Risks Associated with Second-Hand Smoke

"Passive smoking," or environmental tobacco smoke (ETS), has significant health consequences for nonsmokers. Exposure to cigarette smoke at home or at work increases a nonsmoker's risk of coronary artery disease by up to 30%. And each year between 37,000 and 40,000 nonsmokers die of cardiovascular disease caused by cigarette smoke. These sobering statistics have launched many legislative efforts to ban smoking in public places. And two recent studies add weight to those arguments.

Passive Smoking and Heart Disease

Data from the Nurses' Health Study document that regular exposure to cigarette smoke at home or at work nearly doubles a woman's risk of heart disease. Researchers—including *Harvard Heart Letter* editorial board members Walter C. Willett, MD, and Charles H. Hennekens, MD—focused on 32,046 women who were 36-61 years old in 1982. At that time, all of these women reported that they had never smoked, and all were free of known coronary artery disease, stroke, or cancer.

Although all the women were nonsmokers, about 80% of them reported regular or occasional exposure to environmental tobacco smoke at home or work. More than 10,000 of the women reported regular exposure. During the next 10 years, 25 of these women died from

Excerpted from May 1998 issue of *Harvard Heart Letter*, ©1998 President and Fellows of Harvard College; reprinted with permission.

coronary artery disease and another 127 had nonfatal heart attacks. After adjusting for other heart-attack risk factors, researchers found that women reporting regular exposure to cigarette smoke had a 91% increase in the risk of heart disease. Those who reported occasional exposure had a 58% increase in risk. While either workplace or home exposure was associated with an increase in heart-disease risk, that risk was greatly increased for women exposed to cigarette smoke both at home and at work.

In short, regular exposure to passive smoking at work or home increased the risk of coronary artery disease among nonsmoking women—a group generally considered at low risk for heart attack. This study illustrates that environmental tobacco smoke is a significant risk factor for heart disease. (*Circulation*, Vol. 95, No. 10, pp. 2374-2379.)

Cigarette Smoke and Atherosclerosis

The ARIC (Atherosclerosis Risk in Communities) study examined the effects of both "active" and passive smoking on blood vessels in 16,000 people, and the news is disturbing. To assess the effects of cigarette smoke on the progression of atherosclerosis, researchers used ultrasound to measure the thickness of the carotid arteries (the arteries in the neck that carry blood to the brain). This measurement was used to track the progression of atherosclerosis over three years in five groups:

- smokers
- past smokers who were regularly exposed to environmental tobacco smoke (ETS)
- past smokers who had not been exposed to ETS
- people who had never smoked but were exposed to ETS
- never-smokers who did not report ETS exposure

Over the study period, atherosclerosis progressed 50% in current smokers and 25% in past smokers. Compared to those not exposed to ETS, atherosclerosis increased by 20% in those with ETS exposure. That's roughly 34% of the rate for active smokers. And the detrimental effects of smoking proved much worse for people with diabetes or high blood pressure.

Does how much a person smokes influence the progression of atherosclerosis? Researchers also found that the greater the number of cigarettes smoked per day over time, the faster atherosclerosis progressed. But when comparing people who had smoked the same number of cigarettes, it didn't matter whether the study participants were current or past smokers; atherosclerosis progressed at the same rate in both groups. And atherosclerosis progressed 24% faster in former smokers than in never-smokers, implying that some of the smoking's effects on blood vessels may be irreversible. (*Journal of the American Medical Association*, Vol. 279, No. 2, pp. 119-124).

Clearing the Smoke

Data from these studies emphasize the dangers of environmental tobacco smoke and will inform the debate that surrounds banning smoking in public places. The suggestion that some of the effects of passive smoking may be permanent does not mean smokers shouldn't bother kicking the habit. Epidemiological studies continue to show that mortality rates from cardiovascular disease for former smokers return to that of never-smokers within three to five years of quitting. Simply put, cigarette smoke contributes to heart disease and other illnesses in a number of ways, and quitting reduces the risk. If anything, these studies should provide people with another good reason never to start.

Chapter 17

Physical Activity and Cardiovascular Health

Introduction

Over the past 25 years, the United States has experienced a steady decline in the age-adjusted death toll from cardiovascular disease (CVD), primarily in mortality caused by coronary heart disease and stroke. Despite this decline, coronary heart disease remains the leading cause of death and stroke the third leading cause of death. Lifestyle improvements by the American public and better control of the risk factors for heart disease and stroke have been major factors in this decline.

Coronary heart disease and stroke have many causes. Modifiable risk factors include smoking, high blood pressure, blood lipid levels, obesity, diabetes, and physical inactivity. In contrast to the positive national trends observed with cigarette smoking, high blood pressure, and high blood cholesterol, obesity and physical inactivity in the United States have not improved. Indeed automation and other technologies have contributed greatly to lessening physical activity at work and home.

Excerpted from "Physical Activity and Cardiovascular Health." NIH Consensus Statement Online 1995 December 18-20 [cited 1999 September 21]; 13(3):1-33. A complete copy of this report, including a list of the consensus development panel members, speakers, planning committee, conference sponsors and cosponsors, and bibliographic references, is available at http://odp.od.nih.gov/consensus.

The purpose of this conference was to examine the accumulating evidence on the role of physical activity in the prevention and treatment of CVD and its risk factors. [NIH Consensus Statements are prepared by a nonadvocate, non-Federal panel of experts, based on (1) presentations by investigators working in areas relevant to the consensus questions during a 2-day public session; (2) questions and statements from conference attendees during open discussion periods that are part of the public session; and (3) closed deliberations by the panel during the remainder of the second day and morning of the third. This statement is an independent report of the consensus panel and is not a policy statement of the NIH or the Federal Government.]

Physical activity in this statement is defined as "bodily movement produced by skeletal muscles that requires energy expenditure" and produces healthy benefits. Exercise, a type of physical activity, is defined as "a planned, structured, and repetitive bodily movement done to improve or maintain one or more components of physical fitness." Physical inactivity denotes a level of activity less than that needed to maintain good health.

Physical inactivity characterizes most Americans. Exertion has been systematically engineered out of most occupations and lifestyles. In 1991, 54 percent of adults reported little or no regular leisure physical activity. Data from the 1990 Youth Risk Behavior Survey show that most teenagers in grades 9-12 are not performing regular vigorous activity. About 50 percent of high school students reported they are not enrolled in physical education classes.

Physical activity protects against the development of CVD and also favorably modifies other CVD risk factors, including high blood pressure, blood lipid levels, insulin resistance, and obesity. The type, frequency, and intensity of physical activity that are needed to accomplish these goals remain poorly defined and controversial.

Physical activity is also important in the treatment and management of patients with CVD or increased risk, including those who have hypertension, stable angina, a prior myocardial infraction, peripheral vascular disease, or heart failure. Physical activity is an important component of cardiac rehabilitation, and people with CVD may benefit from participation. In addition to potential advantages, questions remain regarding benefits, risks, and costs associated with becoming physically active.

Many factors influence adopting and maintaining a physically active lifestyle, such as socioeconomic status, cultural influences, age, and health status. Understanding is needed on how such variables influence the adoption of this behavior at the individual level. Intervention strategies for encouraging individuals from different backgrounds to adopt and adhere to a physically active lifestyle need to be developed and tested. Different environments such as schools, worksites, health care settings, and the home can play a role in promoting physical activity. These community-level factors also need to be better understood.

What Is the Health Burden of a Sedentary Lifestyle on the Population?

Physical inactivity among the U.S. population is now widespread. National surveillance programs have documented that about one in four adults (more women than men) currently have sedentary lifestyles with no leisure time physical activity. An additional one-third of adults are insufficiently active to achieve health benefits. The prevalence of inactivity varies by gender, age, ethnicity, health status, and geographic region but is common to all demographic groups. Change in physical exertion associated with occupation has declined markedly in this century.

Girls become less active than do boys as they grow older. Children become far less active as they move through adolescence. Obesity is increasing among children. It is related to an energy imbalance (i.e., calories consumed in excess of calorie expenditure [physical activity].) Data indicate that obese children and adolescents have a high risk of becoming obese adults, and obesity in adulthood is related to coronary artery disease, hypertension, and diabetes. Thus, the prevention of childhood obesity has the potential of preventing CVD in adults. At age 12, 70 percent of children report participation in vigorous physical activity; by age 21 this activity falls to 42 percent for men and 30 percent for women. Furthermore, as adults age, their physical activity levels continue to decline.

Although knowledge about physical inactivity as a risk factor for CVD has come mainly from investigations of middle-aged, white men, more limited evidence from studies in women minority groups and the elderly suggests that the findings are similar in these groups. On the basis of current knowledge, we must note that physical inactivity occurs disproportionately among Americans who are not well educated and who are socially or economically disadvantaged.

Physical activity is directly related to physical fitness. Although the means of measuring physical activity have varied between studies (i.e., there is no standardization of measures), evidence indicates that physical inactivity and lack of physical fitness are directly associated with increased mortality from CVD. The increase in mortality is not entirely explained by the association with elevated blood pressure, smoking, and blood lipid levels.

There is an inverse relationship between measures of physical activity and indices of obesity in most U.S. population studies. Only a few studies have examined the relationship between physical activity and body fat distribution, and these suggest an inverse relationship between levels of physical activity and visceral fat. There is evidence that increased physical activity facilitates weight loss and that the addition of physical activity to dietary energy restriction can increase and help to maintain loss of body weight and body fat mass.

Middle-aged and older men and women who engage in regular physical activity have significantly higher high-density lipoprotein (HDL) cholesterol levels than do those who are sedentary. When exercise training has extended to at least 12 weeks, beneficial HDL cholesterol level changes have been reported.

Most studies of endurance exercise training of individuals with normal blood pressure and those with hypertension have shown decreases in systolic and diastolic blood pressure. Insulin sensitivity is also improved with endurance exercise.

A number of factors that affect thrombotic function—including hematocrit, fibrinogen, platelet function, and fibrinolysis—are related to the risk of CVD. Regular endurance exercise lowers the risk related to these factors.

The burden of CVD rests most heavily on the least active. In addition to its powerful impact on the cardiovascular system, physical inactivity is also associated with other adverse health effects, including osteoporosis, diabetes, and some cancers.

What Type, What Intensity, and What Quantity of Physical Activity Are Important to Prevent Cardiovascular Disease?

Activity that reduces CVD risk factors and confers many other health benefits does not require a structured or vigorous exercise program. The majority of benefits of physical activity can be gained by performing moderate-intensity activities. The amount or type of physical activity needed for health benefits or optimal health is a concern due to limited time and competing activities for most Americans. The amount and types of physical activity that are needed to prevent disease and promote health must, therefore, be clearly communicated,

Physical Activity and Cardiovascular Health

and effective strategies must be developed to promote physical activity to the public.

The quantitative relationship between level of activity or fitness and magnitude of cardiovascular benefit may extend across the full range of activity. A moderate level of physical activity confers health benefits. However, physical activity must be performed regularly to maintain these effects. Moderate-intensity activity performed by previously sedentary individuals results in significant improvement in many health-related outcomes. These moderate-intensity activities are more likely to be continued than are high-intensity activities.

We recommend that all people in the United States increase their regular physical activity to a level appropriate to their capacities, needs, and interest. We recommend that all children and adults should set a long-term goal to accumulate at least 30 minutes or more of moderate-intensity physical activity on most, or preferably all, days of the week. Intermittent or shorter bouts of activity (at least 10 minutes), including occupational, nonoccupational, or tasks of daily living, also have similar cardiovascular and health benefits if performed at a level of moderate intensity (such as brisk walking, cycling, swimming, home repair, and yardwork) with an accumulated duration of at least 30 minutes per day. People who currently meet the recommended minimal standards may derive additional health and fitness benefits from becoming more physically active or including more vigorous activity.

Some evidence suggests lowered mortality with more vigorous activity, but further research is needed to more specifically define safe and effective levels. The most active individuals have lower cardiovascular morbidity and mortality rates than do those who are least active; however, much of the benefit appears to be accounted for by comparing the least active individuals to those who are moderately active. Further increases in the intensity or amount of activity produce further benefits in some, but not all, parameters of risk. High-intensity activity is also associated with an increased risk of injury, discontinuation of activity, or acute cardiac events during the activity. Current low rates of regular activity in Americans may be partially due to the misperception of many that vigorous, continuous exercise is necessary to reap health benefits. Many people, for example, fail to appreciate walking as "exercise" or to recognize the substantial benefits of short bouts (at least 10 minutes) of moderate-level activity.

The frequency, intensity, and duration of activity are interrelated. The number of episodes of activity recommended for health depends on the intensity and/or duration of the activity: higher intensity or longer duration activity could be performed approximately three times weekly and achieve cardiovascular benefits, but low-intensity or shorter duration activities should be performed more often to achieve cardiovascular benefits.

The appropriate type of activity is best determined by the individual's preferences and what will be sustained. Exercise, or a structured program of activity, is a subset of activity that may encourage interest and allow for more vigorous activity. People who perform more formal exercise (i.e., structured or planned exercise programs) can accumulate this daily total through a variety of recreational or sports activities. People who are currently sedentary or minimally active should gradually build up to the recommended goal of 30 minutes of moderate activity daily by adding a few minutes each day until reaching their personal goal to reduce the risk associated with suddenly increasing the amount or intensity of exercise. (The defined levels of effort depend on individual characteristics such as baseline fitness and health status.)

Developing muscular strength and joint flexibility is also important for an overall activity program to improve one's ability to perform tasks and to reduce the potential for injury. Upper extremity and resistance (or strength) training can improve muscular function, and evidence suggests that there may be cardiovascular benefits, especially in older patients or those with underlying CVD, but further research and guidelines are needed. Older people or those who have been deconditioned from recent inactivity or illness may particularly benefit from resistance training due to improved ability in accomplishing tasks of daily living. Resistance training may contribute to better balance, coordination, and agility that may help prevent falls in the elderly.

Physical activity carries risks as well as benefits. The most common adverse effects of activity relate to musculoskeletal injury and are usually mild and self-limited. The risk of injury increases with increased intensity, frequency, and duration of activity and also depends on the type of activity. Exercise-related injuries can be reduced by moderating these parameters. A more serious but rare complication of activity is myocardial infraction or sudden cardiac death. Although persons who engage in vigorous physical activity have a slight increase in risk of sudden cardiac death during activity, the health benefits outweigh this risk because of the large overall risk reduction.

In children and young adults, exertion-related deaths are uncommon and are generally related to congenital heart defects (e.g., hypertrophic

Physical Activity and Cardiovascular Health

cardiomyopathy, Marfan's syndrome, severe aortic valve stenosis, prolonged QT syndromes, cardiac conduction abnormalities) or to acquired myocarditis. It is recommended that patients with those conditions remain active but not participate in vigorous or competitive athletics.

Because the risks of physical activity are very low compared with the health benefits, most adults do not need medical consultation or pretesting before starting a moderate-intensity physical activity program. However, those with known CVD and men over age 40 and women over age 50 with multiple cardiovascular risk factors who contemplate a program of vigorous activity should have a medical evaluation prior to initiating such a program.

What Are the Benefits and Risks of Different Types of Physical Activity for People with Cardiovascular Disease?

More than 10 million Americans are afflicted with clinically significant CVD, including myocardial infraction, angina pectoris, peripheral vascular disease, and congestive heart failure. In addition, more than 300,000 patients per year are currently subjected to coronary artery bypass surgery and a similar number to percutaneous transluminal coronary angioplasty. Increased physical activity appears to benefit each of these groups. Benefits include reduction in cardiovascular mortality, reduction of symptoms, improvement in exercise tolerance and functional capacity, and improvement in psychological well-being and quality of life.

Several studies have shown that exercise training programs significantly reduce overall mortality, as well as death caused by myocardial infraction. The reported reductions in mortality have been highest—approximately 25 percent—in cardiac rehabilitation programs that have included control of other cardiovascular risk factors. Rehabilitation programs using both moderate and vigorous physical activity have been associated with reductions in fatal cardiac events, although the minimal or optimal level and duration of exercise required to achieve beneficial effects remain uncertain. Data are inadequate to determine whether stroke incidence is affected by physical activity or exercise training.

The risk of death during medically supervised cardiac exercise training programs is very low. However, those who exercise infrequently and have poor functional capacity at baseline may be at somewhat higher risk during exercise training. All patients with CVD should have a medical evaluation prior to participation in a vigorous exercise program.

Appropriately prescribed and conducted exercise training programs improve exercise tolerance and physical fitness in patients with coronary heart disease. Moderate as well as vigorous exercise training regimens are of value. Patients with low basal levels of exercise capacity experience the most functional benefits, even at relatively modest levels of physical activity. Patients with angina pectoris typically experience improvement in angina in association with a reduction in effort-induced myocardial ischemia, presumably as a result of decreased myocardial oxygen demand and increased work capacity.

Patients with congestive heart failure also appear to show improvement in symptoms, exercise capacity, and functional well-being in response to exercise training, even though left ventricular systolic function appears to be unaffected. The exercise program should be tailored to the needs of these patients and supervised closely in view of the marked predisposition of these patients to ischemic events and arrhythmias.

Cardiac rehabilitation exercise training often improves skeletal muscle strength and oxidative capacity and, when combined with appropriate nutritional changes, may result in weight loss. In addition, such training generally results in improvement in measures of psychological status, social adjustment, and functional capacity. However, cardiac rehabilitation exercise training has less influence on rates of return to work than many nonexercise variables, including employer attitudes, prior employment status, and economic incentives. Multifactorial intervention programs—including nutritional changes and medication plus exercise—are needed to improve health status and reduce cardiovascular disease risk.

Cardiac rehabilitation programs have traditionally been institutional-based and group-centered (e.g., hospitals, clinics, community centers). Referral and enrollment rates have been relatively low, generally ranging from 10 to 25 percent of patients with CHD. Referral rates are lower for women than for men and lower for non-whites than for whites. Home-based programs have the potential to provide rehabilitative services to a wider population. Home-based programs incorporating limited hospital visits with regular mail or telephone followup by a nurse case manager have demonstrated significant increases in functional capacity, smoking cessation, and improvement in blood lipid levels. A range of options exists in cardiac rehabilitation including site, number of visits, monitoring, and other services.

There are clear medical and economic reasons for carrying out cardiac rehabilitation programs. Optimal outcomes are achieved when exercise training is combined with educational messages and feedback about changing lifestyle. Patients who participate in cardiac rehabilitation programs show a lower incidence of rehospitalization and lower charges per hospitalization. Cardiac rehabilitation is a cost-efficient therapeutic modality that should be used more frequently.

What Are the Successful Approaches to Adopting and Maintaining a Physically Active Lifestyle?

The cardiovascular benefits from and physiological reactions to physical activity appear to be similar among diverse population subgroups defined by age, gender, income, region of residence, ethnic background, and health status. However, the behavioral and attitudinal factors that influence the motivation for and ability to sustain physical activity are strongly determined by social experiences, cultural background, and physical disability and health status. For example, perceptions of appropriate physical activity differ by gender, age, weight, marital status, family roles and responsibilities, disability, and social class. Thus, the following general guidelines will need to be further refined when one is planning with or prescribing for specific individuals and population groups, but generally physical activity is more likely to be initiated and maintained if the individual:

- Perceives a net benefit.
- Chooses an enjoyable activity.
- Feels competent doing the activity.
- Feels safe doing the activity.
- Can easily access the activity on a regular basis.
- Can fit the activity into the daily schedule.
- Feels that the activity does not generate financial or social costs that he or she is unwilling to bear.
- Experiences a minimum of negative consequences such as injuries, loss of time, negative peer pressure, and problems with self-identity.
- Is able to successfully address issues of competing time demands.
- Recognizes the need to balance the use of labor-saving devices (e.g., power lawnmowers, golf carts, automobiles) and sedentary

activities (e.g., watching television, use of computers) with activities that involve a higher level of physical exertion.

Other people in the individual's social environment can influence the adoption and maintenance of physical activity. Health care providers have a key role in promoting smoking cessation and other risk-reduction behaviors. Preliminary evidence suggests that this also applies to physical activity. It is highly probable that people will be more likely to increase their physical activity if their health care provider counsels them to do so. Providers can do this effectively by learning to recognize stages of behavior change, to communicate the need for increased activity, to assist the patient in initiating activity, and by following up appropriately.

Family and friends can also be important sources of support for behavior change. For example, spouses or friends can serve as "buddies," joining in the physical activity; or a spouse could offer to take on a household task, giving his or her mate time to engage in physical activity. Parents can support their children's activity by providing transportation, praise, and encouragement, and by participating in activities with their children.

Worksites have the potential to encourage increased physical activity by offering opportunities, reminders, and rewards for doing so. For example, an appropriate indoor area can be set aside to enable walking during lunch hours. Signs placed near elevators can encourage the use of the stairs instead. Discounts on parking fees can be offered to employees who elect to park in remote lots and walk.

Schools are a major community resource for increasing physical activity, particularly given the urgent need to develop strategies that affect children and adolescents. As noted previously, there is now clear evidence that U.S. children and adolescents have become more obese. There is also evidence that obese children and adolescents exercise less than their leaner peers. All schools should provide opportunities for physical activities that:

- Are appropriate and enjoyable for children of all skill levels and are not limited to competitive sports or physical education classes.
- Appeal to girls as well as to boys and youngsters from diverse backgrounds.
- Can serve as a foundation for activities throughout life.
- Are offered on a daily basis.

Successful approaches may involve mass education strategies or changes in institutional policies or community variables. In some environments (e.g., schools, worksites, community centers), policy-level interventions may be necessary to enable people to achieve and maintain an adequate level of activity. Policy changes that increase opportunities for physical activity can facilitate activity maintenance for motivated individuals and increase readiness to change among the less motivated. As in other areas of health promotion, mass communication strategies should be used to promote physical activity. These strategies should include a variety of mainstream channels and techniques to reach diverse audiences that acquire information through different media (e.g., TV, newspaper, radio, Internet).

What Are the Important Considerations for Future Research?

While much has been learned about the role of physical activity in cardiovascular health, there are many unanswered questions.

- Maintain surveillance of physical activity levels in the U.S. population by age, gender, geographic, and socioeconomic measures.

- Develop better methods for analysis and quantification of activity. These methods should be applicable to both work and leisure time measurements and provide direct quantitative estimates of activity.

- Conduct physiologic, biochemical, and genetic research necessary to define the mechanisms by which activity affects CVD including changes in metabolism as well as cardiac and vascular effects. This will provide new insights into cardiovascular biology that may have broader implications than for other clinical outcomes.

- Examine the effects of physical activity and cardiac rehabilitation programs on morbidity and mortality in elderly individuals.

- Conduct research on the social and psychological factors that influence adoption of a more active lifestyle and the maintenance of that behavior change throughout life.

- Carry out controlled randomized clinical trials among children and adolescents to test the effects of increased physical activity on CVD risk factor levels including obesity. The effects of intensity, frequency, and duration of increased physical activity should be examined in such studies.

Conclusions

Accumulating scientific evidence indicates that physical inactivity is a major risk factor for CVD. Moderate levels of regular physical activity confer significant health benefits. Unfortunately, most Americans have little or no physical activity in their daily lives.

All Americans should engage in regular physical activity at a level appropriate to their capacities, needs, and interests. All children and adults should set and reach a goal of accumulating at least 30 minutes of moderate-intensity physical activity on most, and preferably all, days of the week. Those who currently meet these standards may derive additional health and fitness benefits by becoming more physically active or including more vigorous activity.

Cardiac rehabilitation programs that combine physical activity with reduction in other risk factors should be more widely applied to those with known CVD. Well-designed rehabilitation programs have benefits that are lost because of these programs' limited use.

Individuals with CVD and men over 40 or women over 50 years of age with multiple cardiovascular risk factors should have a medical evaluation prior to embarking on a vigorous exercise program.

Recognizing the importance of individual and societal factors in initiating and sustaining regular physical activity, the panel recommends the following:

- Development of programs for health care providers to communicate to patients the importance of regular physical activity.
- Increased community support of regular physical activity with environmental and policy changes at schools, worksites, community centers, and other sites.
- Initiation of a coordinated national campaign involving a consortium of collaborating health organizations to encourage regular physical activity.

The implementation of the recommendations in this statement has considerable potential to improve the health and well-being of American citizens.

Chapter 18

Energize Yourself: Stay Physically Active

Add Activity to Your Daily Routine and Feel More Energetic!

Being physically active is important. It can help you feel better and improve your health. There are many fun things that you can do to be active—by yourself or with family or friends. Children and adults should do 30 minutes or more of moderate physical activity each day. You can do 30 minutes all at once or 10 minutes at a time, three times a day. If you are not used to being active, start out slowly and work up to 30 minutes a day. Add more activities for longer periods of time as you begin to feel more fit, or add some vigorous activity.

Improve Your Outlook!

Physical activity can be your solution to feeling tired, bored, and out of shape. With more physical activity you may feel less stressed!

Physical Activity Can Also

- make you feel more energetic
- help you lose weight and control your appetite
- help you sleep better

National Heart, Lung, and Blood Institute (NHLBI), NIH Pub. No. 97-4059, September 1997.

- lower your chance for diabetes
- lower your chance for a stroke
- lower your blood pressure
- improve your blood cholesterol levels

Move Your Body!

Change your habits by adding activity to your daily routine. Any movement you do burns calories. The more you move, the better. Check out some of these simple activities to get you started today.

To Perk Up

- Get up 15 minutes earlier in the morning and stretch.
- Jog in place.
- Ride your stationary bike while watching TV.
- Workout along with an exercise video.

To Do a Quick Workout

- Use the stairs instead of the elevator.
- Walk to the bus or train stop.
- Walk to each end of the mall when you go shopping.
- Park your car a few blocks away and walk.

To Have Fun

- Play your favorite dance music. Do the old steps you love—add some new moves.
- Jump rope or play tag with your kids or grandkids.
- Use hand-held arm weights during a phone conversation with a friend.

What's the Best Type of Physical Activity for You?

The best type is the one or two that you will do! Pick an activity that you enjoy doing and one that will fit into your daily routine. Start with moderate levels of activity and work your way up!

Energize Yourself: Stay Physically Active

Moderate Level Of Activity

Here's a good place to start. Moderate activities such as walking and climbing stairs for 10 minutes, three times a day can improve your health. Pick a few things to try from the list below.

Moderate Activities

- walking
- dancing
- raking leaves
- bowling
- gardening
- vacuuming
- climbing stairs

Vigorous Level of Activity

You can increase to this higher level as you become more fit. You get additional health benefits from doing vigorous activity. If you are already at this level, keep up the good work!

Vigorous Activities

- bicycling
- swimming
- doing aerobics
- jogging/running
- marching in place
- playing sports (basketball, football, soccer, baseball)

Make Staying Physically Active a Lifelong Habit!

Make It a Family Thing

Work out with your family, friends, or neighbors. Teaming up with a partner keeps you both motivated.

Make It a Religious Thing

Start a physical activity group at your church.

Make It a Work Thing

Keep a pair of walking shoes at your job. Hookup with a coworker and use part of your lunch time or breaks to be active. Challenge each other to better health.

Are You Ready to Get Active?

- You can start being physically active slowly if you do not have a health problem.
- If you have a health problem, check with your doctor before starting a vigorous exercise program.

Create a Healthier You!

Choose one activity from the list of moderate or vigorous activities above and get started for a healthier you! Get a pencil and write your answer below.

My goal is to (write one favorite activity here) for at least (minutes per day) minutes (number of times) times each week.

Make Physical Activity a Habit

Track your daily progress. Start out slowly. Soon you will reach 30 minutes or more a day!

Chapter 19

Lose Weight If You Are Overweight

Maybe you've been thinking about losing weight for some time now. Perhaps you have even tried to lose weight before. Reading this chapter shows you have the motivation to get started again. Follow the steps below to help you form good habits to keep you going until you reach your goal weight.

What Causes a Person to Be Overweight?

Two common reasons for being overweight are eating too much and not being active enough. If you eat more calories than your body burns up, the extra calories are stored as fat. Everyone has some stored fat. Too much fat results in being overweight.

Why Should an Overweight Person Lose Weight?

Losing weight helps you feel better and makes it easier to be more active. Losing weight is not easy but take the challenge. You can do it!

If you are overweight, here are some other good reasons to lose weight.

- Your blood cholesterol levels may improve.
- Your blood pressure levels may go down.
- Your blood sugar level may be better controlled.

National Heart, Lung, and Blood Institute (NHLBI), NIH Pub. No. 97-4063, September 1997.

Even if you don't have health problems due to being overweight, a healthy weight can help you lower your risk of heart disease.

Looking for a Quick and Easy Way to Lose Weight?

Don't be fooled. Be wary of misleading programs that offer quick weight loss. Some famous phrases like, "Eat all you want and still lose weight," or "Melt fat away—while you sleep," may come to mind. Some other phrases to be wary of are:

- Guaranteed
- Easy
- Fast
- Breakthrough
- Miracle Cure
- New Discovery
- Quick
- Immediate
- Effortless
- Magical

Ready, Set ... Lose!

You can make losing weight a family project or set your own personal goal. Pick a day to begin. Focus on making simple changes on a daily basis. Make these changes slowly. Stick to them. Try these tips:

Choose Lower Fat, Lower Calorie Foods

- Prepare food by broiling or baking more often instead of frying.
- Eat fewer breaded and fried foods. Breading and frying foods like fish, shrimp, chicken, and vegetables add fat and calories.
- Eat lean meat, fish, and poultry without skin. Choose poultry breasts and drumsticks more often than the wings and thighs.
- Eat more fruits, whole grain, and vegetables. If you are a nibbler, choose fruit and vegetables as snacks more often.
- Use the food label to choose lower calorie foods.
- Drink fewer alcoholic and high-calorie beverages.
- Drink six to eight glasses of water each day.

Lose Weight If You Are Overweight

Limit Your Portion Size

- Eat smaller portions—do not go back for seconds.
- Try eating only one serving of high-fat, high-calorie foods like pizza, ice cream, or chips. Slowly cut back on your portion size. Substitute with lower fat, lower calorie foods during the rest of the day.

Don't Forget to Exercise

Keep Moving

- Be physically active for at least 30 minutes a day, or as much as you can. It really helps you to lose weight if you are more active.

Table 19.1. How Big Is a Serving? (These serving sizes are the same as those on the Nutrition Facts food label.)

One Portion of:	Serving Size	Is about the Size of:
Meat	3 ounces cooked	a deck of cards
Cheese	1 ounce	a pair of dice
Potato	½ cup	an ice cream scoop
Bread	1 slice	half a bagel, half an English muffin, half a hamburger or hot dog bun
Cereal	1 ounce	½ to 1 cup depending on the type of cereal
Rice or pasta	½ cup cooked	a very small bowl that side dishes are served in at a cafeteria
Salad dressing or gravy	2 tablespoons	half a ladle of dressing at a salad bar
Fruits and vegetables	½ cup chopped, cooked, or canned	a very small bowl that side dishes are served in at a cafeteria
	1 piece	a medium apple or orange
Juice (fruit or vegetable)	3/4 cup	a small juice glass

Heart Diseases and Disorders Sourcebook, Second Edition

Try These to Move More

- Park your car a block or two away and walk.
- Get off one or two bus stops early and walk the rest of the way.
- Use the stairs.
- Dance. See if you remember all the steps or learn some new ones. Add more moves for a personalized workout.

Aim for a Healthy Weight!

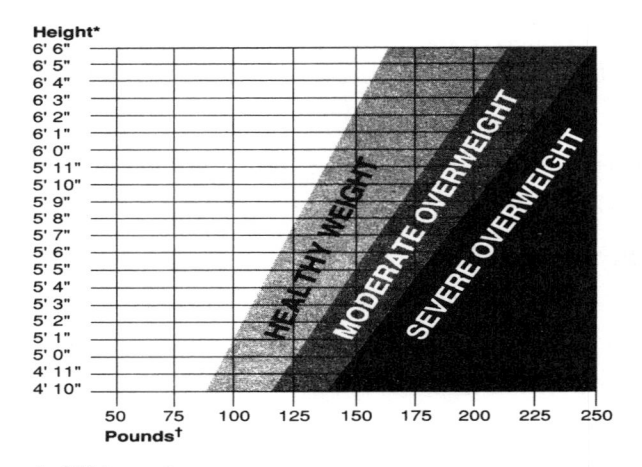

* Without shoes.
† Without clothes. The higher weights apply to people with more muscle and bone, such as many men.

Figure 19.1. Weight Chart. Source: Report of the Dietary Guidelines Advisory Committee on the Dietary Guidelines for Americans, 1995, pages 23-24.

My weight is _____ pounds.

Use the chart shown in Figure 19.1. to find out if your weight is within the healthy weight range suggested for people of your height. Weights above the healthy weight range are less healthy for most people.

Try not to gain extra weight. If you are overweight, try to lose weight slowly. Lose about ½ to 1 pound a week until you reach a healthy weight. Keep track of your progress. To help you lose weight, ask for help from your doctor or a dietitian.

Lose Weight If You Are Overweight

Identify two or three things you will do now to lose weight of to maintain a healthy weight. Your long-term goal should be to do them all.

- Choose lower fat, lower calorie foods more often.
- Eat more slowly.
- Eat more fruits and vegetables for snacks.
- Use the stairs instead of the elevator.
- Drink water instead of soft drinks with sugar.
- Use less high-fat cheeses, cream, shortening, and butter when cooking.
- Limit alcoholic beverages.

Chapter 20

The New Food Label: Help in Preventing Heart Disease

My mother, an on-again, off-again, low-fat, low-cholesterol dieter, rushed up to me in the grocery store one day last year. She was clutching a package of turkey frankfurters. Knowing I'm a registered dietitian, she pointed to the 5 milligrams of cholesterol listed on the package's nutrition panel and said, "Now, tell me: Is this high or low in cholesterol?"

If she had been holding a package with the new Nutrition Facts panel, I wouldn't have had to stand there sputtering and stammering as I did, waiting for the answer to come to me. Instead, I would have quickly referred her to the % Daily Value column on the panel's right side.

There, she would have seen at a glance that a serving of those turkey franks (two of them, about 55 grams) provided only 2 percent of the Daily Value for cholesterol. As a rule of thumb, foods containing 5 percent or less of the Daily Value for a nutrient are low in that nutrient. So, a serving of those franks was low in cholesterol.

Now when my mother and others like her shop for "heart-healthy" foods, they can easily find this information on many products. Regulations requiring it and other labeling changes went into effect for many food products May 1994, and many now carry the new label.

The regulations come from the Food and Drug Administration and the U.S. Department of Agriculture. FDA's rules implement the Nutrition Labeling and Education Act of 1990.

_____
This article originally appeared in the December 1994 *FDA Consumer*. The version reprinted here is from a reprint of the original article and contains revisions made in September 1995 and December 1996, NIH Pub. (FDA) No. 97-2290.

Besides % Daily Values, consumers will find the new label helpful in other ways. For one thing, nutrition information in bigger, more readable type will be on most packaged foods. It also is available at the point of purchase for many fresh foods, like fruits and vegetables and fish and meat.

Second, the information is more complete. In addition to the amount of calories, fat, carbohydrate, protein, iron, calcium, and vitamins A and C on some labels before, most nutrition labels now must include additional information about saturated fat, cholesterol, fiber, calories from fat, and other dietary components important to today's consumers.

Third, the serving sizes are more realistic and thus more useful.

Fourth, nutrient content claims, like "low cholesterol" and "no saturated fat," can be believed because the claims must follow strict government rules.

Consumers also will be able to trust health claims, which describe the relationship of a food or nutrient to a disease or health condition, such as heart disease. Only claims about which there is significant scientific agreement are allowed.

Fat and Cholesterol

Some of the label information, such as that about fat—particularly saturated fat—and cholesterol, will be of special interest to people concerned about high blood cholesterol and heart disease.

High intakes of saturated fat and cholesterol are linked to high blood cholesterol, which in turn is linked to increased risk of coronary heart disease (CHD). CHD is the most common form of heart disease and is caused by narrowing of the arteries that feed the heart.

For the general population, the Dietary Guidelines for Americans recommend that fat intake be limited to no more than 30 percent of the day's total calorie intake. Saturated fat intake should be limited to no more than 10 percent of the day's calories. The Daily Values used in food labeling follow these same guidelines.

Thus, people eating 2,000 calories a day should limit their daily fat intake to no more than 65 grams (g). (30 percent times 2,000 calories = 600 calories divided by 9 calories/gram of fat = 65 g.) They should limit saturated fat intake to no more than 20 grams a day. (10 percent times 2,000 calories = 200 calories divided by 9 calories/gram of fat = 20 g.)

The 2,000-calorie level is the basis on which % Daily Values on the label are calculated. According to Ed Scarbrough, Ph.D., director of

The New Food Label: Help in Preventing Heart Disease

FDA's Office of Food Labeling, FDA and USDA chose this level partly because it is a "user-friendly" number that allows for easy adjustments in Daily Value numbers, if consumers want to figure them to their own diet and calorie intakes.

The Daily Value for cholesterol is 300 milligrams (mg). It remains the same whatever the person's calorie intake. FDA and USDA chose this level because it corresponds to the recommendations of other health organizations, such as the American Heart Association, the National Research Council of the National Academy of Sciences, and

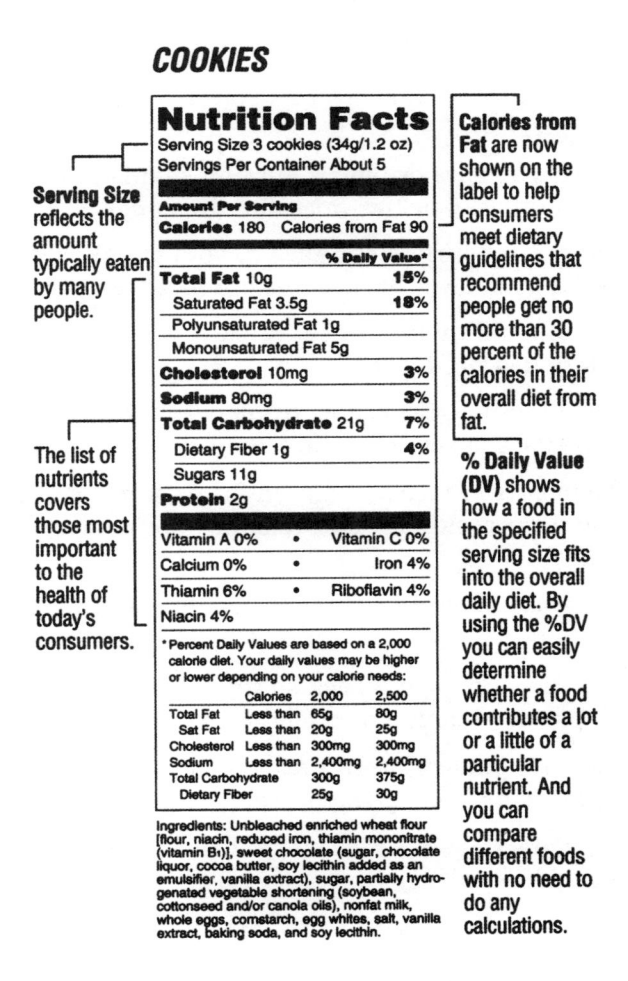

COOKIES

Nutrition Facts
Serving Size 3 cookies (34g/1.2 oz)
Servings Per Container About 5

Serving Size reflects the amount typically eaten by many people.

Amount Per Serving	
Calories 180	Calories from Fat 90

	% Daily Value*
Total Fat 10g	15%
Saturated Fat 3.5g	18%
Polyunsaturated Fat 1g	
Monounsaturated Fat 5g	
Cholesterol 10mg	3%
Sodium 80mg	3%
Total Carbohydrate 21g	7%
Dietary Fiber 1g	4%
Sugars 11g	
Protein 2g	

Vitamin A 0%	•	Vitamin C 0%	
Calcium 0%	•	Iron 4%	
Thiamin 6%	•	Riboflavin 4%	
Niacin 4%			

The list of nutrients covers those most important to the health of today's consumers.

*Percent Daily Values are based on a 2,000 calorie diet. Your daily values may be higher or lower depending on your calorie needs:

	Calories	2,000	2,500
Total Fat	Less than	65g	80g
Sat Fat	Less than	20g	25g
Cholesterol	Less than	300mg	300mg
Sodium	Less than	2,400mg	2,400mg
Total Carbohydrate		300g	375g
Dietary Fiber		25g	30g

Ingredients: Unbleached enriched wheat flour [flour, niacin, reduced iron, thiamin mononitrate (vitamin B1)], sweet chocolate (sugar, chocolate liquor, cocoa butter, soy lecithin added as an emulsifier, vanilla extract), sugar, partially hydrogenated vegetable shortening (soybean, cottonseed and/or canola oils), nonfat milk, whole eggs, cornstarch, egg whites, salt, vanilla extract, baking soda, and soy lecithin.

Calories from Fat are now shown on the label to help consumers meet dietary guidelines that recommend people get no more than 30 percent of the calories in their overall diet from fat.

% Daily Value (DV) shows how a food in the specified serving size fits into the overall daily diet. By using the %DV you can easily determine whether a food contributes a lot or a little of a particular nutrient. And you can compare different foods with no need to do any calculations.

Figure 20.1. Example of Nutrition Facts Label

the National Cholesterol Education Program of the National Institutes of Health.

People with severe high blood cholesterol or heart disease may need to limit their saturated fat and cholesterol intakes even further. Camille Brewer, a registered dietitian and nutritionist in FDA's Office of Food Labeling, advises people with specific health problems that require a low-saturated-fat, low-cholesterol diet to see a physician, registered dietitian, or nutritionist first. These professionals can help tailor a diet to a person's specific health needs.

Tips to Reduce Fat and Cholesterol

- Steam, boil, bake, or microwave vegetables rather than frying.
- Season vegetables with herbs and spices instead of fatty sauces, butter or margarine.
- Try flavored vinegars or lemon juice on salads or use smaller servings of oil-based or low-fat salad dressings.
- Try whole-grain flours to enhance flavors of baked goods made with less fat and fewer or no cholesterol-containing ingredients.
- Replace whole milk with low-fat or skim milk in puddings, soups and baked products.
- Substitute plain low-fat yogurt or blender-whipped low-fat cottage cheese for sour cream or mayonnaise.
- Choose lean cuts of meat, and trim fat from meat and poultry before and after cooking. Remove skin from poultry before or after cooking.
- Roast, bake, broil, or simmer meat, poultry and fish rather than frying.
- Cook meat or poultry on a rack so the fat will drain off. Use a non-stick pan for cooking so added fat is unnecessary.
- Chill meat and poultry broth until the fat becomes solid. Remove the fat before using the broth.
- Limit egg yolks to one per serving when making scrambled eggs. Use additional egg whites for larger servings.
- Try substituting egg whites in recipes calling for whole eggs. Use two egg whites in place of one whole egg in muffins, cookies and puddings.

The New Food Label: Help in Preventing Heart Disease

Fiber and Others

A food's fiber content also may be of interest to consumers seeking "heart-healthy" foods. Some studies suggest that dietary fiber—that is, fiber from foods such as fruits, vegetables and grains—may help lower the risk of heart disease.

The Daily Value for fiber is 25 grams. This is based roughly on FDA and USDA reference amounts of 11.5 grams of fiber per 1,000 calories.

Fiber information is important for weight reduction, too. Overweight is a risk factor for heart disease, and reducing fat while increasing fiber can benefit those who want to lose or maintain their weight.

The reason for fiber's importance, according to FDA's Brewer, is that high-fiber foods tend to be lower in calories because they are mostly carbohydrate and tend to have little, if any, fat. (One gram of carbohydrate and protein each provides 4 calories, while one gram of fat gives 9 calories.)

And, Brewer said, "High-fiber foods take longer to chew and increase the feeling of fullness, which may reduce meal size. Therefore, unless their high-fiber food, like broccoli, is swimming in butter, people are likely to eat fewer calories."

Consumers interested in "heart-healthy" foods who also have high blood pressure should check the label for information about the food's sodium content, too. High blood pressure is another risk factor for heart disease, and in some people, sodium increases the risk of high blood pressure.

% Daily Values

The place to find out whether a food is relatively high or low in a nutrient is the % Daily Value column on the Nutrition Facts panel, usually on the side or back of the food package. For people concerned about high blood cholesterol and heart disease, the % Daily Values for fat (especially saturated fat), cholesterol, and fiber are important.

If, for individual foods, the % Daily Value is 5 or less, the food is generally considered low in that nutrient. The more foods chosen that have a % Daily Value of 5 or less for fat, saturated fat, cholesterol, and sodium, the easier it is to eat a healthier daily diet. Foods with 10 percent or more of the Daily Value for fiber are considered good sources of that dietary component.

The overall goal should be to select foods that together do not exceed 100% of the Daily Value each for fat, saturated fat, cholesterol, and sodium and that will meet or exceed that amount for other nutrients.

Table 20.1. Guide to Label Nutrient Claims

Fat

    Fat-free: less than 0.5 grams (g) per labeled serving size

    Low-fat: 3 g or less per reference amount and, if the serving size is 30 g or less or 2 tablespoons or less, per 50 g of the food

    Reduced or less fat: at least 25 percent less per serving than reference food

Saturated Fat

    Saturated fat free: less than 0.5 g and less than 0.5 g trans fatty acids per serving. (Trans fatty acid is found in solid fat products, like margarine and vegetable shortenings. Evidence suggests that trans fatty acid has the same effect on blood cholesterol as saturated fat; therefore, FDA believes the level of trans fatty acid should be limited in products claiming to be "saturated fat free.")

    Low saturated fat: 1 g or less per serving and not more than 15 percent of calories from saturated fatty acids

    Reduced or less saturated fat: at least 25 percent less per serving than reference food

Cholesterol

    Cholesterol-free: less than 2 milligrams (mg) and 2 g or less of saturated fat per serving

    Low-cholesterol: 20 mg or less and 2 g or less of saturated fat per serving and, if the serving is 30 g or less or 2 tablespoons or less, per 50 g of the food

    Reduced or less cholesterol: at least 25 percent less than reference food and 2 g or less of saturated fat per serving

Meat: The following claims can be used to describe meat, poultry, seafood, and game meats.

    Lean: less than 10 g fat, 4.5 g or less saturated fat, and less than 95 mg cholesterol per reference amount and per 100 g

    Extra lean: less than 5 g fat, less than 2 g saturated fat, and less than 95 mg cholesterol per reference amount and per 100 g

Table 20.1. Guide to Label Nutrient Claims (continued)

Healthy

—"Low-fat," "low saturated fat," with 60 mg or less cholesterol per serving (or, if raw meat, poultry and fish, "extra lean")

—at least 10 percent of Daily Value for one or more of vitamins A and C, iron, calcium, protein, and fiber per serving

—480 mg or less sodium per serving, and, if the serving is 30 g or less or 2 tablespoons or less, per 50 g of the food. (After Jan. 1, 1998, maximum sodium levels drop to 360 mg.)

Fiber

High-fiber: 5 g or more per serving

Good source of fiber: 2.5 g to 4.9 g per serving

More or added fiber: at least 2.5 g more per serving than the reference food. (The label will say the food has 10 percent more of the Daily Value for fiber.)

—Foods making claims about increased fiber content also must meet the definition for "low-fat" or the amount of total fat per serving must appear next to the claim.

Serving Size

The serving size information on the Nutrition Facts panel also is important. It tells the amount of food, stated in both common household and metric measures, to which all other numbers apply.

Unlike before, serving sizes now are more uniform among similar products and reflect the amounts people actually eat. For example, the reference amount for a serving of snack crackers is 30 grams. So, the serving size for soda crackers is 10, while the serving size for Goldfish crackers is 55, because those amounts are the ones that come closest to weighing 30 grams.

This makes it easy to compare the nutritional qualities of related foods.

Front Label Info

On some food packages, short label statements describing the food's nutritional benefits may appear. Often, they will be on the front label, where shoppers can readily see them.

Some statements, like "low in saturated fat" and "no cholesterol," are called nutrient content claims. They are used to highlight foods with desirable levels of nutrients.

Other statements are health claims. FDA approved eight of them, two of which relate to heart disease. These two can state that:

- A diet low in saturated fat and cholesterol may reduce the risk of coronary heart disease.
- A diet high in fruits, vegetables and grain products that contain fiber, particularly soluble fiber, and low in saturated fat and cholesterol may reduce the risk of coronary heart disease.

These health claims also must state that the risk of coronary heart disease depends on many factors. Both types of claims signal that the food contains desirable levels of the stated nutrients.

Other Nutrition Information

"Calories from Fat" appears on the Nutrition Facts panel, listed next to "calories." This information helps people limit their total fat intake to 30 percent or less of their total daily calorie intake.

Here's how to use "Calories from Fat": At the end of the day, add up total calories and then calories from fat eaten. Divide calories from fat by total calories. The answer gives the percentage of calories from fat eaten that day. For example, 450 calories from fat divided by 1,800 calories = 0.25 (25 percent), an amount within the recommended level of not more than 30 percent.

The Nutrition Facts panel also gives the amount by weight, in grams or milligrams, of certain nutrients, including fat, saturated fat, cholesterol, and sodium. These amounts are helpful for people who monitor their daily consumption of these nutrients.

The amount by weight of polyunsaturated and monounsaturated fats also may appear under Nutrition Facts. Information about each is required when a claim is made on the label about the food's saturated fat or cholesterol content. Otherwise, it's voluntary.

If the information is provided, it will appear below saturated fat and be given in grams per serving of the food. This information is

The New Food Label: Help in Preventing Heart Disease

helpful for people who closely monitor their fat intake to reduce their risk of heart disease. Polyunsaturated fats, when substituted for saturated fats in the diet, tend to lower blood cholesterol levels. Monounsaturated fats are considered neutral in terms of increasing the risk of fatty deposits in the arteries.

Look to the Label

Whenever my mother and other consumers check the label for the nutritional qualities of the foods they eat, they'll find plenty of information to help them choose foods that may help reduce their risk of heart disease.

On the Nutrition Facts panel, % Daily Values will tell them at a glance whether a food has desirable levels of cholesterol, saturated fat, fiber, and other nutrients that may be beneficial for them.

Claims, usually on the front of labels, will signal to them right away that the food contains appropriate levels of certain nutrients.

And all of the information will be easy for them to read and use so, like my mother, they won't have to rely on a dietitian or nutritionist to help them out.

As FDA Commissioner David A. Kessler, M.D., says about the new label: "You don't have to be a nutritionist to understand. Just take a minute to find the % Daily Values on the label. They really tell you what's in a food."

—by Paula Kurtzweil

Paula Kurtzweil is a member of FDA's public affairs staff.

Chapter 21

Keeping Your Cholesterol under Control

Cholesterol is the Jekyll and Hyde of the body.

Like the literary split personality, it has a good side because it is needed for certain important body functions. But for many Americans, cholesterol also has an evil side. When present in excessive amounts, it can injure blood vessels and cause heart attacks and stroke.

The body needs cholesterol for digesting dietary fats, making hormones, building cell walls, and other important processes. The bloodstream carries cholesterol in particles called lipoproteins that are like blood-borne cargo trucks delivering cholesterol to various body tissues to be used, stored or excreted. But too much of this circulating cholesterol can injure arteries, especially the coronary ones that supply the heart. This leads to accumulation of cholesterol-laden "plaque" in vessel linings, a condition called atherosclerosis.

When blood flow to the heart is impeded, the heart muscle becomes starved for oxygen, causing chest pain (angina). If a blood clot completely obstructs a coronary artery affected by atherosclerosis, a heart attack (myocardial infarction) or death can occur.

Heart disease is the number one killer of both men and women in this country. More than 90 million American adults, or about 50 percent, have elevated blood cholesterol levels, one of the key risk factors for heart disease, according to the National Heart, Lung, and Blood Institute's National Cholesterol Education Program.

While the institute estimates that heart disease killed nearly half a million in 1996, the most recent year for which figures are available,

FDA Consumer, January 1999, vol. 33, p. 23(1).

a study published in the *New England Journal of Medicine* in September 1998 says heart disease deaths have declined steadily over the last 30 years. Indeed, between 1990 and 1994, heart disease deaths decreased by 10.3 percent, the study says. From this and other studies, it appears that this is due largely to improvements in medical care after heart attack, a reduction in the number of repeat heart attacks, and better prevention of heart disease development.

A key factor in this drop is that the public, patients and doctors today are better informed about the risks associated with elevated cholesterol and the benefits of lifestyle changes and medical measures aimed at lowering blood cholesterol. "Public health initiatives such as the National Cholesterol Education Program have raised consumer awareness, promoted effective interventions, and have likely contributed to the reduction in heart disease deaths," says David Orloff, M.D., of the Food and Drug Administration's division of metabolic and endocrine drug products.

Another factor in the drop may be a relatively new class of drugs called statins. These have provided doctors with an arsenal of therapies to lower elevated blood cholesterol levels, often dramatically. To date, FDA has approved six statin drugs.

How to Know When Cholesterol Becomes a Problem

Two types of lipoproteins and their quantity in the blood are main factors in heart disease risk:

- Low-density lipoprotein (LDL)—This "bad" cholesterol is the form in which cholesterol is carried into the blood and is the main cause of harmful fatty buildup in arteries. The higher the LDL cholesterol level in the blood, the greater the heart disease risk.

- High-density lipoprotein (HDL)—This "good" cholesterol carries blood cholesterol back to the liver, where it can be eliminated. HDL helps prevent a cholesterol buildup in blood vessels. Low HDL levels increase heart disease risk.

One of the primary ways LDL cholesterol levels can become too high in blood is through eating too much of two nutrients: saturated fat, which is found mostly in animal products, and cholesterol, found only in animal products. Saturated fat raises LDL levels more than anything else in the diet (see "Food for Thought").

Several other factors also affect blood cholesterol levels:

Keeping Your Cholesterol under Control

- Heredity—High cholesterol often runs in families. Even though specific genetic causes have been identified in only a minority of cases, genes still play a role in influencing blood cholesterol levels.
- Weight—Excess weight tends to increase blood cholesterol levels. Losing weight may help lower levels.
- Exercise—Regular physical activity may not only lower LDL cholesterol, but it may increase levels of desirable HDL.
- Age and gender—Before menopause, women tend to have total cholesterol levels lower than men at the same age. Cholesterol levels naturally rise as men and women age. Menopause is often associated with increases in LDL cholesterol in women.
- Stress—Studies have not shown stress to be directly linked to cholesterol levels. But experts say that because people sometimes eat fatty foods to console themselves when under stress, this can cause higher blood cholesterol.

Though high total and LDL cholesterol levels, along with low HDL cholesterol, can increase heart disease risk, they are among several other risk factors. These include cigarette smoking, high blood pressure, diabetes, obesity, and physical inactivity. If any of these is present in addition to high blood cholesterol, the risk of heart disease is even greater.

The good news is that all these can be brought under control either by changes in lifestyle—such as diet, losing weight, or an exercise program—or quitting a tobacco habit. Drugs also may be necessary in some people. Sometimes one change can help bring several risk factors under control. For example, weight loss can reduce blood cholesterol levels, help control diabetes, and lower high blood pressure.

But some risk factors cannot be controlled. These include age (45 or older for men and 55 or older for women) and family history of early heart disease (father or brother stricken before age 55; mother or sister stricken before age 65).

What Is High Blood Cholesterol?

Cholesterol levels are determined through chemical analysis of a blood sample taken from a finger prick or from a vein in the arm. Home cholesterol kits, first approved in 1993, test only for total cholesterol levels but are as accurate as tests done in a doctor's office, says Steven Gutman, M.D., director of FDA's division of clinical laboratory devices.

"These tests can give a consumer very valuable information when screening for high cholesterol," he says. "But they shouldn't be considered substitutes for a test conducted in a doctor's office." He adds that if test results are elevated, consumers should see a doctor right away for a more refined blood analysis. The National Cholesterol Education Program considers cholesterol testing in a doctor's office to be the preferred way because the patient can get advice immediately about the meaning of the results and what to do.

Besides determining total cholesterol levels, doctors often order a lipoprotein profile that shows the amounts of LDL, HDL, and another type of blood fat called triglycerides. This information gives doctors a better idea of heart disease risk and helps guide any treatment.

Cholesterol levels are measured in milligrams per deciliter (mg/dL). The National Cholesterol Education Program developed the following classifications for people over age 20 who do not have heart disease:

- Desirable blood cholesterol—Total blood cholesterol is less than 200 mg/dL; LDL is lower than 130 mg/dL.

- Borderline high cholesterol—Total level is between 200 and 239 mg/dL or LDL is 130 to 159 mg/dL.

- High blood cholesterol—Total level is greater than 240 mg/dL or LDL is 160 mg/dL or higher. For patients with heart disease, LDL above 100 mg/dL is too high. In addition, an HDL level less than 35 mg/dL is considered low and increases the risk of heart disease.

The main goal of cholesterol treatment is to lower LDL in people without heart disease. If the LDL level is in the "high" category and fewer than two other risk factors for heart disease are present, the goal is an LDL level lower than 160 mg/dL. If two or more risk factors are present, the goal is less than 130 mg/dL. If a patient already has heart disease, LDL levels should be 100 mg/dL or less. By reducing LDL, heart disease patients may prevent future heart attacks, prolong their lives, and slow down or even reverse cholesterol buildup in the arteries, according to the National Heart, Lung, and Blood Institute.

Treating High Blood Cholesterol

When a patient without heart disease is first diagnosed with elevated blood cholesterol, doctors often prescribe a program of diet, exercise, and weight loss to bring levels down. National Cholesterol Education Program guidelines suggest at least a six-month program of reduced dietary saturated fat and cholesterol, together with physical activity and weight control, as the primary treatment before resorting to drug therapy. Typically, doctors prescribe the Step I/Step II diet (see "Food for Thought") to lower dietary fat, especially saturated fat. Many patients respond well to this diet and end up sufficiently reducing blood cholesterol levels. Study data reinforce these benefits. For example, a 1998 Columbia University study examined 103 male and female patients of diverse ages and ethnic backgrounds and found that reducing dietary saturated fat directly affected blood cholesterol. For every 1 percent drop in saturated fat, the study showed a 1 percent lowering of LDL in patients.

But sometimes diet and exercise alone are not enough to reduce cholesterol to goal levels. Perhaps a patient is genetically predisposed to high blood cholesterol. In these cases, doctors often prescribe drugs. The National Cholesterol Education Program estimates that as many as 9 million Americans take some form of cholesterol-lowering drug therapy. The most prominent cholesterol drugs are in the statin family, an array of powerful treatments that includes Mevacor (lovastatin), Lescol (fluvastatin), Pravachol (pravastatin), Zocor (simvastatin), Baycol (cervastatin), and Lipitor (atorvastatin). Many doctors say statin drugs have revolutionized patient care.

"These drugs have had a fantastic impact on cholesterol treatment," says Redonda Miller, M.D., assistant professor of medicine at Johns Hopkins University School of Medicine. "They all lower cholesterol levels, but the side effects are minimal."

A study published in the medical journal *Circulation* in 1998 showed that statins dramatically lower the risk of dying from heart disease. Research found that for every 10 percentage points cholesterol was reduced, the risk of death from heart disease dropped by 15 percent.

So far, only three of the drugs—Zocor, Mevacor and Pravachol—have been studied in long-term, controlled trials. "Based on existing evidence, [statin drugs] all have similar safety profiles and are effective at lowering cholesterol in appropriately selected patients," says FDA's Orloff. "The difference between drugs lies mainly in their absolute capacity to lower cholesterol—that is, at the highest approved daily doses."

One landmark study completed in 1994, the Scandinavian Simvastatin Survival Study, or 4S, showed a 42 percent reduction in deaths from heart disease and a 30 percent drop in death from all causes over five years in patients with coronary heart disease whose high LDL levels were lowered with Zocor. The West of Scotland study, reported in 1995, revealed similar benefits from lowering LDL levels with Pravachol in patients without heart disease. And the Cholesterol and Recurrent Events (CARE) study, reported in 1996, showed that lowering LDL levels with Pravachol reduced heart attacks and deaths in patients with a previous heart attack but with cholesterol levels relatively average for the general population. This study showed that Pravachol treatment not only reduced death from heart disease but also death from all causes in a group of heart disease patients with average cholesterol levels.

A 1997 study, the Air Force/Texas Coronary Atherosclerosis Prevention Study, showed that Mevacor helped prevent a first heart attack or unstable angina in men and women with average cholesterol levels but with below-average HDL.

Statins work by interfering with the cholesterol-producing mechanisms of the liver and by increasing the capacity of the liver to remove cholesterol from circulating blood. Statins can lower LDL cholesterol by as much as 60 percent, depending on the drug and dosage.

Heart patient Norbert Hoffmann, 65, of Northfield, Minn., saw what he calls "a dramatic drop" in cholesterol levels after taking Zocor for three months. For example, his total cholesterol went from 270 to 145 mg/dL and LDL from 182 to 82 mg/dL.

But patients can respond differently to drugs. Some patients may have fewer side effects with one drug than another. "I had problems such as stomach cramps with Zocor," says Oklahoma patient Linden Gilbert, 50. His doctor ultimately switched him to Lipitor, which he credits with lowering his total cholesterol from 230 to 150 mg/dL.

Other Drug Treatments

These include:

- Nicotinic acid (niacin)—This lowers total and LDL cholesterol and raises HDL cholesterol. It also can lower triglycerides. Because the dose needed for treatment is about 100 times more than the Recommended Daily Allowance for niacin and thus can potentially be toxic, the drug must be taken under a doctor's care.
- Resins—Doctors have been prescribing Questran (cholestyramine) and Colestid (colestipol) for about 20 years. These "resins" bind bile acids in the intestine and prevent their recycling through

the liver. Because the liver needs cholesterol to make bile, it increases its uptake of cholesterol from the blood.

- Fibric acid derivatives—Used mainly to lower triglycerides, Lopid (gemfibrozil) and Tricor (fenofibrate) can also increase HDL levels.

- Aspirin—Because studies have shown that aspirin can have a protective effect against heart attacks in patients with clogged blood vessels, doctors often prescribe the drug to patients with heart disease.

The decision of which drug to prescribe is one the doctor makes based on factors such as degree of cholesterol lowering desired, side effects, and cost. "If a patient has only a modest cholesterol elevation, I might prescribe Mevacor," says Johns Hopkins' Miller. "But if a more drastic reduction is needed, especially of LDL, I'll prescribe Lipitor."

The potential for drug interaction is a crucial concern, says FDA's Orloff. "Some statin drugs are known to interact adversely with other drugs, and that information may guide a decision about which statin to use." In June 1998, FDA announced the withdrawal of the drug Posicor (mibefradil), used to treat high blood pressure and stable angina, because it caused adverse reactions in patients taking various other drugs, including Mevacor and Zocor.

Though it is impossible to know yet just how many lives cholesterol-lowering therapies have saved, public health experts say awareness efforts such as the National Cholesterol Education Program are getting the word out to Americans about heart disease, its prevention and management. Reflecting on his own experience with elevated cholesterol, Hoffmann says, "Get informed [about cholesterol]. Read books, search the Internet, look at your risk factors, and, most of all, don't wait to do something about it if you have a [cholesterol] problem."

Food for Thought

One of the main ways blood cholesterol can reach undesirable levels is through a diet high in saturated fat and cholesterol. Fatty cholesterol deposits can collect in blood vessels, raising the risk of heart disease.

Drugs, exercise, and other therapies may be prescribed. But in many cases, cholesterol levels can be lowered by revising dietary habits and limiting the kinds of foods known to boost cholesterol, such as those high in saturated fat. This doesn't mean totally eliminating all your favorite foods, such as desserts, says the National Cholesterol Education Program (NCEP). It means taking a more prudent approach to the kinds and amounts of foods you eat.

When elevated cholesterol is first discovered in a person without heart disease, doctors often start patients on the Step I diet recommended by the American Heart Association and NCEP. On this program, patients should eat: 8 to 10 percent of the day's total calories from saturated fat, 30 percent or less of total calories from fat, less than 300 milligrams of dietary cholesterol a day, and just enough calories to achieve and maintain a healthy weight. A doctor or a registered dietitian can suggest a reasonable calorie level. Food labels also are very helpful in determining how much saturated fat, cholesterol, and calories are in various foods.

If the Step I diet doesn't result in desirable cholesterol levels, doctors may try the Step II diet, which changes the daily saturated fat limits to below 7 percent of daily calories and dietary cholesterol to below 200 milligrams. Step II also is the diet for people with heart disease.

In many patients, blood cholesterol levels should begin to drop a few weeks after starting on a cholesterol-lowering diet. Just how much of a drop depends on factors such as how high the cholesterol level is and how each person's body responds to changes made. With time, cholesterol levels may be reduced 10 to 50 milligrams per deciliter or more, a clinically significant amount.

For more information on lowering blood cholesterol through diet or other means, contact:

National Cholesterol Education Program NHLBI Information Center
P.O. Box 30105
Bethesda, MD 20824-0105
www.nhlbi.nih.gov

—by John Henkel

John Henkel is a staff writer for *FDA Consumer*.

Chapter 22

Get Your Blood Pressure Checked

Anyone can develop high blood pressure, also called hypertension. African Americans are at higher risk for this serious disease than any other race or ethnic group. High blood pressure tends to be more common, happens at an earlier age, and is more severe for many African Americans. The good news is that high blood pressure can be controlled—and better yet, it can be prevented!

What Is Blood Pressure?

Blood pressure is the force of blood pushing against your blood vessels. Your blood pressure is at its greatest when your heart contracts and is pumping blood. This is systolic blood pressure. When your heart rests between beats, your blood pressure falls. This is called diastolic blood pressure. Blood pressure is always given as these two numbers: the systolic and diastolic pressures. The numbers are usually written one above or before the other, with systolic first, for example, 120/80.

Is High Blood Pressure Really a Big Deal?

Yes! When your blood pressure is high, your heart has to work harder than it should to pump blood to all parts of the body. High blood pressure is called the "silent killer" because most people feel healthy

---

National Heart, Lung, and Blood Institute (NHLBI), NIH Pub. No, 97-4062, September 1997.

and don't even know that they have it. If it is not treated, high blood pressure can cause:

- stroke
- heart attack
- kidney problems
- eye problems
- death

Know Your Number

- Have your blood pressure checked. It is easy, quick, and painless.
- Your blood pressure should be checked by your health care provider at least once each year.
- If you have high blood pressure, it should be checked more often. You can have your blood pressure checked at your doctor's office, your neighborhood clinic, health fairs at your church, or some shopping malls.

Check Table 22.1. to see where you fit in.

Table 22.1. Blood pressure categories (adults age 18 and over)

Category	Systolic (mm/Hg)	Diastolic (mm/Hg)
Normal	130 or less	85 or less
High normal	130-139	85-89
High blood pressure	140 or more	90 or more

Strive for an optimal blood pressure of 120/80 or less.

Prevent High Blood Pressure

If your blood pressure is not high now, take steps to prevent it from becoming high. Here's how:

Aim for a Healthy Weight

- Choose foods lower in fat and calories.

Get Your Blood Pressure Checked

- Eat smaller portions.
- Try not to gain extra weight. Lose weight if you are overweight. Try losing weight slowly, about ½ to 1 pound each week until you reach a healthy weight.
- Be physically active every day.

Eat Less Salt and Sodium

- Read the food label. Choose foods with less salt and sodium.
- Prepare lower sodium meals from scratch instead of using convenience foods that are high in sodium.
- Use spices, herbs, and salt free seasoning blends instead of salt.
- Use only small amounts of cured or smoked meats for flavor.
- Use less salt when cooking.

What Else Can You Do? Add Spice to Your Life

When you cook, try adding herbs and spices instead of salt.

Poultry, Fish, Meat:

- Poultry: Ginger, rosemary, thyme, curry powder, dill, sage, tarragon, oregano, cloves, orange rind
- Fish: Curry powder, pepper, lemon juice, ginger, marjoram, onion, paprika
- Pork: Garlic, onion, sage, ginger, curry, cloves, bay leaf, oregano

Vegetables:

- Greens: Thyme, ginger, onion, dill, garlic
- Potatoes: Garlic, pepper, paprika, thyme, onion, sage
- Beans: Thyme, onion, dill, cumin, oregano, garlic, tarragon, rosemary
- Okra: Garlic, pepper, thyme, onion

Eat More Fruits and Vegetables

- Eat more fruits and vegetables in meals and as snacks.

- Add more vegetables to stews and casseroles.
- Serve fruit as a dessert more often.

Be Active Every Day

- Walk a little further each day or walk to the bus stop.
- Dance, skip, jump, run ... take every opportunity to move your body.
- Use the stairs instead of the elevator.

Cut Back on Alcoholic, Beverages.

- Alcohol raises blood pressure. Alcohol also adds calories and may make it harder to lose weight. Men who drink should have no more than two drinks a day. Women who drink should have no more than one drink a day. Pregnant women should not drink any alcohol.

Lower Your High Blood Pressure

If you have high blood pressure, you may be able to lower or keep your high blood pressure down. Practice these steps.

- Maintain a healthy weight.
- Be more active every day.
- Eat fewer foods high in salt and sodium.
- Cut back on alcoholic beverages.

You may also need medicine to lower your high blood pressure. Tell your doctor about any medicine you are already taking.

Follow these tips if you take medicine:

- Take your medicine the way your doctor tells you. To help you remember, plan to take your medicine at the same time every day.
- Tell the doctor night away if the medicine makes you feel strange or sick. The doctor may make changes in your medicine.
- Make sure you don't miss any days. Refill your prescription before you use up your medicine.

Get Your Blood Pressure Checked

- Have your blood pressure checked often to be sure your medicine is working the way you and your doctor planned.
- Don't stop taking your medicine if your blood pressure is okay—that means the medicine is working.

Empower Yourself

Check what you will do to prevent or lower your high blood pressure. Try to do them all.

- Maintain a healthy weight.
- Be more active every day.
- Eat fewer foods high in salt and sodium.
- Eat more fruits and vegetables.
- Cut back on the number of alcoholic beverages, if you drink.
- Have blood pressure checked.
- Take medicine the way the doctor says.

Chapter 23

How to Take Your Own Blood Pressure

Home monitoring of blood pressure is useful for both patient and physician. By keeping track of daily or weekly changes in blood pressure, you can help your doctor determine whether you should take medication to lower it or if the drugs you are already taking are working. Often, blood pressure readings taken in a doctor's office or clinic will be higher than those taken at home. Once a person has learned to monitor her own blood pressure, it may not be necessary to make repeated trips to a doctor's office or clinic simply for a blood pressure measurement. Most people can quickly learn to take their own blood pressure, especially if one of the several automated sphygmomanometers is used. These devices have a built-in sensing device that removes the need to use a stethoscope.

Following is a step-by-step procedure for taking your blood pressure using a nonautomated sphygmomanometer and stethoscope. A similar procedure is followed if you use an automated device except you do not use a stethoscope and the blood pressure will appear on a digital readout.

- Pick a quiet spot. You have to use your ears to "hear" the blood pressure. Anything that diminishes your hearing will alter the true reading.

"How to Take Your Own Blood Pressure," by J. Thomas Bigger, Jr., in *The Columbia University College of Physicians and Surgeons Complete Home Medical Guide*, Third Ed., 1995, p. 408. Copyright © 1985, 1987, and 1995 by G.S. Sharpe Communications, Inc. and the Trustees of Columbia University in the City of New York. Reprinted by permission of Crown Publishers, Inc.

- It is customary to take the pressure seated and most information on treatment is taken from seated measurements. Blood pressure will vary in the lying, sitting, and standing positions.

- Sit next to a table so that when you rest your forearm flat on the table, your upper arm (where the cuff will be placed) is at about the same level as your heart. Having your arm above your heart will lower the reading (and vice versa), but the changes are relatively minor.

- Use your fingertips to locate the brachial artery in the crook of your elbow by feeling for the pulse, a little to the inside of the center of the elbow's crease. Get to know this spot, since it is the best place for the stethoscope. If you can't feel it, just set the stethoscope in the general area just above the elbow crease, to the inside of center.

- Slip on the deflated cuff, placing the stethoscope over the artery. Use the ring and Velcro wrap to make the cuff snug.

- Place the stethoscope in your ears. Most people need to have the tips tilted slightly forward, but you may have to experiment to find the position that gives the loudest sound. You can test this before putting on the cuff by gently tapping the stethoscope with your finger and finding the best position for the ear pieces.

- Once the cuff and stethoscope are set, get the manometer (pressure gauge) in a good viewing position and you are ready to inflate the cuff.

- You will want to inflate the cuff roughly 30 points (millimeters of mercury [mmHg]) above your expected systolic pressure in order to get the most accurate readings. This value has been determined by trial and error. Since most people know about where their pressure is, it is easy for them to decide how high to inflate.

- Once the cuff pressure is greater than your systolic pressure, you should not hear any sound in the stethoscope. In effect, you have made a tourniquet for your arm and cut off all of the blood supply. This is why it feels uncomfortable.

- Now, keeping your eyes on the gauge, gradually release the pressure in the cuff using the release on the bulb. It takes practice to learn how to release slowly so that the pressure falls 2 to 3 points with each heartbeat.

How to Take Your Own Blood Pressure

- As the pressure in the cuff falls, it will continue to act as a tourniquet as long as its pressure is greater than the pressure in the artery. As soon as the cuff pressure drops below the arterial pressure, a pulse beat gets through, and you hear the sound of that pulse in your stethoscope. Read the gauge level when you hear the first sound. The first recorded sound is the systolic pressure. If you also concentrate on feeling, you can learn to sense this first beat. It gives a good check on your sound readings.

- Continue to let air out. The thumping sound, corresponding to the amount of the pulse wave that gets through the tourniquet, will first get louder as more blood gets by. Then, as the cuff pressure approaches diastolic pressure, the sounds gets faint. Listen carefully until the sounds disappear. The gauge reading at the time of the last sound is the diastolic pressure. Note at this time, you no longer feel a pulse in your arm inside the cuff. This is because the tourniquet effect of the cuff disappears when its pressure is the same as or less than the diastolic pressure.

- Optional check. Wait a minute and repeat the measurement. This time, readjust your initial cuff pressure to exactly 30 points above your previous systolic pressure. Slow the pressure fall to as close to 2 points per beat as you can.

- Record date, time, systolic, and diastolic pressures.

- You can increase the value of the data by also measuring your weight and your pulse. This helps you and your doctor to interpret any changes in pressure. So will notes on any unusual related events such as menstrual periods, taking of other medicines, a recent argument, or physical exertion.

Chapter 24

Managing Stress

You can have a healthier heart when you make changes in your lifestyle. Managing your emotions better may help, because some people respond to certain situations in ways that can cause health problems for them. For instance, someone feeling pressured by difficult circumstances might start smoking or smoke more, overeat and become overweight. Finding more satisfactory ways to respond to pressure will help protect their health.

What Is Stress?

Stress is your body's response to change. It's a very individual thing. A situation that one person finds stressful may not bother someone else. For example, one person may become tense when driving; another person may find driving a source of relaxation and joy. Something that causes fear in some people, such as rock climbing, may be fun for others. There's no way to say that one thing is "bad" or "stressful" because everyone's different.

Not all stress is bad, either. Speaking to a group or watching a close football game can be stressful, but they can be fun, too. Life would be dull without some stress. The key is to manage stress properly, because too much of it may lead to health problems in some people.

Reproduced with permission of American Heart Association World Wide Web Site. Copyright 1998 American Heart Association.

How Does Stress Make You Feel?

- It can make you feel angry, afraid, excited or helpless.
- It can make it hard to sleep.
- It can give you aches in your head, neck, jaw and back.
- It can lead to habits like smoking, drinking, overeating or drug abuse.
- You may not even feel it at all, even though your body suffers from it.

How Can I Cope With It?

Outside events (like problems with your boss, preparing to move or worrying about a child's wedding) can be upsetting. But remember that it's not the outside force, but how you react to it inside that's important. You can't control all the outside events in your life, but you can change how you handle them emotionally and psychologically. Here are some good ways to cope:

- Take 15 to 20 minutes a day to sit quietly, breath deeply, and think of a peaceful picture.
- Try to learn to accept things you can't change. You don't have to solve all of life's problems. Talk out your troubles and look for the good instead of the bad in situations.
- Exercise regularly. Do what you enjoy—walk, swim, ride a bike or jog to get your big muscles going. Letting go of the tension in your body will help you feel a lot better.
- Limit caffeine (coffee, tea and soft drinks). Also limit alcohol and don't smoke.

How Can I Live a More Relaxed Life?

- Think ahead about what may upset you. Some things you can avoid. For example, spend less time with people who bother you or avoid driving in rush-hour traffic.
- Think about problems and try to come up with good solutions. You could talk to your boss about difficulties at work, talk with your neighbor if the dog next door bothers you, or get help when you have too much to do.

Managing Stress

- Change how you respond to difficult situations. Be positive, not negative.
- Learn to say no. Don't promise too much. Give yourself enough time to get things done.

How Can I Learn More?

- Talk to your doctor, nurse or health care professional. Or call your local American Heart Association at 1-800-242-8721.
- If you have heart disease, members of your family also may be at higher risk. It's very important for them to make changes now to lower their risk.

Do You Have Questions or Comments for Your Doctor?

- Take a few minutes to write your own questions for the next time you see your doctor.

Chapter 25

The Effects of Mental Health on Heart Health

Hearts and Minds, Part 1

In the constant search for ways to thwart heart disease, physicians and scientists have repeatedly examined the effects of mental states. Anything that might throw light on the causes or treatment of myocardial infarction (heart attacks) and coronary artery disease would be of enormous medical significance. Researchers are especially interested in learning whether psychotherapy may be useful, either to prolong life and maintain health in patients with these disorders or to prevent the disorders from developing in the first place. The main subjects under investigation have been depression and anxiety, personality, anger, stress, loneliness, and the suppression or repression of feelings. The findings present many problems of interpretation because the relationships are so complex and difficult to unravel. Both credulity and incredulity must be avoided in considering claims about the influence of our emotions on the chief killer in the industrial world.

The Role of Depression

In the United States, 2% of the population is depressed at any given time, but in patients with heart disease the number is closer to 20%. One in six people in the general population but (according to some

---

"Hearts and Minds" part 1 and part 2. Excerpted from July 1997 and August 1997 issues of *Harvard Mental Health Letter*, © 1997 President and Fellows of Harvard College; reprinted with permission.

estimates) nearly 50% of heart patients have suffered an episode of major depression. In a recent large survey, the Center for Health Statistics found that even moderate depression was associated with a 60% greater likelihood of high blood pressure. In another study, depression raised the rate of ischemic heart disease (caused by obstructed coronary arteries) by 60% and the rate of heart attacks by 50% after adjustment for smoking, drinking, poor nutrition, and lack of exercise. In another survey of 3,000 subjects, the National Health and Nutrition Examination Epidemiological Follow-up Study, researchers recently found that after adjustment for age, sex, weight, diabetes, and stroke, depression and anxiety significantly raised the risk that high blood pressure would develop within 7 to 16 years.

In 1996, researchers in Baltimore presented the results of a 10-year study with 1,500 participants. They found that after statistical correction for age, sex, high blood pressure, and other health risks, people with a history of depression were four times more likely to have a heart attack. The flaws in this study were a high dropout rate and reliance for evidence of past depression on the subjects' memories, which might have been biased by present poor health.

A 1992 study of 1,200 middle-age Finnish men indicated that although mild to moderate depression alone was not directly associated with arteriosclerosis, men who smoked were three and a half times more likely to suffer from arteriosclerosis if they suffered from depression as well. The depressed men also had twice the average level of low density lipoprotein (LDL, the dangerous kind), even when they had no symptoms of heart disease. In a 1988 report, members of the Harvard classes of 1939 to 1944 were evaluated as pessimistic or optimistic on the basis of essays they had written in college. The more pessimistic they had been, the greater the chance that they would develop atherosclerosis and other chronic diseases by age 45.

A 27-year study of more than 700 Danish men and women suggests that depressive symptoms, even in the absence of clinical depression, can play a role in a person's first heart attack or first symptoms of heart disease. The risk of a heart attack rose steadily with ratings for depression on the Minnesota Multiphasic Personality Inventory (MMPI), a personality questionnaire. People whose scores stood in the top 15% were 71% more likely to have a heart attack and 59% more likely to die than those in the lowest 15%. The association persisted even after statistical correction for physical symptoms (loss of appetite, insomnia, backaches, headaches, chronic fatigue) that might have resulted from either depression or a heart condition. As further evidence that the symptoms were not just signs of incipient heart disease, the researchers found that the subjects had no heart attacks in the first year after the original evaluation.

Depression also seems to affect the chance of survival after a heart attack. Researchers in St. Louis found that patients with recently diagnosed heart disease who had symptoms of major depression in the hospital were more likely to suffer a "cardiac event" (heart attack, surgery, or death) in the next year. In fact, major depression was more highly associated with cardiac events than age, high cholesterol, smoking, high blood pressure, or diabetes.

Canadian researchers studying 200 patients who had recently had heart attacks came to similar conclusions. After six months, 12 had died, and 6 of them were among the 35 who had been seriously depressed at the original interview. At 18 months, the death rate in the most depressed was 20%, as compared with an average of 6%. Depression predicted death as well as previous heart attacks or poor heart functioning did. Of patients with a previous history of depression who were also depressed after their heart attack, 50% died within 18 months, compared with 10% of patients who became depressed in the hospital for the first time in their lives. Pessimism at the time of the heart attack was also an accurate predictor of death—in fact, better than artery blockage, high blood pressure, cholesterol, and damage to the heart muscle. Eight years after their heart attack, 21 of the 25 most pessimistic and only 6 of the 25 most optimistic patients had died.

Anxiety and Panic Disorder

Anxiety has also been associated with heart disease and death from heart attacks. In a long-term study of the population of Framingham, Massachusetts, men with high levels of anxiety early in life—as indicated by their own reports of tension, tightness, restlessness, headaches, and other symptoms—had twice the average rate of high blood pressure 20 years later. None of the standard dietary and health risk factors predicted the development of high blood pressure. In the same study, researchers found that high anxiety more than tripled the risk of a fatal heart attack over a 32-year period. But highly anxious men did not have a higher rate of angina (chest pain caused by obstructed coronary arteries) or nonfatal heart disease, and neither anxiety nor any other psychological state in youth was associated with later high blood pressure in women.

Panic disorder is another condition sometimes associated with heart disease. A British study of 1,500 middle-age men found that those with symptoms of panic, although otherwise healthy, had an increased risk of dying from heart disease. In a two-year Harvard study of 34,000 men, those with a high rating for phobic symptoms were more likely to die from heart attacks (although not more likely to have heart attacks). Overlapping symptoms present a problem here, since chest pain, shortness of breath, and dizzy spells can be warning signs of a heart problem as well as symptoms of a panic attack.

Type A Personality

Much research and analysis has been devoted to the subject of heart disease and the Type A personality. A 1964 study found that middle-age people considered Type A—ambitious, competitive, workaholic, sometimes irritable and impatient—had a much greater risk of heart disease than calmer, more passive or even-tempered personalities, even after correction for standard medical risk factors. But results since then have been inconclusive and mostly negative. In a recent 22-year study of 750 subjects, men described as "pressured" and "socially dominant" had a higher death rate from heart disease than those who were more placid. But other studies have found no relationship, and a 1995 meta-analysis (compilation and statistical re-analysis) of nearly 300 studies including 25,000 subjects suggests that Type A personality is not associated with high blood pressure.

One problem is that the traits described as Type A may have different meanings in different circumstances; for example, the personality style is less distinctive in a culture that values and promotes individualism and achievement. There may be class differences as well. In the Framingham Heart Study, the risk of heart disease was high for Type A personalities not among blue-collar men but only among middle-class. The concept of Type A itself has been challenged as obscuring more than it explains. It is not a personality disorder or even a term ordinarily used by psychiatrists to describe a personality type. Critics believe the label has been applied to a mixture of traits and symptoms that are better analyzed separately. For example, Type A personality is sometimes associated with emotional distress, neurosis, and anger, but these are not necessary correlates of drive and ambition or even of a tendency toward impatience.

High levels of hostility alone may better indicate both the danger of developing heart disease and the chance that a person with a heart condition will suffer sudden death. In a seven-year study of men over 60, those who showed the highest level of anger on the MMPI had three times the average risk of a heart attack and fatal heart disease.

The Effects of Mental Health on Heart Health

In a study of 800 subjects, Yale researchers found that students who scored high in hostility on a personality test as freshmen had higher levels of cholesterol and were more likely to be smokers 20 years later. A study of 1,300 men in Boston revealed that those with high scores for anger on a questionnaire (with such statements as "At times I feel like picking a fistfight" and "I have been so angry that I felt as if I would explode") were three times more likely than low scorers to develop heart disease in the next seven years (after correction for the usual medical risk factors).

In the long-term Finnish study of 1,200 middle-age men, those who admitted to being argumentative, irritable, or easily angered were considerably more likely to die if they had both high blood pressure and ischemic heart disease (the result of narrowed and inflexible arteries). Angina was almost three times more common in the 5% with the highest level of hostility than in the 35% with the lowest level. The overall death rate of the most hostile was three times higher, and their death rate from heart disease 2.4 times higher. Among men with high blood pressure and heart disease, those with the highest hostility levels had 13 times the death rate of men with more placid temperaments.

Anger and Heart Disease

Anger can also be dangerous once heart disease sets in. When people with heart disease are asked to recall an incident that made them angry, their blood pressure rises and the amount of blood pumped by the heart at each beat (the ventricular ejection fraction) falls significantly. In a Harvard study of 1,600 men and women who had had a heart attack, 2% said they had been enraged, with such symptoms as clenched fists and table pounding, at some time in the two hours before the attack. The researchers estimated that the risk of a heart attack was doubled in the two hours following one of these episodes.

The findings on this subject are not entirely consistent. In the Framingham Heart Study, a high level of anger at the original interview was not associated with high blood pressure 20 years later. In a 20-year study at the Mayo Clinic, researchers found that high hostility believing others to be dishonest or immoral) raised the risk of heart disease and death, but the correlations vanished after corrections for age, sex, and weight. The weaknesses of this study included a high dropout rate and a lack of information on smoking and cholesterol.

Suppressing anger may also be risky. A Belgian study found that heart attack survivors with a strong tendency to suppress their feelings were 27% more likely to die within ten years (after correction for the usual medical risk factors). In another study, women who indicated at age 18 that they often suppressed anger were three times more likely to have died than women who either expressed their anger or rarely became angry. In this study, competitiveness and work addiction alone were not dangerous to the heart.

Chronic resentment, grudge carrying, cynicism, and mistrust are difficult to judge and measure and are not necessarily correlated with overt rage. Another possibly related condition is alexithymia (the Greek means "no words for emotions"), or an inability to identify and describe one's feelings, even after an outburst of anger or tears (see *Mental Health Letter*, June 1989). Alexithymic persons are often said to be unimaginative, boring, and lacking in empathy; some studies suggest that individuals with this personality type have an increased susceptibility to heart disease and other illnesses. The 1996 meta-analysis of 300 studies revealed an association between high blood pressure and what the reviewers interpreted as defensiveness (presumably unfelt or denied anger), but no association with conscious anger, either expressed or suppressed.

Stress Takes a Toll

The cardiac effects of stress have been studied apart from specific feelings and personality traits. Acute stress raises blood pressure and can be especially dangerous for people with heart conditions. In an experiment at Duke University, researchers induced mental stress in patients with coronary artery disease by asking them to perform arithmetic calculations, draw from a reflected image, and make a public speech. After adjustment for age and prior heart condition, patients who developed angina during the experiment had three times the average rate of heart attacks, surgery, or death from heart disease in the next five years. That was higher than the rate of cardiac events among patients who developed angina during a bicycle exercise test. In another experiment, 63 patients with atherosclerosis were asked to wear devices that recorded the heart's activity for a day or two while they made notes on their physical activities and emotional states. Recordings indicating ischemia (an insufficient supply of blood to the heart muscle, sometimes resulting in chest tension or angina) were just as closely associated with intense anger or anxiety as with strenuous physical activities like climbing stairs.

Chronic stress, like chronic hostility and resentment, is more difficult to identify and measure. A study of more than 2,400 Danish bus drivers found a high risk of heart disease among those with more traffic congestion on their routes. In another study, the risk for Italian railway workers was found to rise with greater job responsibility as well as less physical activity. In contrast, Swedish researchers found a higher rate of heart disease in men who lacked decision-making power and discretion in their work than in those who had some control and independence (independence and discretion were judged by the job description). But work that was mentally strenuous or performed under time pressure did not raise the risk of heart disease.

Most researchers have not found a strong relationship between death from chronic physical illness and "objectively" stress-provoking events—those that most people would regard as disturbing, disappointing, or demoralizing. One exception is a study in which Swedish researchers followed the lives of 750 50-year-old men for seven years, during which 41 died—13 from heart disease, 18 from cancer, and 11 from alcohol-related illnesses. The chance of dying was not affected by a man's cholesterol level, weight, or blood pressure at 50, nor by his stated belief that he was under stress. Men were more likely to die if their marriages had broken up or they had financial troubles or had lost a job in the previous year.

Hearts and Minds, Part 2

In Part 1 we discussed ways in which the heart and its disorders are affected by depression and anxiety, anger, stress, and the Type A personality. In this part we discuss cardiac effects of isolation and suppression of feelings, the physiological basis of the relationship between emotions and heart disease, and the psychotherapeutic treatment of heart patients.

Loneliness or social isolation is one possible source of acute and chronic stress that may lead to depression, anxiety, and heart disease. In many studies, strong support from friends and family has been associated with lower blood pressure and other signs of good heart functioning. In six large studies with more than 20,000 participants, researchers found a death rate two to four times higher among the socially isolated (after adjustment for age and physical health).

The presence of a familiar person lowers blood pressure under stress. Experimental subjects have a lower heart rate when they perform a stress-provoking action in the presence of a friend, rather than a stranger; this effect is greatest when the situation is most threatening. According to one study, people whose heart rates rise most in these experiments have higher blood pressure 10 to 15 years later, whether or not they acknowledge being under stress or feeling intense emotion.

Widows and widowers have a high rate of heart attacks in the year after the death, and people who live alone are more likely to die after a heart attack. In a study of 500 Californians, people were more than twice as likely to die over a nine-year period, even after correction for their physical condition, when they had limited social affiliations. They were classified as socially isolated when they said they did not talk to their doctors after the heart attack, rarely visited friends or family members in their homes, and did not belong to a church or other voluntary group.

In a study conducted at Duke, the five-year survival rate among 1,300 people with coronary heart disease was 82% among those who had a confidant (husband, wife, or close friend) and only 50% of those who did not. In a study of 1,200 heart attack survivors, men who lived alone had twice the average death rate in the first year (12% versus 6%) after adjustment for physical health. Some kinds of cultural cohesion may protect against heart disease. In a 1976 study of Japanese-Americans in San Francisco, those who preserved their traditional customs had a lower rate of coronary artery disease, even after their lower fat diet was taken into account.

Although the simple presence of another person (or even a pet) can be comforting, what counts in the long run may not be the people one knows or the groups one belongs to but the belief that someone is there to help. In other words, isolation is partly subjective. A recent study conducted at Yale indicates that people who say they lack friends in times of need are more likely to die of a later heart attack even if they are not living alone. Nearly 3,000 participants, all over 65, were asked whether there was someone they could turn to with problems or ask for help in making decisions. After adjustment for medical risk factors, those who said they lacked that kind of support were twice as likely to die of heart disease in the next six months.

The results of research on hearts and minds are sometimes unsatisfactory or difficult to interpret because of the need to sort out cause and effect among so many biological feedback systems and interdependent physical and emotional conditions, events, and social circumstances. Depression, anger, and anxiety can be early signs of physical illness or results of physical illness, besides exacerbating the symptoms and complicating the treatment. Ill health and emotional disturbance may come from the same underlying physiological processes, and physical health can be affected either by behavior rooted in emotional disorder or by the effects of emotions on the body. Since psychiatric

The Effects of Mental Health on Heart Health

disorders make physical suffering worse and people with these disorders use more medical services, a doctor may be more likely to take notice if they show signs of heart disease. Conversely, doctors are more likely to recognize and treat a psychiatric disorder in someone who is using medical services because of heart disease. The relationship among circumstances, events, and states of mind is equally complicated. People who say that no one cares for them may have lost friends because they are depressed, may have become depressed because of loneliness, or may have wrongly come to regard themselves as friendless because of depression.

Some ways in which emotional states affect the preservation of health and resistance to disease are obvious. People who live alone may have no one to remind them to take their medications. People who are depressed and anxious may not eat or sleep well or exercise adequately. They may also become discouraged and stop following medical instructions. In clinical experiments on antihypertensive drugs, patients who take their pills conscientiously and consistently are more likely to improve even when the pill is a placebo.

Biological Connections

The main biological pathways through which emotions and physical processes interact are the hypothalamic pituitary axis (HPA) and the sympathetic nervous system. These systems originate in the same region of the brain (the hypothalamus), activate each other, and respond to many of the same chemical transmitters. The HPA regulates body functions by releasing hormones into the bloodstream. The sympathetic nervous system, part of the circuitry controlling the body's involuntary functions (including the cardiovascular system), heightens activity in preparation for emergencies.

When an organism is endangered by external threat or internal stress, the hypothalamus stimulates the pituitary gland to produce hormones that travel to the adrenal glands, causing the release of cortisol and other steroids as well as epinephrine and its chemical relative norepinephrine (NE), which is also a neurotransmitter in the sympathetic system. Blood flow, heart rate, and breathing rate rise as the body mobilizes for fighting or fleeing. Appetite is suppressed and sleep is delayed. The blood becomes stickier to clot a potential wound (aspirin, which tends to prevent clotting, was found to neutralize the effects of an angry disposition in one experiment on patients with heart disease). The associated state of mind is alert, vigilant, attentive, and sometimes hostile or fearful.

Mental and physical stress may not have exactly the same effects on the heart. In a recent study, 200 people with coronary artery disease were asked to take a bicycle exercise test and speak before an audience. Using devices that measured not only their blood pressure and heart rate but also movements of their artery walls, researchers found that strenuous physical activity made the coronary arteries more flexible and allowed the heart to pump more blood at each beat. Under mental stress, the arteries became more rigid and resistant, and less blood was pumped with each beat. In effect, anxiety caused by public speaking raised the body's demand for oxygen (delivered by the bloodstream) while reducing the supply.

Feedback mechanisms normally prevent the stress response from spiraling out of control and ensure that it is temporary; for example, the hypothalamus reacts to high cortisol levels in the blood by instructing the pituitary to stop releasing hormones. These control mechanisms can fail for many reasons, including organic malfunction, traumatic events or circumstances, and a genetic predisposition to instability. Then the emergency response may be activated inappropriately or transformed into a debilitating persistent condition. Sudden, intense discharges of the sympathetic system sometimes take the form of panic attacks. Chronic stress may transmute alertness, vigilance, and rational fear into insomnia and pervasive anxiety.

The hearts of depressed patients often beat faster than normal, and their heart rhythms may adjust poorly to new circumstances. They often have abnormalities in the production of the stress hormones NE and cortisol which constrict arteries, force the heart to contract more strongly, and raise the level of low density lipoprotein in the blood by reducing the secretion of growth hormone. Stress or anger can also disrupt activity in the sympathetic nerves controlling the heart and cause the often deadly rapid twitching of individual muscle fibers known as ventricular fibrillation.

These parallel processes in the brain (or mind) and cardiovascular system, once activated, are mutually reinforcing. High blood pressure can cause a rise in sympathetic activity that produces behavior or emotions that further excite the sympathetic system. The knowledge of having an illness, or a potential illness, may be a source of stress that leads to further physiological reactions. Some studies suggest that people with high blood pressure show a higher than average rate of anxiety mainly when they are aware of the physical condition. Heart attack survivors who live alone may be terrified by the prospect of dying suddenly with no one to help, and that fear may react upon the heart.

Immunity and Heart Disease

The connections between the immune system and heart disease are more obscure and doubtful. Emotional states certainly affect health through their influence on the immune system, which has extensive connections with the HPA axis and the sympathetic nervous system. Infant monkeys who are separated from their mothers generate fewer leukocytes (white blood cells) and antibodies, and friendly monkeys have stronger immune responses under stress than hostile ones. In one study, medical students with closer family relationships were found to have a stronger immune response to vaccination. In another study of medical students, the activity of natural killer cells, an important part of the immune system, was lower in those who said they were lonely. Researchers in several studies have found that in severely depressed patients the immune system is impaired in various ways, and the leukocytes of widows and widowers have been found to respond more slowly than average. Much research suggests that family support is associated with better immune functioning in older people.

But little research has been done on this subject in people with heart disease, and it is not clear how immune responses would affect the illness. The influence of changes in immune function associated with emotional disturbances is rarely dramatic, even in patients with cancer and infectious disease, where the significance of immunity is more obvious The immune system is complicated, with many different kinds of cells and many paths of influence radiating to, from, and within it. The effects of stress vary in different parts of the system and at different stages of hormone release and sympathetic activity. Skeptics have also criticized the research on emotions and immunity for uncertain diagnoses and unreliable or partial measures of immune function.

Psychotherapies

The successful treatment of psychiatric disorders or even help with milder emotional problems can be as useful for people with heart disease as for anyone else. Standard psychotherapies are often effective. Among antidepressant drugs, selective serotonin reuptake inhibitors such as fluoxetine (Prozac) are most helpful because they have fewer physical side effects. Less is known about whether mental health treatment, beyond improving the quality of life in patients with actual or potential heart disease, can prevent the development of illness or preserve and prolong life in people who are already ill. Learning how psychotherapy works in patients with heart disease (and which therapies work for which symptoms) might also suggest some ideas about how emotion affects the heart; for example, it would be interesting to know whether the most important effect of psychotherapy is a change in physiological responses or an improvement in the ability of patients to care for themselves.

People with or without serious psychiatric disorders can use various techniques such as muscle relaxation (alternately relaxing and tensing the body's muscles), autogenic training (scanning the body and imagining parts of it becoming heavy and relaxed), biofeedback (the use of signaling electrodes to provide information on the state of the body and allow correction), and cultivation of serenity through meditation (sitting still and silently repeating a syllable or paying calm attention to one's breathing). Aside from the psychological benefits, these techniques have been shown to relieve angina and may also lower blood pressure, at least for a time.

In a recent study, patients with high blood pressure were given muscle relaxation training, transcendental meditation, or standard care for three months. Transcendental meditation was most effective in reducing both systolic and diastolic blood pressure. Researchers in another study found that yoga and meditation combined with a low-fat diet reversed hardening of the arteries; it is not clear which part of the treatment was more important. One meta-analysis found that meditation and relaxation training had only slightly more effect than a placebo on blood pressure in general, but defenders of these techniques say that they should be expected to affect only abnormally high blood pressure.

Cognitive-behavioral therapy may lower blood pressure in the short run, although meta-analysis has not shown significant long-term effects. Group therapy has produced good results in four out of six controlled experiments. In one study, for example, small group discussions among older people who said they were lonely lowered blood pressure. In a study at Stanford, heart attack survivors were divided into three groups. One received standard care alone; the second also participated in discussions of medication, exercise, and diet; and the third received small group counseling sessions as well. During the next four and a half years, the patients who received counseling had 44% fewer heart attacks than the others. In a study of patients with chronic illnesses including heart disease, researchers found that when depression was treated and improved, yearly disability days associated with physical illness fell from 79 to 57 in cases of major depression and from 62 to 18 in cases of milder depression.

A recent meta-analysis of 23 controlled studies indicates that patients with coronary artery disease who were given psychosocial treatment had significantly reduced blood pressure, heart rate, and cholesterol levels, as well as less need for surgery and fewer heart attacks and deaths in the two years of follow-up. After adjustment for other health risks, their death rate was 1.7 times lower during that period.

But critics insist that the importance of feelings and attitudes as causes of physical illness in general and heart disease in particular should not be exaggerated. Emotions may be minor factors compared to exercise, diet, smoking, and drinking. Some commentators have pointed out that if patients are told that their feelings are a source of their illness, they may hear an implicit suggestion, hardly therapeutic, that they are to blame if they do not recover. Providers of psychological treatment for patients with physical illness must be careful not to make excessive claims or minimize the importance of standard medical treatment.

In the future, physicians will devote more attention to evaluating heart patients for depression and other psychiatric symptoms. There will be more research on the biological features of heart disease related to psychiatric symptoms. Studies will be enhanced by new medical technology, including brain scans, heart scans, and the methods of molecular biology. More studies will consider the interactions of cardiovascular, immune, sympathetic, and hormonal systems. Both life and health will be served by this clarification of the complex relationship between states of mind and the state of the heart.

For Further Reading

George C. Chrousos and Philip W. Gold. The concepts of stress and stress system disorders: Overview of physical and behavioral homeostasis. *Journal of the American Medical Association* 267:1244-1252 (March 4, 1992).

Catherine Frank and Stephen Smith. Stress and the heart: Biobehavioral aspects of sudden cardiac death. *Psychosomatics* 31:255-264 (1990).

Randall S. Jorgensen, Blair T. Johnson, Monika E. Kolodziej, and George E. Schreer. Elevated blood pressure and personality: A meta-analytic review. *Psychological Bulletin* 120:293-320 (1996).

W. Linden, C. Stossel, and J. Maurice. Psychosocial intervention for patients with coronary artery disease: A meta-analysis. *Archives of Internal Medicine* 156: 745-752 (April 8, 1996).

Bert N. Uchino, John T. Cacioppo, and Janice K. Kiecolt-Glaser. The relationship between social support and physiological processes: A review with emphasis on underlying mechanisms and implications for health. Psychological Bulletin 119: 488-531 (1996).

Chapter 26

An Aspirin a Day... Just Another Cliche?

Or Should You Take This Advice to Heart?

"DOES NOT AFFECT THE HEART." That assurance in the Bayer aspirin ads of the 1920s spoke to concerns of the day that some drugs could damage the life-sustaining organ. Today it's clear that aspirin can affect the heart. Ironically, it turns out the effects are beneficial, so much so that some aspirin ads now carry the American Heart Association's seal to highlight the cardiovascular effects.

In fact, of the 80 million aspirin tablets Americans take each day, most are taken not for everyday aches and pains but to reduce the risk of heart disease, according to aspirin manufacturer Bayer Corp. (See Table 26.1.)

Based on studies showing aspirin's usefulness in treating cardiovascular disease, including heart attack and stroke, the Food and Drug Administration has approved its use to treat some of these serious conditions. Most recently, last October [1998], FDA finalized a rule to give doctors updated information about the use of aspirin for men and women who have had a heart attack or stroke or are at high risk for them.

"Used the way it should be, the information should save a lot of lives," says Debra Bowen, M.D., deputy director of an FDA drug review office. "In addition," she says, "the information should reduce adverse reactions and allow doctors to better target those who need to use the product."

U.S. Food and Drug Administration, *FDA Consumer*, March-April 1999.

Table 26.1. The Popular Uses of Aspirin

Used for	Percent
Heart Disease	37.6
Arthritis	23.3
Headache	13.8
Body Ache	12.2
Other	14.1

Figures rounded to nearest tenth

Beyond Pain Relief

As summarized in FDA's October rule and in the updated professional labeling for aspirin, the 100-plus-year-old drug has been shown to reduce the risk of the following medical problems:

- stroke in those who have had a previous stroke or who have had a warning sign called a transient ischemic attack (mini-stroke)
- heart attack in those who have had a previous heart attack or experience angina (chest pain)
- death or complications from a heart attack if the drug is taken at the first signs of a heart attack
- recurrent blockage for those who have had heart bypass surgery or other procedures to clear blocked arteries, such as balloon angioplasty or carotid endarterectomy.

Under the rule, the recommended doses for cardiovascular uses are lower than those doctors had been prescribing since this new use became popular: generally, 50 to 325 milligrams once daily (75 to 325 milligrams for angina and previous heart attack).

Scientists believe that aspirin's ability to reduce the body's production of hormone-like "prostaglandins" is both the reason for its effectiveness in relieving pain and reducing inflammation and its protective effects against heart attacks and strokes. Prostaglandins, it seems, can cause platelets in the blood to stick together, which can eventually lead to blocked blood vessels and prevent delivery of oxygen-rich blood to the tissues.

"When a clot forms in the brain, it can cause a stroke, and in the heart, a heart attack," explains George Sopko, M.D., the head of the Interventional Cardiology Scientific Research Group at the National Institutes of Health. Reduce the prostaglandins, and you reduce the risk of dangerous blood clots, heart attacks, and strokes.

"Aspirin is a great drug: effective, cheap, and relatively safe," Sopko says. "The drug has been used by just about everybody, so it may not have the sex appeal of newer drugs, but it can have a huge beneficial impact if used properly. Looking at aspirin's impact, on heart attacks for example, it may be equal to or better than some drug therapies that cost thousands of dollars."

Other pain relievers and fever-reducing drugs, such as acetaminophen, ibuprofen, naproxyn sodium, and ketoprofen, have not been shown to have aspirin's beneficial impact on cardiovascular health. "It's not the pain-relieving quality that is the major thrust of aspirin's beneficial cardiovascular effects," Sopko explains, "but its pharmacological effect on platelets."

Not for Everyone

Although aspirin is a familiar and readily available drug, people shouldn't take it for its cardiovascular benefits without discussing the risks of long-term use with a doctor, cautions Charles H. Hennekens, M.D., chief of preventive medicine at Brigham and Women's Hospital in Boston. "If someone feels they're a candidate, they should talk to their doctor in making the judgment if the benefits outweigh the risks."

The same quality that gives aspirin its potential benefit—its ability to inhibit clotting of the blood—may increase the risk of excessive bleeding, including the possibility of bleeding in the brain. Some other possible risks are:

- **Stomach irritation.** Aspirin can irritate the stomach lining and cause heartburn, pain, nausea, vomiting, and, over time, more serious consequences such as internal bleeding, ulcers, and holes in the stomach or intestines. Chronic alcohol users may be at increased risk of stomach bleeding, as well as liver damage, from aspirin use.
- **Ringing in the ears.** At high doses, aspirin may cause temporary ringing in the ears and hearing loss, which usually disappear when the dose is lowered.

- **Allergy.** Facial swelling and sometimes an asthma attack may occur in the two out of 1,000 people who are allergic to aspirin, according to the Mayo Clinic in Rochester, Minn.
- **In children, Reye syndrome.** While not a problem among candidates for cardiovascular aspirin use, aspirin should not be used for children's flu-like symptoms or chickenpox because of the risk of this rare but serious disease.

Because of its risks, aspirin is not approved for decreasing the risk of heart attack in healthy individuals. Even Hennekens isn't ready to recommend an aspirin a day for everyone, although he headed up the celebrated 1988 "Physicians' Health Study," which showed aspirin's protective effects in healthy people.

Why *can't* this so-called "wonder drug" help everyone? Hennekens' example: A 30-year-old woman's risk of a heart attack is typically "very small," even over the next 30 years. "It would be unfortunate if such a young woman was taking aspirin," he explains, "because it would give no benefit and could cause gastrointestinal effects or dangerous bleeding."

Three Drinks = No Pain Relievers

Aspirin and all other over-the-counter pain relievers and fever reducers for adults will soon carry a warning to people who drink three or more alcoholic beverages a day: Talk with your doctor before using these drugs. Heavy drinkers may have an increased risk of liver damage and stomach bleeding from these medicines, which contain aspirin, other salicylates, acetaminophen, ibuprofen, naproxen sodium, or ketoprofen.

The alcohol warning is required under an FDA rule (distinct from the aspirin labeling rule) finalized last October [1998]. Some newer over-the-counter pain relievers, including Aleve (naproxyn sodium), Orudis KT and Actron (ketoprofen), Advil Liquigels (solubilized ibuprofen), and Tylenol Extended Release (acetaminophen), have already been required to carry a warning for heavy drinkers but were not required to include the specific risks. These products, too, will need to comply with the October rule.

Head Start

In the wide range of patients who could see large benefits, aspirin, regrettably, is not used nearly enough, according to Hennekens.

An Aspirin a Day... Just Another Cliche?

Studies bear this out, including a survey last year of elderly heart attack survivors entering nursing homes, which found that fewer than one in five were taking aspirin.

According to the American Heart Association, 5,000 to 10,000 of the 900,000 lives lost each year to cardiovascular disease could be saved if more people took aspirin upon the first signs of a heart attack. Some typical signs are an uncomfortable pressure or pain in the center of the chest (sometimes along with lightheadedness, fainting, shortness of breath, nausea, or sweating) or a pain going to the shoulders, neck and arms.

Aspirin should be used by "just about everyone" who has survived a heart attack or stroke due to a blocked blood vessel, Hennekens emphasizes, or who within the previous 24 hours has had symptoms of an evolving heart attack.

While appropriate aspirin use is important, experts say it is by no means a cure-all. "In the time crunch surrounding a heart attack, taking an aspirin provides you a head-start therapy and a better chance for a good outcome, Sopko says. "But it should never be a substitute for a physician's attention."

And aspirin should not replace a healthy lifestyle or other helpful medical steps, FDA's Bowen says. "Physicians really need to look at aspirin in the context of complete care, as part of a whole treatment plan for people at risk of heart attack or stroke."

For More Information on Aspirin and the Heart

Aspirin Foundation of America
1-800-432-3247
aspirin@aspirin.org
www.aspirin.org

American Heart Association
1-800-242-8721
www.amhrt.org

—by Tamar Nordenberg

Tamar Nordenberg is a staff writer for *FDA Consumer.*

Chapter 27

Coenzyme Q10: The Next Aspirin?

Coenzyme Q10—also known as ubiquinone—is a natural substance readily available without a prescription. It is described in books and pamphlets as a "miracle nutrient" and possible "fountain of youth" that can alleviate problems ranging from heart failure to high blood pressure to high cholesterol to diabetes. Research studies in basic-science laboratories support possible mechanisms by which coenzyme Q10 could help people with these problems, and a few researchers, themselves, are actually taking this substance every day because they believe that the potential benefits exceed any risks.

Why, then, is coenzyme Q10 something about which most physicians are unaware? Is this a drug that readers of the *Harvard Heart Letter* should be taking now? Is there a conspiracy to suppress knowledge about alternative-medicine therapies that might reduce the market for products of conventional pharmaceutical companies?

The easiest of these questions to answer is the last—there is no conspiracy. Physicians and patients are so anxious to find effective treatments for cardiovascular and other health problems that no conspiracy could ever suppress knowledge of an important treatment. Witness, for example, how rapidly cardiologists adopted the cheapest of medications—aspirin. The more important issue is whether coenzyme Q10 is the next aspirin, a relatively safe drug that offers benefits for people with heart disease.

Excerpted from October 1996 issue of *Harvard Heart Letter*, © 1996 President and Fellows of Harvard College; reprinted with permission.

The Orange Extract

Although coenzyme Q10 was discovered in 1940, more is known about what it might do than what it actually does when taken as a pill by a human being. In the 1950s, coenzyme Q10 was identified as an orange substance found in the cells of cows' heart muscle, and within a few years researchers realized that it existed in many other organs, including the human heart, liver, kidney, and pancreas—thus, the name "ubiquinone."

In biology, substances that exist everywhere tend to be particularly important, since they are essential for the health of many different types of cells. Coenzyme Q10 turns out to be an important factor in helping cells turn food into energy. Researchers therefore theorized that a deficiency of this substance might weaken cells—such as heart cells. Some studies showed that coenzyme Q10 might help prevent harmful effects that occur when the body's cells consume oxygen—in short, it might be an antioxidant analogous to some vitamins that have captured so much attention in recent years (see March 1993 *Harvard Heart Letter*). In fact, some of the most impressive data on coenzyme Q10 come from animal studies that show coenzyme Q10 can help protect hearts against some effects of ischemia—transient decreases in the amount of oxygen that the cells receive.

Tough Challenge

However, what works in animals does not always lead to better health for people trying to live with a disease. One reason is that people use many strategies to improve their health, including medications, while animals or cells in a laboratory dish do not. Even if coenzyme Q10 does offer some protection to the hearts of animals against ischemia or helps to strengthen contractions, that does not mean that coenzyme Q10 is actually going to benefit people.

In short, to be useful to people, coenzyme Q10 must both provide demonstrated health benefits to humans and add to the beneficial effects of therapies that are already proven to be valuable. As an analogy, think of coenzyme Q10 as a bicycle. It may help a person get from one place to another more quickly if that person has no other transportation. But if a person also has a car—in this case, effective conventional drugs—then the addition of the bicycle is not of any particular use. To take this analogy one step further, someone who already lives near a desired destination needs neither a bike nor a car. Thus, someone who is at low risk for coronary disease might get little or no benefit from coenzyme Q10.

If coenzyme Q10 provided additional benefits beyond the drugs available in 1996, it would be a cause for considerable rejoicing and for the addition of this substance to the treatment regimens of patients. However, convincing studies to prove that coenzyme Q10 does offer such benefits have not been performed. Such trials would require that researchers randomly assign thousands of patients who were receiving ideal medical treatment to receive, in addition, either coenzyme Q10 or a placebo tablet. Studies of this type are extremely expensive to perform and would take years to complete.

One reason researchers have not performed such studies is that the existing evidence indicates that the benefits of coenzyme Q10, if real, are modest at best. Another may be that no pharmaceutical company has an interest in promoting this product. The lack of a private-sector "champion" for a drug does not stand in the way of its evaluation, however, since the National Heart, Lung, and Blood Institute often sponsors major trials of medical interventions. However, for the Institute to sponsor such research—and spend millions of taxpayer dollars—there must be convincing pilot data to suggest that such an investment is worthwhile. So far, there have been no such studies, and the prospects for a large-scale research study of coenzyme Q10 are slim.

Tantalizing Hints

In the absence of definitive studies, interest in coenzyme Q10 has been kept alive by small studies that suggest benefit in a variety of diseases. Advocates for coenzyme Q10 believe it can help people with angina by allowing their heart-muscle cells to use oxygen more efficiently. Angina is the chest pain or discomfort that occurs when the heart muscle is not receiving enough blood from the coronary arteries. One study of 18 patients with stable angina showed that the amount of time they could exercise increased when they received coenzyme Q10. Other studies have found similar results, but also in small numbers of patients. These studies would not be sufficiently convincing for the Food and Drug Administration to approve the drug because they involve too few subjects.

There are also studies that indicate coenzyme Q10 may enhance the benefits of lipid-lowering drugs, help lower blood pressure, protect the heart from damage during surgery, and improve cardiac function for patients with congestive heart failure (a condition in which the heart is unable to pump enough blood to maintain the normal circulation). But the studies that have rigorously compared coenzyme Q10 to a placebo all had just 10 to 20 patients. The larger studies that demonstrate improvement for patients taking coenzyme Q10 had no comparison group, and therefore the possibility that the researchers or patients imagined the benefit because of the power of suggestion cannot be excluded.

Safe but Effective?

Overall, research has not proven coenzyme Q10 effective, but it has not proven it ineffective either. People who are living with angina or heart failure may not wish to wait for the definitive study of coenzyme Q10—particularly since it may never be performed. The question for these patients is whether they should go to the health store now and pick up coenzyme Q10. The answer is probably not.

An important issue in this decision is the cost of the drug. Coenzyme Q10 is not as cheap as aspirin—prices in Boston are between $8 and $10 per week if a person takes 100 mg per day. On the other hand, most studies demonstrate that coenzyme Q10 is fairly free of major side effects, with less than 1% of patients reporting an upset stomach, loss of appetite, or nausea—at least in the dosages used in the studies. Advocates point to this lack of side effects as a reflection of the natural mechanisms of coenzyme Q10. Skeptics say that coenzyme Q10 is doing nothing. Since coenzyme Q10 has been studied only in small trials, it is not possible to say with absolute certainty that it is safe. Just because a substance is "natural" does not mean it cannot have adverse effects. For example, high doses of vitamin A taken by pregnant women were recently found to contribute to birth defects.

Nevertheless, the most likely "side effect" of coenzyme Q10 is dollar depletion. None of the physicians consulted in the preparation of this article recommend the use of coenzyme Q10.

For the foreseeable future, the decision of whether to use coenzyme Q10 will be a personal one in which patients assess whether their out-of-pocket costs are justified by the benefits of coenzyme Q10—which can best be described as unproven and, if real, not likely to be dramatic.

Chapter 28

Postmenopausal Estrogen/Progestin Interventions Trial (PEPI)

Heart disease is the leading cause of death and illness for women and men. But unlike men, women usually don't suffer the effects of heart disease until after age 60.

This is thought to be related to women's production of estrogen, which changes with menopause. Estrogen is believed to affect factors that lead to heart disease. If it does, its use during menopause might help women stay healthy and avoid heart disease.

Hormone replacement therapies (HRT) have long been used to treat the symptoms of menopause, such as hot flashes and flushes, sweats, and sleep disturbances. A woman takes an estrogen alone or in combination with another hormone, progestin (progesterone).

Although evidence has accumulated supporting the benefits of HRT, there are still concerns about its risks, particularly whether it increases the likelihood of breast cancer. The lack of definite answers about HRT creates a tough decision for postmenopausal women and their doctors: Should they use it or not?

Finding Answers

To offer guidance to women and their doctors, the National Heart, Lung, and Blood Institute (NHLBI) and other units of the National Institutes of Health (NIH) started a major clinical trial in 1987—the "Postmenopausal Estrogen/Progestin Interventions Trial," known as PEPI.

News and Features, National Institutes of Health, Fall 1997.

PEPI's other sponsors are the National Institute of Child Health and Human Development, the National Institute of Arthritis and Musculoskeletal and Skin Diseases, the National Institute of Diabetes and Digestive and Kidney Diseases, and the National Institute on Aging.

PEPI was conducted at seven clinical centers across the United States and followed 875 women for 3 years. At the start of the trial, the women were ages 45-64. All were healthy and postmenopausal; about a third had had a hysterectomy (removal of the uterus). Participants were of various races but mostly white. All were closely monitored.

PEPI's main goal was to see what effects different regimens of estrogen alone or in combination with progestin or a placebo would have on key risk factors for heart disease, such as increased cholesterol and high blood pressure. (A placebo looks like a drug but has no biological effect.) It also was not clear whether a progestin would reduce or enhance estrogen's positive effects on cardiovascular health, and if it would protect the uterus from bad effects.

PEPI also examined HRT's effects on bone mass (mineral density) and quality of life. Decrease in bone mass is called osteoporosis, a severe thinning of the bones that can cause fractures, a serious problem for older women. About 20 percent of women over age 50 are at risk of developing osteoporosis.

Additionally, PEPI compared the effects of cyclic and continuous use of progestin. Cyclic use means taking a medication for only some days of each month, while continuous use means taking the drug daily throughout the month. These use options are important for women who may want to use HRT but not have the bleeding problems that can result from the cyclic use of progestin.

PEPI tested four hormone regimens: estrogen alone, taken daily; estrogen taken daily and a synthetic progestin, MPA (medroxyprogesterone acetate), taken 12 days a month; estrogen and MPA taken daily; and estrogen taken daily plus micronized progesterone (a natural progesterone), taken 12 days a month.

Results for heart disease risk factors, endometrial cancer risk, and bone mass are given below; other results are still being analyzed and have not yet been published.

Heart Disease Risk Factors

PEPI found that each of the active hormone therapies improved key heart disease risk factors:

Postmenopausal Estrogen/Progestin Interventions Trial (PEPI)

- All hormone regimens raised levels of high-density lipoprotein (HDL), also called the "good cholesterol" because it helps remove cholesterol from the bloodstream.
- All hormone regimens decreased about equally the levels of low-density lipoprotein termed the "bad cholesterol" because it carries most cholesterol and fat through blood vessels, where they can build up.
- No hormone regimen increased blood pressure or caused weight gain.
- All active regimens lowered fibrinogen levels. Fibrinogen allows blood to clot more readily, increasing the risk of heart disease and stroke.

Endometrial (Uterine Lining) Changes

All three estrogen plus progestin therapies prevented overgrowth of the uterine lining, which is called hyperplasia. Women with a uterus who took estrogen alone had a higher risk of hyperplasia.

Bone Density

PEPI found that HRT not only slows the bone loss that occurs with menopause, but also significantly increases bone mass. These effects on bone were strongest among older women and those who had not recently used hormones. All of the hormone regimens increased bone density. Smokers, who generally lose bone mass more quickly than nonsmokers, gained as much bone mass on average as non-smokers.

Deciding on HRT

PEPI cannot answer every question about HRT. For instance, the trial was not large enough and did not last long enough to examine breast cancer issues. However, other research suggests HRT slightly increases that risk and perhaps only in women who take it for 5 or more years.

PEPI will release findings in the future about HRT's effects on quality of life. But more research is needed to provide women with more definitive guidelines about HRT. Questions remain about when to start and how long to continue HRT, the minimum dose of progestin needed to prevent hyperplasia, and differences in effects among estrogens and progestins, and from various regimens. Studies under way at NIH and elsewhere are trying to find more answers. (See next two sections for more information on HRT and research).

*— by Louise Williams, writer/editor,
National Heart, Lung, and Blood Institute.*

How to Decide

To decide whether or not to use HRT, a woman should talk with her health care provider about her risk of heart disease, osteoporosis, and cancer, her family medical history and quality of life issues of importance to her.

Theses guidelines may help in selecting a type of HRT:

- Postmenopausal women who have not had a hysterectomy should consider taking a therapy that combines estrogen with progestin or natural progesterone. A woman with a uterus who decides to take estrogen alone should have a yearly endometrial biopsy (examination of the uterine lining).

- Postmenopausal women who have had a hysterectomy get no added cardiovascular or bone-mass benefit from adding a progestin. These women are not at risk for endometrial hyperplasia and they can use estrogen alone.

Talking with Your Doctor about HRT

If a woman is considering HRT, she should talk to her doctor about whether HRT is right for her. It is important to ask questions and express concerns. Here are some sample questions:

- Should I take hormones? Why?
- How could hormone therapy improve my heart disease risk factor profile?
- At what age should I begin?
- What is the best regimen for me? Why?
- How long should I stay on the therapy?
- If breast cancer has occurred in my family, should I consider HRT?
- If I have had breast cancer, should I consider HRT?

Postmenopausal Estrogen/Progestin Interventions Trial (PEPI)

- What follow-up tests will I need? How often will I need to take each test?

Check in with your doctor on a regular basis to review your health status and your risk profile, which may change over time.

Part Four

Common Types of Heart Problems

Chapter 29

Angina

Questions and Answers about Angina

What is angina?

Angina pectoris ("angina") is a recurring pain or discomfort in the chest that happens when some part of the heart does not receive enough blood. It is a common symptom of coronary heart disease (CHD), which occurs when vessels that carry blood to the heart become narrowed and blocked due to atherosclerosis.

Angina feels like a pressing or squeezing pain, usually in the chest under the breast bone, but sometimes in the shoulders, arms, neck, jaws, or back. Angina is usually precipitated by exertion. It is usually relieved within a few minutes by resting or by taking prescribed angina medicine.

What brings on angina?

Episodes of angina occur when the heart's need for oxygen increases beyond the oxygen available from the blood nourishing the heart. Physical exertion is the most common trigger for angina. Other triggers can be emotional stress, extreme cold or heat, heavy meals, alcohol, and cigarette smoking.

National Heart, Lung, and Blood Institute (NHLBI), NIH Pub. No. 95-2890, September 1995.

Does angina mean a heart attack is about to happen?

An episode of angina is not a heart attack. Angina pain means that some of the heart muscle in not getting enough blood temporarily—for example, during exercise, when the heart has to work harder. The pain does NOT mean that the heart muscle is suffering irreversible, permanent damage. Episodes of angina seldom cause permanent damage to heart muscle.

In contrast, a heart attack occurs when the blood flow to a part of the heart is suddenly and permanently cut off. This causes permanent damage to the heart muscle. Typically, the chest pain is more severe, lasts longer, and does not go away with rest or with medicine that was previously effective. It may be accompanied by indigestion, nausea, weakness, and sweating. However, the symptoms of a heart attack are varied and may be considerably milder.

When someone has a repeating but stable pattern of angina, an episode of angina does not mean that a heart attack is about to happen. Angina means that there is underlying coronary heart disease. Patients with angina are at an increased risk of heart attack compared with those who have no symptoms of cardiovascular disease, but the episode of angina is not a signal that a heart attack is about to happen. In contrast, when the pattern of angina changes—if episodes become more frequent, last longer, or occur without exercise—the risk of heart attack in subsequent days or weeks is much higher.

A person who has angina should learn the pattern of his or her angina—what cause an angina attack, what it feels like, how long episodes usually last, and whether medication relieves the attack. If the pattern changes sharply or if the symptoms are those of a heart attack, one should get medical help immediately, perhaps best done by seeking an evaluation at a nearby hospital emergency room.

Is all chest pain "angina?"

No, not at all. Not all chest pain is from the heart, and not all pain from the heart is angina. For example, if the pain lasts for less that 30 seconds or if it goes away during a deep breath, after drinking a glass of water, or by changing position, it almost certainly is NOT angina and should not cause concern. But prolonged pain, unrelieved by rest and accompanied by other symptoms may signal a heart attack.

How is angina diagnosed?

Usually the doctor can diagnose angina by noting the symptoms and how they arise. However one or more diagnostic tests may be

Angina

needed to exclude angina or to establish the severity of the underlying coronary disease. These include the electrocardiogram (ECG) at rest, the stress test, and x-rays of the coronary arteries (coronary "arteriogram" or "angiogram").

The ECG records electrical impulses of the heart. These may indicate that the heart muscle is not getting as much oxygen as it needs ("ischemia"); they may also indicate abnormalities in heart rhythm or some of the other possible abnormal features of the heart. To record the ECG, a technician positions a number of small contacts on the patient's arms, legs, and across the chest to connect them to an ECG machine.

For many patients with angina, the ECG at rest is normal. This is not surprising because the symptoms of angina occur during stress. Therefore, the functioning of the heart may be tested under stress, typically exercise. In the simplest stress test, the ECG is taken before, during, and after exercise to look for stress related abnormalities. Blood pressure is also measured during the stress test and symptoms are noted.

A more complex stress test involves picturing the blood flow pattern in the heart muscle during peak exercise and after rest. A tiny amount of a radioisotope, usually thallium, is injected into a vein at peak exercise and is taken up by normal heart muscle. A radioactivity detector and computer record the pattern of radioactivity distribution to various parts of the heart muscle. Regional differences in radioisotope concentration and in the rates at which the radioisotopes disappear are measures of unequal blood flow due to coronary artery narrowing, or due to failure of uptake in scarred heart muscle.

The most accurate way to assess the presence and severity of coronary disease is a coronary angiogram, an x-ray of the coronary artery. A long thin flexible tube (a "catheter") is threaded into an artery in the groin or forearm and advanced through the arterial system into one of the two major coronary arteries. A fluid that blocks x-rays (a "contrast medium" or "dye") is injected. X-rays of its distribution show the coronary arteries and their narrowing.

How is angina treated?

The underlying coronary artery disease that causes angina should be attacked by controlling existing "risk factors." These include high blood pressure, cigarette smoking, high blood cholesterol levels, and excess weight. If the doctor has prescribed a drug to lower blood pressure, it should be taken as directed. Advice is available on how to eat to control weight, blood cholesterol levels, and blood pressure. A physician can also help patients to stop smoking. Taking these steps reduces the likelihood that coronary artery disease will lead to a heart attack.

Most people with angina learn to adjust their lives to minimize episodes of angina, by taking sensible precautions and using medications if necessary.

Usually the first line of defense involves changing one's living habits to avoid bringing on attacks of angina. Controlling physical activity, adopting good eating habits, moderating alcohol consumption, and not smoking are some of the precautions that can help patients live more comfortably and with less angina. For example, if angina comes on with strenuous exercise, exercise a little less strenuously, but do exercise. If angina occurs after heavy meals, avoid large meals and rich foods that leave one feeling stuffed. Controlling weight, reducing the amount of fat in the diet, and avoiding emotional upsets may also help.

Angina is often controlled by drugs. The most commonly prescribed drug for angina is nitroglycerin, which relieves pain by widening blood vessels. This allows more blood to flow to the heart muscle and also decreases the work load of the heart. Nitroglycerin is taken when discomfort occurs or is expected. Doctors frequently prescribe other drugs, to be taken regularly, that reduce the heart's workload. Beta blockers slow the heart rate and lessen the force of the heart muscle contraction. Calcium channel blockers are also effective in reducing the frequency and severity of angina attacks.

What if medication fails to control angina?

Doctors may recommend surgery or angioplasty if drugs fail to ease angina or if the risk of heart attack is high. Coronary artery bypass surgery is an operation in which a blood vessel is grafted onto the blocked artery to bypass the blocked or diseased section so that blood can get to the heart muscle. An artery from inside the chest (an "internal mammary" graft) or long vein from the leg (a "saphenous vein" graft) may be used.

Balloon angioplasty involves inserting a catheter with a tiny balloon at the end into a forearm or groin artery. The balloon is inflated briefly to open the vessel in places where the artery is narrowed. Other catheter techniques are also being developed for opening narrowed coronary arteries, including laser and mechanical devices applied by means of catheters.

Angina

Can a person with angina exercise?

Yes. It is important to work with the doctor to develop an exercise plan. Exercise may increase the level of pain-free activity, relieve stress, improve the heart's blood supply, and help control weight. A person with angina should start an exercise program only with the doctor's advice. Many doctors tell angina patients to gradually build up their fitness level—for example, start with a 5-minute walk and increase over weeks or months to 30 minutes or 1 hour. The idea is to gradually increase stamina by working at a steady pace, but avoiding sudden bursts of effort.

What is the difference between "stable" and "unstable" angina?

It is important to distinguish between the typical stable pattern of angina and "unstable" angina.

Angina pectoris often recurs in a regular or characteristic pattern. Commonly a person recognizes that he or she is having angina only after several episodes have occurred, and a pattern has evolved. The level of activity or stress that provokes the angina is somewhat predictable, and the pattern changes only slowly. This is "stable" angina, the most common variety.

Instead of appearing gradually, angina may first appear as a very severe episode or as frequently recurring bouts of angina. Or, an established stable pattern of angina may change sharply; it may by provoked by far less exercise than in the past, or it may appear at rest. Angina in these forms is referred to as "unstable angina" and needs prompt medical attention.

The term "unstable angina" is also used when symptoms suggest a heart attack but hospital tests do not support that diagnosis. For example, a patient may have typical but prolonged chest pain and poor response to rest and medication, but there is no evidence of heart muscle damage either on the electrocardiogram or in blood enzyme tests.

Are there other types of angina?

There are two other forms of angina pectoris. One, long recognized but quite rare, is called Prinzmetal's or variant angina. This type is caused by vasospasm, a spasm that narrows the coronary artery and lessens the flow of blood to the heart. The other is a recently discovered type of angina called microvascular angina. Patients with this condition experience chest pain but have no apparent coronary artery blockages. Doctors have found that the pain results from poor function of tiny blood vessels nourishing the heart as well as the arms and legs. Microvascular angina can be treated with some of the same medications used for angina pectoris.

Additional Resources:

- *Facts About Blood Cholesterol* (revised 1994), NIH Publication No. 94-2696
- *Facts About Coronary Heart Disease* (reprinted 1993), NIH Publication No. 93-2265
- *Facts About Heart Failure* (reprinted 1995) NIH Publication No. 95-923
- *Facts About Heart Disease and Women: So You Have Heart Disease*, NIH Publication No. 95-2645
- *High Blood Pressure and What You Can Do About It*, No. 55-222A
- *So You Have High Blood Cholesterol* (revised 1993), NIH Publication No. 93-2922
- *Step by Step: Eating to Lower Your High Blood Cholesterol* (revised 1994) NIH Publication No. 94-2920

For Further Information

Call or write:

National Heart, Lung, and Blood Institute
Information Office
P.O. Box 30105
Bethesda, MD 20892-0105
Telephone: (301) 251-1222

Chapter 30

Unstable Angina

What Is Unstable Angina?

Unstable angina is a type of coronary artery disease. The coronary arteries bring oxygen-rich blood to your heart. Because your heart is a muscle, it needs oxygen to work well. In coronary artery disease, one or more of these arteries may be partially or even completely blocked.

The type of coronary artery disease you have usually depends on the amount of blockage in your arteries. A heart attack, called a myocardial infarction, means the heart muscle has been damaged by not getting enough blood. Stable angina usually does not damage the heart. Unstable angina is worse than stable angina and may progress to a heart attack if not treated.

Angina is caused by a lack of oxygen in the heart muscle. The symptoms of angina include pain or discomfort in the chest, arms, back, neck, or jaw. Sometimes, anginal pain may feel like a tightness or crushing sensation, or it may be a stabbing pain or seem like numbness. Some people mistake anginal pain as indigestion or gas pain.

Having either stable or unstable angina does not always mean you will have a heart attack. But, unstable angina can be serious and should be treated by a doctor.

Agency for Health Care Policy and Research (AHCPR), AHCPR Pub. No. 94-0604, March 1994.

Purpose of This Chapter

The purpose of this chapter is to describe unstable angina and how it relates to other heart conditions, answer some common questions about this condition, and describe the main types of treatments available.

This chapter is written for people who have been told they have unstable angina, have been treated before for coronary artery disease, or think they might have coronary artery disease. It is also for people with a family member or friend who has unstable angina or stable angina.

This chapter also suggests some questions to ask your doctor, as well as the best time to ask them.

How Are Stable and Unstable Angina Different?

Anginal discomfort may be different for different people. Some people have anginal discomfort when they over-exert themselves (for example, when they shovel snow). Other people feel anginal pain when they get very upset or excited. Over time, they can usually tell which

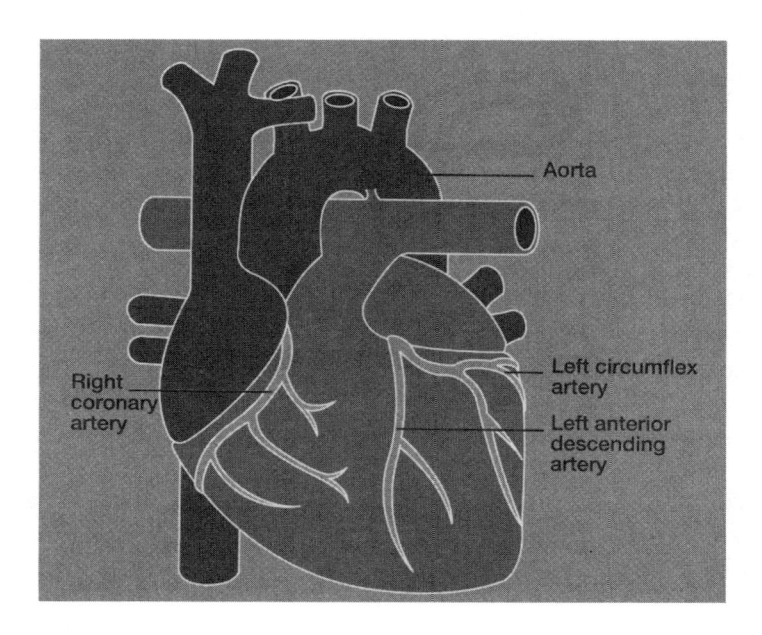

Figure 30.1. Outer view of heart showing the coronary arteries.

activities will give them discomfort. Usually, the discomfort will go away in a few minutes. This type of chest discomfort is called stable angina.

Stable angina attacks usually have a regular pattern. But in some people the pattern of angina is different—it becomes unstable.

People with unstable angina include those who:

- Have anginal discomfort when they resting or that awakens them from sleep.
- Suddenly develop moderate or severe discomfort on exertion when they have never had angina before.
- Have a marked increase in the frequency or severity of their discomfort.

Unstable angina is more serious than stable angina because the risk of having a heart attack is greater.

What Causes Unstable Angina?

In coronary artery disease, blockages—made up of fats, such as cholesterol, and other debris—form on the inside walls of the coronary arteries. In patients who have stable angina, the blockages may not seriously block the flow of blood.

In unstable angina, the blockages may be large. Sometimes, the blockage cracks open. When this happens, your body tries to heal the crack in the blockage by making a blood clot around the damage. If the clot is big enough to block the artery, the clot will keep blood flow from getting through. This can cause a heart attack.

Do I Need to See a Doctor?

This may depend on whether or not your doctor has ever told you that you have coronary artery disease.

If you have chest pain like that described in the section "Chest Pain Can Be An Emergency," you should call an ambulance and then your doctor.

People without Known Coronary Artery Disease

Many people do not know if they have heart disease. Any new or severe chest discomfort that is not related to an injury, such as a pulled muscle, could be unstable angina or a heart attack.

Unstable angina is not dangerous to most people who get medical care right away, but it can be very serious if it is not treated. Even anginal pain that goes away with rest can be serious. Only your doctor will be able to tell how serious it is and what should be done.

People with Known Coronary Artery Disease

If you have coronary artery disease, your past symptoms are the best guide to whether you should call your doctor about new symptoms. Call your doctor if the discomfort you are having is more severe or lasts longer than the discomfort you have had before, has

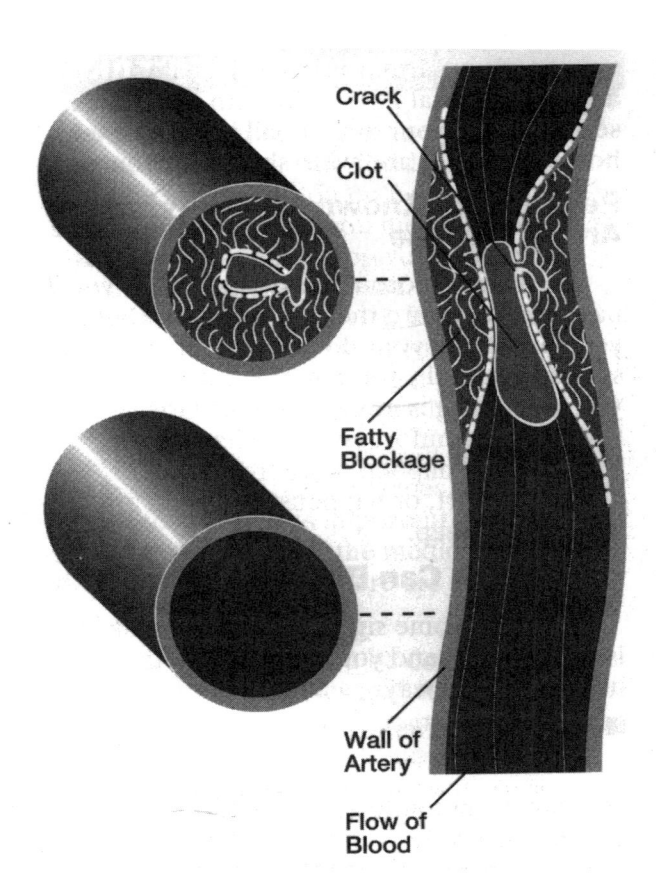

Figure 30.2. Cross-section of a coronary artery showing blocked and normal sections.

begun to happen more frequently or with less effort, or happens when you are resting or asleep.

Chest Pain Can Be an Emergency

Here are some signs that your angina is very serious and you should go to the hospital right away:

- Pain or discomfort that is very bad, gets worse, and lasts longer than 20 minutes.
- Pain or discomfort along with weakness, feeling sick to your stomach, or fainting.
- Pain or discomfort that does not go away when you take three nitroglycerin tablets (see the section, "Nitrates" later in the chapter).
- Pain or discomfort that is worse than you have ever had before.

If you live in an area where ambulance service is not quickly available, have someone drive you to the nearest hospital. You should not drive yourself to the hospital.

It is a good idea to talk with your family, friends, or neighbors about your heart condition and have them read this information. They should be familiar with warning signs that signal when you should go to the hospital. You also may want to tell them which medicines you are taking and where you keep them.

What Will Happen in the Emergency Room?

At your hospital emergency room, the doctors and nurses will decide if you have unstable angina. If you do have unstable angina, they will give you medicines through a vein in your arm to stop your pain and prevent injury to your heart. These medicines will help prevent blood clots and help your heart work more easily. You probably will be given oxygen to help you breathe and get more oxygen in your blood.

The doctors and nurses will ask how you are feeling and if the medicines have stopped your discomfort. It is important to tell them how you really feel. If the medicines do not stop your discomfort, there are other things they can do to help you.

These things need to be done quickly. The doctors and nurses may not be able to explain everything as it is happening. There will be time for you to ask questions after your doctor finds out how serious your condition is.

What Is an Electrocardiogram?

When you are in the emergency room you may have an electrocardiogram, called an ECG or EKG. An ECG records on paper the electrical activity of your heart beat. The ECG may show your doctor if your heart muscle is getting enough oxygen-rich blood.

Will I Have to Stay in the Hospital?

Your ECG, past medical history, and the nature of your pain tell your doctor how serious your problem is.

If your doctor does not consider your condition to be serious enough to admit you to the hospital, he or she may make an appointment to see you in a day or two for more tests. If your chest discomfort comes back before this appointment and is like that described in, "Chest Pain Can Be an Emergency," you should return immediately to the hospital.

It is not easy to accurately diagnose unstable angina, and your doctor may need to see you more than once to be sure.

If your doctor suggests admission to a hospital, you may be put in a regular bed or in an intensive care unit. In either case, treatment will continue while your doctor does more tests.

The tests you have will depend on how serious your condition is and how well the medicines control your discomfort.

What Tests Will I Have?

There is more than one kind of test your doctor can do to decide how badly your coronary arteries are blocked. Some of these tests are usually done while you are in the hospital. Other tests can be done in the hospital, but you do not have to stay overnight. Some tests can be done in your doctor's office.

Stress Tests

You may have an exercise tolerance test. In this test you will be asked to ride a stationary bicycle or walk on a treadmill while a doctor takes an ECG. Your doctor may give you an injection of a radioactive drug that shows up on special cameras. This allows your doctor to make pictures of how your heart moves and the way your blood flows.

This test will let the doctor see the changes that take place in your heart when you exercise. Trained personnel or the doctor will watch your condition by asking how you are feeling during the test. Be sure to follow their instructions carefully and tell them exactly how you feel.

If you have other health problems, you may be given another kind of stress test that does not use exercise. If you have this test, you will be given a special type of drug that makes your heart beat faster and opens your coronary arteries. An ECG will be taken at the same time. This test gives the doctor the same type of information as the exercise tolerance test.

The exercise tolerance test or other stress test will help your doctor tell how well your heart is functioning. Although stress tests are useful, they cannot tell your doctor exactly where your arteries are blocked or how bad the blockages may be. Also, these tests are accurate no more than 90 percent of the time. In some cases, doctors will want to do a cardiac catheterization.

Cardiac Catheterization

An angiogram or cardiac catheterization (sometimes called a cath) lets the doctor see the coronary arteries. A thin tube, called a catheter, is placed in an artery in either your arm or leg. The catheter is threaded up to your heart while your doctor watches on a screen.

The catheter will measure the blood pressure in your heart to see how well it is pumping blood. Then, a liquid is injected through the catheter into the artery, and x-rays are taken. The x-rays allow the doctor to see how much blockage there is and where it is located.

Cardiac catheterization is a test and not a treatment for unstable angina. A treatment called angioplasty looks and feels a lot like cardiac catheterization.

What Can These Tests Show?

Stress testing may help your doctor decide how much of the heart could be in danger from blockages in your arteries. An angiogram shows how severe the blockages are and where they are. If you are told that you have single, two, or three-vessel disease, it means that one, two, or three of the major coronary arteries have a blockage. Your doctor may also talk about the percentage of blockage in the vessel.

The number of blocked arteries and the percentage of blockage are used to measure the severity of your coronary artery disease. Generally, the greater the number of vessels that are blocked, the higher the percentage of blockage, and the more poorly your heart pumps blood, the more severe the disease.

These tests will give your doctor a lot of information about your condition. At this point, he or she can start to give you more information about how serious your condition is and the types of treatment available.

Treatment of Unstable Angina

After your tests, you and your doctor can decide on which treatment you should have. The treatment that is best for you will depend on the results of your tests, whether or not you are still having discomfort, and your own preferences. In general you will have three choices: medical therapy, angioplasty, or bypass surgery.

Medical Therapy

You may have been given medicine in the hospital or emergency room. Some of these medicines, such as heparin which is used to decrease blood clotting, are given to you only in the hospital.

Many other medicines used to treat unstable angina can be taken at home. They come in the form of pills or creams that you can use by yourself.

Many people do very well on medicine alone. If you decide to use medicine to treat your unstable angina, and it does not control all your discomfort, you can still have bypass surgery or angioplasty later.

Almost everyone who has unstable angina will be given some type of medicine. The nurses or doctors caring for you will explain how and when to take all your medicines.

Several types of medicine can help to relieve the discomfort of unstable angina. Many of these drugs also make it easier for the heart to work. Medical therapy may be used alone or in combination with the other treatments described later in this chapter.

Medical therapy alone also may be the right treatment for people with other illnesses and people who do not want to have surgery or other procedures.

Medical therapy alone may benefit patients who:

- Have a blockage or blockages in only one vessel.
- Have a less severe blockage.
- Do not have severe anginal discomfort
- Have stabilized in the hospital

Unstable Angina

Here are some questions to ask your doctor about medical treatment.

- What side effects will I have from the medicine?
- Will I have to take medicine for the rest of my life?

Some people have uncomfortable side effects from the medicine, but most people feel better because they have less anginal discomfort. If you do have a reaction to a medicine, be sure to tell your doctor about it. Often the reaction goes away or becomes less severe with time. If not, your doctor may be able to change your medicine to make you more comfortable.

Remember, none of these drugs removes any of the blockages from your arteries. They do relieve anginal discomfort by bringing more blood to your heart or by making it easier for your heart to work.

Some of the most common medicines given to patients with unstable angina include aspirin, nitrates, and beta blockers.

Aspirin

How it works: Most people think of aspirin as something to relieve a headache or a fever. But aspirin also can prevent blood clots from forming. These are the same kind of blood clots that can block the coronary arteries and cause a heart attack.

Research in patients with unstable angina has proven that taking an aspirin every day reduces the risk of heart attack or death. Acetaminophen (for example, Tylenol®) and ibuprofen (for example, Advil®) are not the same as aspirin and should not be used in place of aspirin.

Side effects: Most patients with unstable angina will be told to take aspirin every day. Your doctor will tell you how much to take. When coated or buffered aspirin is used there are few major side effects. Aspirin should not be used if you are allergic to it or if you have had an ulcer or any other bleeding problem.

Nitrates

How they work: Nitrates (usually nitroglycerin and isosorbide) are used to open blood vessels. Nitrates increase blood flow to the heart muscle and the blood vessels and make it easier for the heart to work. Nitrates can relieve most anginal discomfort very quickly.

Nitrates come in tablets that you put under your tongue or a different type of tablet that you swallow, as a patch that you wear on your skin, or as a cream that you apply on your skin.

Nitrate tablets, cream, and patches all have a limited shelf life after which they will no longer work. Ask your pharmacist how long they will last and when you should replace them.

Nitrate cream and patches are for maintenance therapy only. If you are using a nitrate patch or cream, you should still use nitrate tablets if you have anginal discomfort.

Take one nitroglycerin tablet as soon as you feel discomfort. If the discomfort does not go away in 5 minutes, take a second tablet. If the discomfort does not go away after 5 more minutes, take a third tablet.

If the discomfort has not gone away after taking three tablets in 15 minutes, go to the hospital immediately. Do not wait!

Persistent discomfort that does not go away could be a sign that you are having a heart attack. You should see a doctor immediately.

Side effects: You may feel dizzy or lightheaded right after taking nitrates. Patients are usually told to take nitrate tablets while sitting down. Some people may also get a headache when they take nitrates.

Beta Blockers

How they work: This drug decreases the amount of work your heart has to do and the amount of oxygen your heart needs.

Side effects: Beta blockers are very powerful drugs that can have many side effects. About 10 percent of patients taking beta blockers will feel tired or dizzy. Depression, diarrhea, or skin rash may also happen in about 5 percent of patients. Mental confusion, headaches, heartburn, and shortness of breath are much less common.

Angioplasty

This procedure is done like an angiogram. A thin tube called a catheter is inserted into an artery in the groin and threaded up to the blocked artery. This catheter has a very small balloon attached on the end. When the catheter gets to the blockage, the doctor inflates the balloon. When the balloon is deflated, the blockage should be open enough for the blood to get through, stopping the anginal discomfort.

Unstable Angina

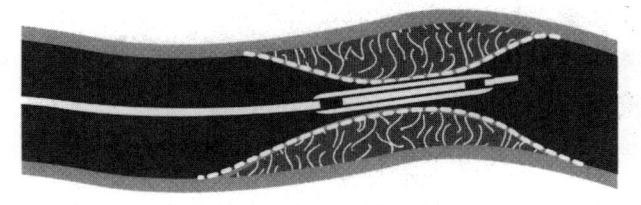

Balloon catheter placed in blocked area of artery

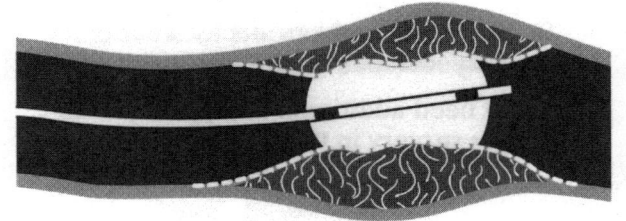

Balloon catheter inflated

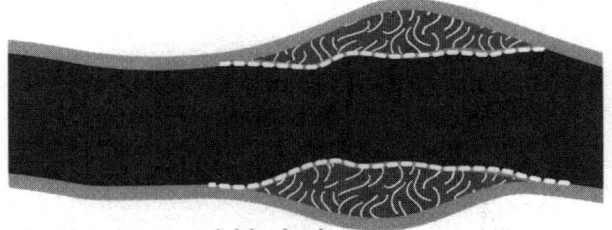

Catheter removed, blocked area open

Figure 30.3. Cross-section of an artery showing how balloon angioplasty opens a blockage.

Possible benefits of angioplasty:

- Relieve anginal pain
- Increase activity/exercise
- Allow return to former activities
- Reduce amount of medicine
- Decrease anxiety/fear

Possible risks of angioplasty

- Worsened angina

Heart Diseases and Disorders Sourcebook, Second Edition

- Emergency bypass surgery
- Heart attack
- Damage to the artery
- Re-blockage of the artery
- Death

Questions to ask your doctor about angioplasty include:

- Will I need additional angioplasty or bypass surgery in the future?
- What will it feel like to have angioplasty?
- What is the chance that I might die during the angioplasty procedure or have other problems?

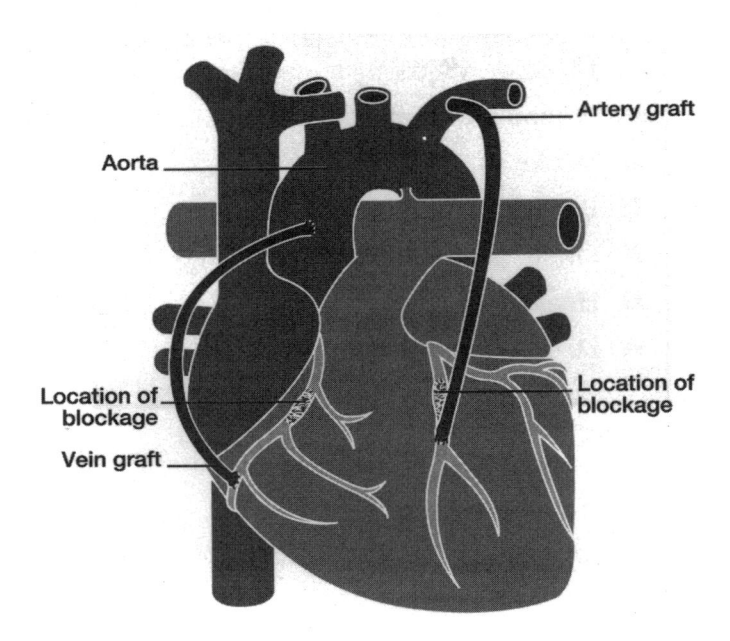

Figure 30.4. Outer view of heart showing how grafts are used to "bypass" blocked arteries.

Unstable Angina

Bypass Surgery

Surgery is usually recommended for patients who have severe blockages in the left main coronary artery or disease in several vessels. Surgery is also an option when medicines do not control anginal symptoms.

Coronary artery bypass surgery can be a very effective way to increase the amount of blood getting to your heart and stop your discomfort.

In this operation, a piece of a vein, usually from your leg or an artery from your chest, is removed and used to "bypass" the section of your artery that has the most blockage. One end of the blood vessel is placed into your aorta. The aorta is the artery that supplies all the blood going out of your heart into your body. The other end is sewn into the artery below the blocked section to bypass the blockage.

Here are some questions to ask your doctor about bypass surgery:

- What will it feel like to have bypass surgery?
- Is it normal to be afraid of having surgery?
- What is the chance that I might die during surgery or have other problems?
- Will I need more surgery in the future?

Possible benefits of coronary bypass surgery:

- Prolong life
- Relieve anginal pain
- Increase activity/exercise
- Allow return to former activities
- Reduce need for medicine
- Decrease anxiety/fear

Possible risks of coronary bypass surgery:

- Bleeding, requiring more surgery
- Wound infection
- Stroke
- Blood clots
- Organ failure (fiver, kidney, lung)

- Heart attack
- Death

Angioplasty or Bypass Surgery?

Both angioplasty and bypass surgery are designed to do the same thing. They both can increase the supply of blood to your heart muscle. Depending on the severity of your disease, you may have a choice between the two.

How will you know which one is right for you? Your doctor will help you make this decision. But in general, angioplasty:

- Is not as major a procedure as bypass surgery.
- Results in a shorter hospital stay.
- Will allow you to return to normal activities sooner.

You should also know that:

- In about 2 to 5 percent of cases, angioplasty does not work, and emergency bypass surgery will be necessary.
- About 40 percent of the time, the arteries become blocked again within 6 months of the angioplasty. If this happens, you may have to have angioplasty again or have bypass surgery.

Talking with Your Health Care Team

Some people think that their doctors are too busy to answer questions. Other people do not know how to ask their questions. But talking with the doctors, nurses, and other health care providers is an important part of your care.

Your questions are important, and the people taking care of you should make the time to answer your questions and listen to what you have to say. Your preferences for the type of treatment you receive are very important.

You may feel more comfortable if a family member or friend is there when you talk to your doctors, nurses, and other health care providers. This person can help to make sure that you understand what is happening, ask questions, and tell the doctor your concerns and preferences for care.

Here are some questions to ask your doctor before you decide what the best treatment might be for you.

Unstable Angina

- Am I a candidate for medical treatment, angioplasty, or bypass surgery?
- What are the chances that my arteries will become blocked again if I have angioplasty or bypass surgery? How soon might this happen?
- Will I have to change my job or retire?
- How soon can I resume my normal activities? What about resuming sexual activity?
- How much will my treatment cost?
- Do I have to go on a low-sodium or low-fat diet? If so, for how long?
- Will I have a heart attack? Will I always have chest pain?

Can Blockages Come Back?

Neither angioplasty nor bypass surgery is a cure for coronary artery disease. Blockages continue to build up on artery walls even after angioplasty or bypass surgery.

Both angioplasty and bypass surgery can be repeated if the arteries become blocked again. The only way to stop coronary artery disease is to prevent the blockages from building up.

Although doctors do not know for sure why blockages form, they do know, from studies of large numbers of patients, that some people are more likely to have blocked arteries than others.

Your doctor may recommend that you attend a cardiac rehabilitation program. These programs usually are offered by local hospitals and very often they are covered by insurance. In a rehabilitation program, nurses, exercise specialists, and doctors will help you to change behaviors that put you at higher risk. They will also teach you how to exercise safely and help you gain confidence in your ability to live with heart disease.

Preventing Blockages

The best way to prevent blockages from forming is to:

- Take aspirin every day
- Stop smoking
- Eat foods that are lower in fat
- Keep weight down

- Increase physical activity
- Control blood pressure if it is high
- Lower stress

Living with Coronary Artery Disease

It is normal for you to worry about your health and your future. But, you should know that most people with unstable angina do not have heart attacks. Usually, angina becomes more stable within 8 weeks. In fact, people who are treated for their unstable angina can live productive lives for many years.

Coronary artery disease does not go away. Your behavior and lifestyle will affect your condition. This is why it is so important to follow the advice of your doctor and the other health care professionals who treat you.

Every year, thousands of people are told they have coronary artery disease. This may come as a shock, especially if they have never felt ill before. Often, they become anxious about their future and wonder if they will still be able to take care of their families or other responsibilities. It is normal to feel a loss of control, as if something has taken over your life.

Doctors, nurses, members of the clergy, and counselors all have experience in helping people with coronary artery disease. They can help you and your family. It is important to talk about how you feel, not just physically, but emotionally.

The best way to feel like you are in control is to learn more about coronary artery disease—what it is and the choices you have. When you see your doctor or other health care provider, be prepared to ask questions.

How Can I Learn More about Unstable Angina?

Organizations that can provide additional information include:

American Heart Association
7272 Greenville Avenue
Dallas, TX 75231-4596
Phone: (800) AHA-USA1

National Heart, Lung, and Blood Institute Information Center
P.O. Box 30105
Bethesda, MD 20824
Phone: (301) 251-1222

The Mended Hearts, Inc.
7272 Greenville Avenue
Dallas, TX 75231-4596
Phone: (214) 706-1442

For Further Information

The information in this chapter was based on the *Clinical Practice Guideline on Unstable Angina*. The guideline was developed by a private-sector panel of experts, including physicians, surgeons, nurses, and people with unstable angina.

Support for this guideline was provided by the Agency for Health Care Policy and Research and the National Heart, Lung, and Blood Institute. Other guidelines on common health problems are available, and more are being developed.

For more information on guidelines or to receive another copy of this information, call toll free (800) 358-9295 or write to:

Agency for Health Care Policy and Research
Publications Clearinghouse
P.O. Box 8547
Silver Spring, MD 20907

Chapter 31

Arrhythmias/Rhythm Disorders

Questions and Answers about Arrhythmias

What Is an Arrhythmia?

An arrhythmia is a change in the regular beat of the heart. The heart may seem to skip a beat or beat irregularly or very fast or very slowly.

Does Having an Arrhythmia Mean That a Person Has Heart Disease?

No, not necessarily. Many arrhythmias occur in people who do not have underlying heart disease.

What Causes Arrhythmias?

Many times, there is no recognizable cause of an arrhythmia. Heart disease may cause arrhythmias. Other causes include: stress, caffeine, tobacco, alcohol, diet pills, and cough and cold medicines.

Are Arrhythmias Serious?

The vast majority of people with arrhythmias have nothing to fear. They do not need extensive exams or special treatments for their condition.

National Heart, Lung, and Blood Institute (NHLBI), NIH Pub. No. 95-2264, September 1995.

In some people, arrhythmias are associated with heart disease. In these cases, heart disease, not the arrhythmia, poses the greatest risk to the patient.

In a very small number of people with serious symptoms, arrhythmias themselves are dangerous. These arrhythmias require medical treatment to keep the heartbeat regular. For example, a few people have a very slow heartbeat (bradycardia), causing them to feel lightheaded or faint. If left untreated, the heart may stop beating and these people could die.

How Common Are Arrhythmias?

Arrhythmias occur commonly in middle-age adults. As people get older, they are more likely to experience an arrhythmia.

What Are the Symptoms of an Arrhythmia?

Most people have felt their heart beat very fast, experienced a fluttering in their chest, or noticed that their heart skipped a beat. Almost everyone has also felt dizzy, faint, or out of breath or had chest pains at one time or another. One of the most common arrhythmias is sinus arrhythmia, the change in heart rate that can occur normally when we take a breath. These experiences may cause anxiety, but for the majority of people, they are completely harmless.

You should not panic if you experience a few flutters or your heart races occasionally. But if you have questions about your heart rhythm or symptoms, check with your doctor.

What Happens in the Heart during an Arrhythmia?

Describing how the heart beats normally helps to explain what happens during an arrhythmia.

The heart is a muscular pump divided into four chambers—two atria located on the top and two ventricles located on the bottom (see Figure 31.1.).

Normally each heartbeat starts in the right atrium. Here, a specialized group of cells called the sinus node, or natural pacemaker, sends an electrical signal. The signal spreads throughout the atria to the area between the atria called the atrioventricular (AV) node.

The AV node connects to a group of special pathways that conduct the signal to the ventricles below. As the signal travels through the heart, the heart contracts. First the atria contract, pumping blood into

Arrhythmias/Rhythm Disorders

the ventricles. A fraction of a second later, the ventricles contract, sending blood throughout the body.

Usually the whole heart contracts between 60 and 100 times per minute. Each contraction equals one heartbeat.

An arrhythmia may occur for one of several reasons:

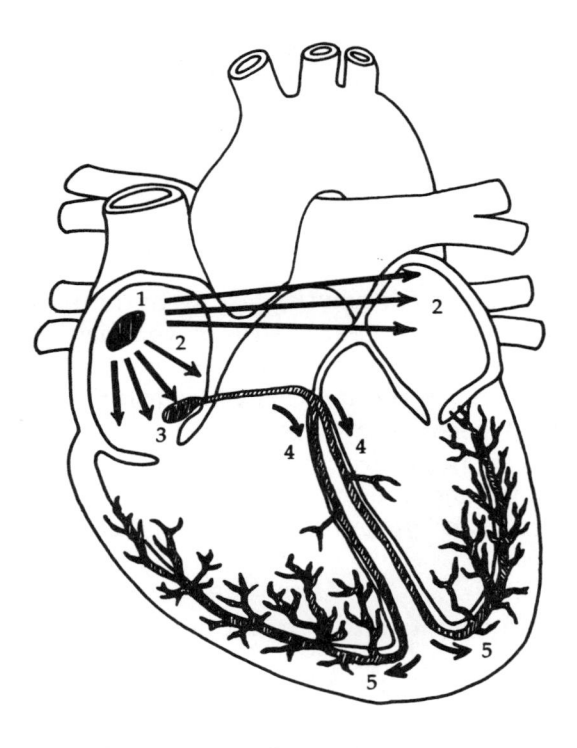

What Makes a Heart Beat

The heartbeat usually starts in the sinus node (1) located in the right atrium.

The sinus node sends an electrical signal throughout the atria (2) and to the atrioventricular (AV) node (3).

The signal then travels down special pathways that conduct it to the ventricles (4,5).

As the signal travels through the heart, the heart contracts or beats.

Figure 31.1. *The Anatomy of a Heart Beat*

- Instead of beginning in the sinus node, the heartbeat begins in another part of the heart.
- The sinus node develops an abnormal rate or rhythm.
- A patient has a heart block.

What Is a Heart Block?

Heart block is a condition in which the electrical signal cannot travel normally down the special pathways to the ventricles. For example, the signal from the atria to the ventricles may be (1) delayed, but each one conducted; (2) delayed with only some getting through; or (3) completely interrupted. If there is no conduction, the beat generally originates from the ventricles and is very slow.

What Are the Different Types of Arrhythmias?

There are many types of arrhythmias. Arrhythmias are identified by where they occur in the heart (atria or ventricles) and by what happens to the heart's rhythm when they occur.

Arrhythmias arising in the atria are called atrial or supraventricular (above the ventricles) arrhythmias. Ventricular arrhythmias begin in the ventricles. In general, ventricular arrhythmias caused by heart disease are the most serious.

Different types of arrhythmias are described below in the section "Arrhythmia Types."

How Does the Doctor Know That I Have an Arrhythmia?

Sometimes an arrhythmia can be detected by listening to the heart with a stethoscope. However, the electrocardiogram is the most precise method for diagnosing the arrhythmia.

An arrhythmia may not occur at the time of the exam even though symptoms are present at other times. In such cases, tests will be done if necessary to find out whether an arrhythmia is causing the symptoms.

What Tests Can Be Done?

First the doctor will take a medical history and do a thorough physical exam. Then one or more tests may be used to check for an arrhythmia and to decide whether it is caused by heart disease. The section below titled "Tests for Detecting Arrhythmias" gives details about these tests.

Arrhythmias/Rhythm Disorders

How Are Arrhythmias Treated?

Many arrhythmias require no treatment whatsoever.

Serious arrhythmias are treated in several ways depending on what is causing the arrhythmia. Sometimes the heart disease is treated to control the arrhythmia. Or, the arrhythmia itself may be treated using one or more of the following treatments.

Drugs. There are several kinds of drugs used to treat arrhythmias. One or more drugs may be used.

Drugs are carefully chosen because they can cause side effects. In some cases, they can cause arrhythmias or make arrhythmias worse. For this reason, the benefits of the drug are carefully weighed against any risks associated with taking it. It is important not to change the dose or type of your medication unless you check with your doctor first.

If you are taking drugs for an arrhythmia, one of the following tests will probably be used to see whether treatment is working: a 24-hour electrocardiogram (ECG) while you are on drug therapy, an exercise ECG, or a special technique to see how easily the arrhythmia can be caused. Blood levels of antiarrhythmic drugs may also be checked.

Cardioversion. To quickly restore a heart to its normal rhythm, the doctor may apply an electrical shock to the chest wall. Called cardioversion, this treatment is most often used in emergency situations. After cardioversion, drugs are usually prescribed to prevent the arrhythmia from recurring.

Automatic implantable defibrillators. These devices are used to correct serious ventricular arrhythmias that can lead to sudden death. The defibrillator is surgically placed inside the patient's chest. There, it monitors the heart's rhythm and quickly identifies serious arrhythmias. With an electrical shock, it immediately disrupts a deadly arrhythmia.

Artificial pacemaker. An artificial pacemaker can take charge of sending electrical signals to make the heart beat if the heart's natural pacemaker is not working properly or its electrical pathway is blocked. During a simple operation, this electrical device is placed under the skin. A lead extends from the device to the right side of the heart, where it is permanently anchored.

Surgery. When an arrhythmia cannot be controlled by other treatments, doctors may perform surgery. After locating the heart tissue that is causing the arrhythmia, the tissue is altered or removed so that it will not produce the arrhythmia.

How Can Arrhythmias Be Prevented?

If heart disease is not causing the arrhythmia, the doctor may suggest that you avoid what is causing it. For example, if caffeine or alcohol is the cause, the doctor may ask you not to drink coffee, tea, colas, or alcoholic beverages.

Is Research on Arrhythmias Being Done?

The National Heart, Lung, and Blood Institute (NHLBI) supports basic research on normal and abnormal electrical activity in the heart to understand how arrhythmias develop. Clinical studies with patients aim to improve the diagnosis and management of different arrhythmias. These studies will someday lead to better diagnostic and treatment strategies.

Where Can I Find Publications about Heart Disease?

To obtain publications about heart disease, you may want to contact your:

- local American Heart Association chapter.
- local or state health department.

The National Heart, Lung, and Blood Institute also has publications about heart disease. For more information, contact:

NHLBI Information Center
P.O. Box 30105
Bethesda, MD 20892-0105
Telephone: (301) 251-1222

Arrhythmia Types

Originating in the Atria

Sinus arrhythmia. Cyclic changes in the heart rate during breathing. Common in children and often found in adults.

Arrhythmias/Rhythm Disorders

Sinus tachycardia. The sinus node sends out electrical signals faster than usual, speeding up the heart rate.

Sick sinus syndrome. The sinus node does not fire its signals properly, so that the heart rate slows down. Sometimes the rate changes back and forth between a slow (bradycardia) and fast (tachycardia) rate.

Premature supraventricular contractions or premature atrial contractions (PAC). A beat occurs early in the atria, causing the heart to beat before the next regular heartbeat.

Supraventricular tachycardia (SVT), paroxysmal atrial tachycardia (PAT). A series of early beats in the atria speed up the heart rate (the number of times a heart beats per minute). In paroxysmal tachycardia, repeated periods of very fast heartbeats begin and end suddenly.

Atrial flutter. Rapidly fired signals cause the muscles in the atria to contract quickly, leading to a very fast, steady heartbeat.

Atrial fibrillation. Electrical signals in the atria are fired in a very fast and uncontrolled manner. Electrical signals arrive in the ventricles in a completely irregular fashion, so the heart beat is completely irregular.

Wolff-Parkinson-White syndrome. Abnormal pathways between the atria and ventricles cause the electrical signal to arrive at the ventricles too soon and to be transmitted back into the atria. Very fast heart rates may develop as the electrical signal ricochets between the atria and ventricles.

Originating in the Ventricles

Premature ventricular complexes (PVC). An electrical signal from the ventricles causes an early heart beat that generally goes unnoticed. The heart then seems to pause until the next beat of the ventricle occurs in a regular fashion.

Ventricular tachycardia. The heart beats fast due to electrical signals arising from the ventricles (rather than from the atria).

Ventricular fibrillation. Electrical signals in the ventricles are fired in a very fast and uncontrolled manner, causing the heart to quiver rather than beat and pump blood.

Heart Diseases and Disorders Sourcebook, Second Edition

Tests for Detecting Arrhythmias

Electrocardiogram (ECG or EKG). A record of the electrical activity of the heart. Disks are placed on the chest and connected by wires to a recording machine. The heart's electrical signals cause a pen to draw lines across a strip of graph paper in the ECG machine (see diagram below). The doctor studies the shapes of these lines to check for any changes in the normal rhythm. The types of ECGs are:

- *Resting ECG.* The patient lies down for a few minutes while a record is made. In this type of ECG, disks are attached to the patient's arms and legs as well as to the chest.

- *Exercise ECG (stress test).* The patient exercises either on a treadmill machine or bicycle while connected to the ECG machine. This test tells whether exercise causes arrhythmias or makes them worse or whether there is evidence of inadequate blood flow to the heart muscle ("ischemia").

- *24-hour ECG (Holter) monitoring.* The patient goes about his or her usual daily activities while wearing a small, portable tape recorder that connects to the disks on the patient's chest. Over time, this test shows changes in rhythm (or "ischemia") that may not be detected during a resting or exercise ECG.

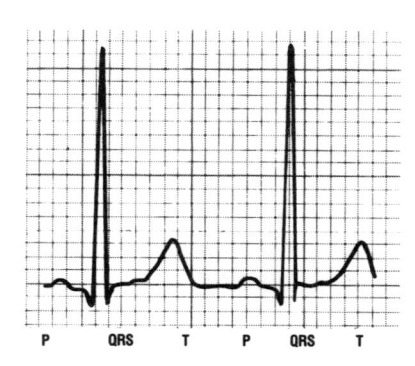

Figure 31.2. Electrocardiogram (ECG or EKG). This ECG shows two complete normal heart cycles. P shows the electrical signal that causes the contraction of the atria. QRS shows the signal of the ventricles. T is the heart's return to its resting state.

Arrhythmias/Rhythm Disorders

- *Transtelephonic monitoring.* The patient wears the tape recorder and disks over a period of a few days to several weeks. When the patient feels an arrhythmia, he or she telephones a monitoring station where the record is made. If access to a telephone is not possible, the patient has the option of activating the monitor's memory function. Later, when a telephone is accessible, the patient can transmit the recorded information from the memory to the monitoring station. Transtelephonic monitoring can reveal arrhythmias that occur only once every few days or weeks.

Electrophysiologic study (EPS). A test for arrhythmias that involves cardiac catheterization. Very thin, flexible tubes (catheters) are placed in a vein of an arm or leg and advanced to the right atrium and ventricle. This procedure allows doctors to find the site and type of arrhythmia and how it responds to treatment.

Chapter 32

Heart Attack (Myocardial Infarction)

- A heart attack is caused by a blood clot obstructing a coronary artery that supplies blood to the heart muscle, causing death of muscle.
- Cholesterol plaque accumulated on the inner wall of a coronary artery is usually the site of blood clot formation.
- A heart attack can cause chest pain and electrical instability of the heart.
- Electrical instability of the heart can cause life threatening abnormal heart rhythm.
- Treatment of heart attack include prompt administration of medications to dissolve and prevent blood clots, balloon angioplasty (PTCA) to open obstructed artery, and medications that open (dilate) blood vessels.
- Early reopening of a blocked coronary artery reduces amount of heart muscle damage, and improves prognosis.
- Patients suffering a heart, attack are hospitalized for several days to detect heart rhythm disturbance, and observe for shortness of breath, and chest pain.

Copyright Medicine Net, Inc. Reprinted with permission. For more health information please visit Medicinenet at www.medicinenet.com.

What Is a Heart Attack?

A heart attack (myocardial infarction) is the death of heart muscle due to the loss of blood supply. Usually, the loss of blood supply is caused by a complete blockage of a coronary artery by a blood clot. A coronary artery is an artery that supplies blood to the heart muscle. Death of the heart muscle causes chest pain and electrical instability of the heart muscle tissue. Electrical instability of the heart causes ventricular fibrillation (chaotic electrical disturbance). Orderly transmission of electrical signals in the heart is important for the regular beating (pumping) of the heart. A heart undergoing ventricular fibrillation simply quivers, and cannot pump or deliver oxygenated blood to the brain. Permanent brain damage and death can occur unless oxygenated blood flow is restored within five minutes.

Approximately one million Americans suffer a heart attack annually. Four hundred thousand of these victims die as a result. Many of the heart attack deaths are due to ventricular fibrillation of the heart that occurs before the victim can reach any medical assistance or the emergency room. These electrical disturbances of the heart can be treated with medications once the patient reaches the hospital. Therefore, 90% to 95% of heart attack victims who make it to the hospital survive. The 5% to 10% who later die are those who have suffered major heart muscle damage.

Early heart attack deaths can be avoided if a bystander starts CPR (cardiopulmonary resuscitation) within five minutes of the onset of ventricular fibrillation. CPR involves breathing for the victim and applying external chest compression to make the heart pump. When paramedics arrive, medications and/or electrical shock (cardioversion) to the heart can be administered to convert ventricular fibrillation to a normal heart rhythm. Therefore, prompt CPR and rapid paramedic response can improve the survival chances from a heart attack.

What Causes a Heart Attack?

A heart attack is caused by the formation of a blood clot on a cholesterol plaque located on the inner wall of an artery to the heart (coronary artery). Cholesterol is a fatty chemical which is part of the outer lining of cells in the body. Cholesterol plaque is the formation of a hard, thick substance on the artery walls which is caused by deposits of cholesterol on the artery walls; a process that begins in the late teens. Over time, the accumulation of cholesterol plaque causes thickening of the artery walls and narrowing of the arteries; a process called atherosclerosis. Plaque accumulation can be accelerated by

Heart Attack (Myocardial Infarction)

smoking, high blood pressure, elevated cholesterol, and diabetes. Ultimately, atherosclerosis causes significant narrowing of the coronary arteries. During exercise or excitement, the narrowed coronary arteries cannot increase the blood supply to meet the increased oxygen demand of the heart muscle.

Heart muscle which is starved of blood oxygen, a condition called ischemia causes chest pain (angina). Chest pain that occurs with exercise is called exertional angina. Exertional angina is reversible, and subsides with rest. Occasionally, for unknown reasons, the surface of the cholesterol plaque can become sticky, causing blood clotting. When a blood clot forms on top of this plaque, the artery becomes completely blocked, causing death of the heart muscle (heart attack).

Unlike exertional angina, death of the heart muscle from a heart attack is permanent.

What Are the Symptoms of a Heart Attack?

Chest pain or pressure is a common symptom of heart attack. Heart attacks most frequently occur from 4:00 A.M. to 10:00 A.M. due to higher adrenaline amounts released from the adrenal glands during the morning hours. Interestingly, heart attacks do not usually happen during exercise, although exercise is commonly associated with exertional angina. One quarter of all heart attacks are silent, without chest pain.

Heart attack victims may complain of:

- chest pressure
- sweating
- jaw pain
- heartburn
- arm pain
- indigestion
- back pain
- general malaise
- nausea
- shortness of breath

How Is a Heart Attack Diagnosed?

The initial diagnosis of a heart attack is made by a combination of clinical symptoms and characteristic electrocardiogram (EKG) changes. An EKG is a recording of the electrical activity of the heart, and can detect areas of muscle ischemia (muscle which is deprived of oxygen) and/or dead tissue in the heart. However, confirmation of a heart attack can only be made hours later through detection of elevated creatinine phosphokinase (CPK) in the blood. CPK is a muscle protein enzyme which is released into the blood circulation by dying heart muscles when their surrounding membranes dissolve.

What Are the Treatment Options for a Heart Attack?

The immediate goal of treatment is to quickly open blocked arteries and restore blood flow to the heart muscles; a process called "reperfusion." Once the artery is open, the heart attack is generally halted and the patient becomes pain free. Early reperfusion minimizes the extent of heart muscle damage and preserves the pumping function of the heart. Delay in establishing reperfusion can result in irreversible death to the heart muscle cells and reduced pumping force of the remaining heart muscle. The amount and health of the remaining heart muscle is the major determinant of the future quality of life and longevity for the patient after a heart attack.

The fastest method of opening a blocked artery, provided the hospital has a cardiac catheterization facility, is to perform an immediate PTCA (percutaneous transluminal coronary angioplasty). Under X-ray guidance, a tiny plastic catheter with a balloon at the end is advanced over a fine guide wire to the blockage site and inflated, thus pushing the clot and plaque out of the way. PTCA can be effective in opening up to 95% of arteries, usually within 60 minutes.

Medications, if given early, are also effective in opening arteries. Clot-dissolving medications (thrombolytic agents) such as tissue plasminogen-activator (t-PA) and streptokinase given intravenously can open 80% of the blocked arteries within 90 minutes. The earlier they are administered, the better the chance of an early artery opening. If thrombolytic agents are given too late (greater than 6 hours after the onset of chest pain), most of the muscle damage has already occurred.

Anti-platelet agents, like aspirin, reduce the tendency of platelets in the blood to clump and clot. This decreases the possibility of recurrent closure of the artery and improves the chances of survival.

An anti-coagulant, heparin, is given intravenously in the hospital as a blood-thinning agent to prevent blood clots and to maintain an open artery during the initial 24 hours.

Nitroglycerin, a blood vessel dilator or vasodilator (which opens the blood vessel by relaxing the muscular wall of the blood vessel) is given either under the tongue or intravenously to prevent blood vessel spasm and to minimize the area of the heart attack.

Heart Attack (Myocardial Infarction)

ACE (angiotensin converting enzyme) inhibitors, another class of vasodilators, are given orally after a heart attack to improve the heart muscle healing process. Examples of ACE inhibitors include captopril (Capoten), enalapril (Vasotec), lisinopril (Zestril and Prinvil). These medications reduce the stress load to the heart, thereby allowing the damaged muscles to recover.

In some patients, PTCA can be technically difficult to perform. In others, PTCA and medications fail to achieve reperfusion or maintain open arteries. These patients may be considered for coronary artery bypass graft (CABG) surgery.

How Does a Patient Recover From a Heart Attack?

Heart attack patients are monitored in the hospital for 3 to 6 days prior to discharge home. Rhythm disturbances, shortness of breath due to heart failure, or recurrent pain are indications for further therapy such as balloon angioplasty, medications, or bypass surgery. Patients gradually increase their activity under observation. Before discharge, low level stress tests are useful for detecting significant residual narrowing in the coronary arteries, rhythm changes, and heart muscle failure. They also guide the physicians in prescribing activity regimens after discharge.

Before resuming full activity or work, several weeks are needed for the area of the heart attack to heal. After a small heart attack, which is measured by the size of heart muscle damage, patients can resume normal activities after two weeks. These activities include returning to work as well as normal sexual activity. A moderate heart attack requires limited, gradually increasing activity for four weeks, while a large heart attack results in a six week recovery period. These time frames are necessary for the dead heart muscle to substantially complete the scarring process. During this healing period, patients should avoid vigorous exertion and heavy lifting (over 20 pounds) or any activity which causes shortness of breath or sweating.

How Can I Prevent a Second Heart Attack?

Aspirin and beta blockers (propranolol, metoprolol, atenolol, timolol) have been shown to reduce chances of a second heart attack and improve future survival. Beta blockers antagonize the action of adrenaline and relieve stress to the heart muscles. Stopping smoking, reducing weight and dietary fat, controlling blood pressure and diabetes, and a reduction of serum cholesterol, along with regular, carefully prescribed exercise can all improve the quality of life and longevity after a heart attack. ACE inhibitor medication (mentioned above) aids in the healing process and improves long-term survival.

A full stress test, often with nuclear isotope imaging or soundwave testing (echocardiography), is usually done at 4 to 8 weeks after the original heart attack to determine whether further treatment is needed, such as a coronary artery bypass graft surgery. Favorable stress testing results permit initiation of a program of cardiac rehabilitation.

What Is in the Future for Heart Attack Sufferers?

Greater public awareness and lifestyle changes have contributed to a dramatic reduction in the incidence of heart attacks over the last 4 decades. Improved blood-thinning agents, such as Hirudin and Hirulog, derived from leech proteins, are being tested to complement current therapies. Newer versions of t-PA are being developed to achieve a higher percentage of open arteries. Work is being done with direct laser energy and ultrasound waves to attack both the blood clot and the underlying plaque. Emergency medical teams which rapidly respond, and are able to diagnose heart attacks and administer emergency drugs in non-hospital settings, as well as performing electrical defibrillation, have been shown in test cities, such as Seattle, to improve outcome and save heart muscle.

Chapter 33

Heart Failure

What Is Heart Failure?

Heart failure occurs when the heart loses its ability to pump enough blood through the body. Usually, the loss in pumping action is a symptom of an underlying heart problem, such as coronary artery disease.

The term heart failure suggests a sudden and complete stop of heart activity. But, actually, the heart does not suddenly stop. Rather, heart failure usually develops slowly, often over years, as the heart gradually loses its pumping ability and works less efficiently. Some people may not become aware of their condition until symptoms appear years after their heart began its decline.

How serious the condition is depends on how much pumping capacity the heart has lost. Nearly everyone loses some pumping capacity, as he or she ages. But the loss is significantly more in heart failure and often results from a heart attack or other disease that damages the heart.

The severity of the condition determines the impact it has on a person's life. At one end of the spectrum, the mild form of heart failure may have little effect on a person's life; at the other end, severe heart failure can interfere with even simple activities and prove fatal. Between those extremes, treatment often helps people lead full lives.

National Heart, Lung, and Blood Institute (NHLBI), 97-923, May 1997.

But all forms of heart failure, even the mildest, are a serious health problem, which must be treated. To improve their chance of living longer, patients must take care of themselves, see their physician regularly, and closely follow treatments.

Is There Only One Type of Heart Failure?

The term congestive heart failure is often used to describe all patients with heart failure. In reality, congestion (the buildup of fluid) is just one feature of the condition and does not occur in all patients. There are two main categories of heart failure although within each category, symptoms and effects may differ from patient to patient. The two categories are:

- Systolic heart failure—This occurs when the heart's ability to contract decreases. The heart cannot pump with enough force to push a sufficient amount of blood into the circulation. Blood coming into the heart from the lungs may back up and cause fluid to leak into the lungs, a condition known as pulmonary congestion.

- Diastolic heart failure—This occurs when the heart has a problem relaxing. The heart cannot properly fill with blood because the muscle has become stiff, losing its ability to relax. This form may lead to fluid accumulation, especially in the feet, ankles, and legs. Some patients may have lung congestion.

How Common Is Heart Failure?

Between 2 to 3 million Americans have heart failure, and 400,000 new cases are diagnosed each year. The condition is slightly more common among men than women and is twice as common among African Americans as whites. Heart failure causes 39,000 deaths a year and is a contributing factor in another 225,000 deaths. The death rate attributed to heart failure rose by 64 percent from 1970 to 1990, while the death rate from coronary heart disease dropped by 49 percent during the same period. Heart failure mortality is about twice as high for African Americans as whites for all age groups. In a sense, heart failure's growing presence as a health problem reflects the nation's changing population: More people are living longer. People age 65 and older represent the fastest growing segment of the population, and the risk of heart failure increases with age. The condition affects 1 percent of people age 50, but about 5 percent of people age 75.

What Causes Heart Failure?

As stated, the heart loses some of its blood-pumping ability as a natural consequence of aging. However, a number of other factors can lead to a potentially life-threatening loss of pumping activity.

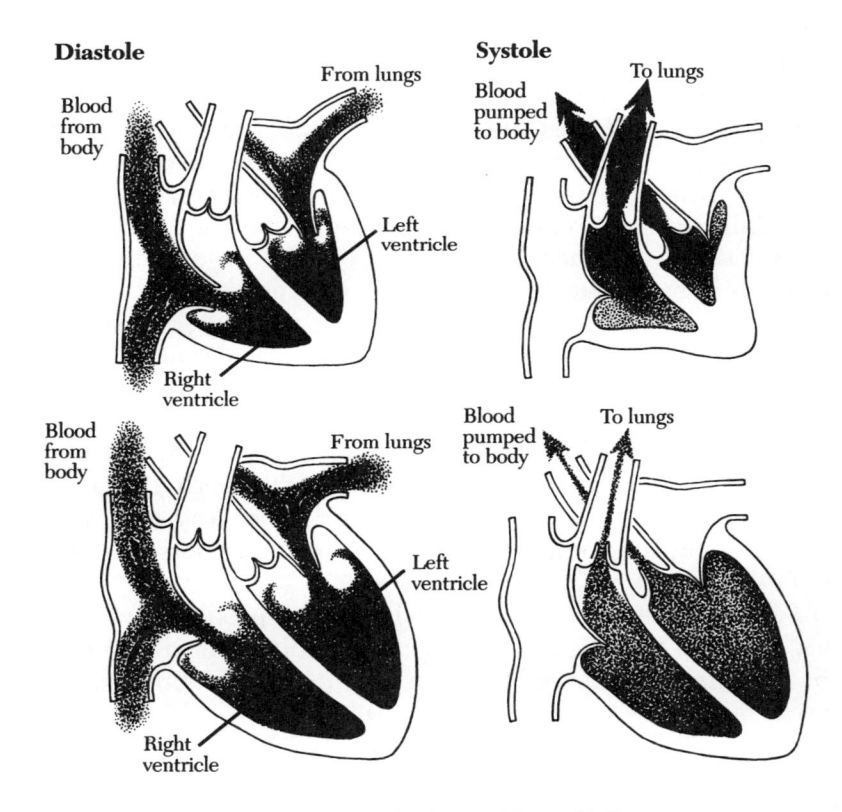

Figure 33.1. Loss of Pumping Action in Heart Failure.

Healthy Heart Muscle [top]. Normally, the heart pumps blood by relaxing and then contacting its chambers. When the chambers relax, blood comes in; when the chambers contract, blood is pushed out, carrying oxygen and nutrients to the rest of the body.

Weakened Heart Muscle [bottom]. Heart failure occurs when the heart muscle loses its ability to pump. The chambers cannot relax and contract well. Less blood moves through the chambers and more blood stays in the heart.

As a symptom of underlying heart disease, heart failure is closely associated with the major risk factors for coronary heart disease: smoking, high cholesterol levels, hypertension (persistent high blood pressure), diabetes and abnormal blood sugar levels, and obesity. A person can change or eliminate those risk factors and thus lower their risk of developing or aggravating their heart disease and heart failure.

Among prominent risk factors, hypertension (high blood pressure) and diabetes are particularly important. Uncontrolled high blood pressure increases the risk of heart failure by about 200 percent, compared with those who do not have hypertension. Moreover, the degree of risk appears directly related to the severity of the high blood pressure.

Persons with diabetes have about a two- to eightfold greater risk of heart failure than those without diabetes. Women with diabetes have a greater risk of heart failure than men with diabetes. Part of the risk comes from diabetes' association with other heart failure risk factors, such as high blood pressure, obesity, and high cholesterol levels. However, the disease process in diabetes also damages the heart muscle.

The presence of coronary disease is among the greatest risks for heart failure. Muscle damage and scarring caused by a heart attack greatly increase the risk of heart failure. Cardiac arrhythmias, or irregular heartbeats, also raise heart failure risk. Any disorder that causes abnormal swelling or thickening of the heart sets the stage for heart failure.

In some people, heart failure arises from problems with heart valves, the flap-like structures that help regulate blood flow through the heart. Infections in the heart are another source of increased risk for heart failure.

A single risk factor may be sufficient to cause heart failure, but a combination of factors dramatically increases the risk. Advanced age adds to the potential impact of any heart failure risk.

Finally, genetic abnormalities contribute to the risk for certain types of heart disease, which in turn may lead to heart failure. However, in most instances, a specific genetic link to heart failure has not been identified.

What Are the Symptoms?

A number of symptoms are associated with heart failure, but none is specific for the condition. Perhaps the best known symptom is shortness of breath ("dyspnea"). In heart failure, this may result from excess

Heart Failure

fluid in the lungs. The breathing difficulties may occur at rest or during exercise. In some cases, congestion may be severe enough to prevent or interrupt sleep.

Fatigue or easy tiring is another common symptom. As the heart's pumping capacity decreases, muscles and other tissues receive less oxygen and nutrition, which are carried in the blood. Without proper "fuel," the body cannot perform as much work, which translates into fatigue.

Fluid accumulation, or edema, may cause swelling of the feet, ankles, legs, and occasionally, the abdomen. Excess fluid retained by the body may result in weight gain, which sometimes occurs fairly quickly.

Persistent coughing is another common sign, especially coughing that regularly produces mucus or pink, blood-tinged sputum. Some people develop raspy breathing or wheezing.

Because heart failure usually develops slowly, the symptoms may not appear until the condition has progressed over years. The heart hides the underlying problem by making adjustments that delay—but do not prevent—the eventual loss in pumping capacity. The heart adjusts, or compensates, in three ways to cope with and hide the effects of heart failure:

- Enlargement ("dilatation"), which allows more blood into the heart;
- Thickening of muscle fibers ("hypertrophy") to strengthen the heart muscle, which allows the heart to contract more forcefully and pump more blood; and
- More frequent contraction, which increases circulation.

By making these adjustments, or compensating, the heart can temporarily make up for losses in pumping ability, sometimes for years. However, compensation has its limits. Eventually, the heart cannot offset the lost ability to pump blood, and the signs of heart failure appear.

How Do Doctors Diagnose Heart Failure?

In many cases, physicians diagnose heart failure during a physical examination. Readily identifiable signs are shortness of breath, fatigue, and swollen ankles and feet. The physician also will check for the presence of risk factors, such as hypertension, obesity, and a history of heart problems. Using a stethoscope, the physician can listen to a patient breathe and identify the sounds of lung congestion. The stethoscope also picks up the abnormal heart sounds indicative of heart failure.

If neither the symptoms nor the patient's history point to a clear-cut diagnosis, the physician may recommend any of a variety of laboratory tests, including, initially, an electrocardiogram, which uses recording devices placed on the chest to evaluate the electrical activity of a patient's heartbeat.

Echocardiography is another means of evaluating heart function from outside the body. Sound waves bounced off the heart are recorded and translated into images. The pictures can reveal abnormal heart size, shape, and movement. Echocardiography also can be used to calculate a patient's ejection fraction, a measure of the amount of blood pumped out when the heart contracts.

Another possible test is the chest x-ray, which also determines the heart's size and shape, as well as the presence of congestion in the lungs.

Tests help rule out other possible causes of symptoms. The symptoms of heart failure can result when the heart is made to work too hard, instead of from damaged muscle. Conditions that overload the heart occur rarely and include severe anemia and thyrotoxicosis (a disease resulting from an overactive thyroid gland).

What Treatments Are Available?

Heart failure caused by an excessive workload is curable by treating the primary disease, such as anemia or thyrotoxicosis. Also curable are forms caused by anatomical problems, such as a heart valve defect. These defects can be surgically corrected.

However, for the common forms of heart failure—those due to damaged heart muscle—no known cure exists. But treatment for these forms may be quite successful. The treatment seeks to improve patients' quality of life and length of survival through lifestyle change and drug therapy.

Patients can minimize the effects of heart failure by controlling the risk factors for heart disease. Obvious steps include quitting smoking, losing weight if necessary, abstaining from alcohol, and making dietary changes to reduce the amount of salt and fat consumed. Regular, modest exercise is also helpful for many patients, though the amount and intensity should be carefully monitored by a physician.

Heart Failure

But, even with lifestyle changes, most heart failure patients must take medication. Many patients receive two or more drugs.

Several types of drugs have proven useful in the treatment of heart failure:

- Diuretics help reduce the amount of fluid in the body and are useful for patients with fluid retention and hypertension.
- Digitalis increases the force of the heart's contractions, helping to improve circulation.
- Results of recent studies have placed more emphasis on the use of drugs known as angiotensin converting enzyme (ACE) inhibitors. Several large studies have indicated that ACE inhibitors improve survival among heart failure patients and may slow, or perhaps even prevent, the loss of heart pumping activity.

Originally developed as a treatment for hypertension, ACE inhibitors help heart failure patients by, among other things, decreasing the pressure inside blood vessels. As a result, the heart does not have to work as hard to pump blood through the vessels. Patients who cannot take ACE inhibitors may get a nitrate and/or a drug called hydralazine, each of which helps relax tension in blood vessels to improve blood flow.

Sometimes, heart failure is life-threatening. Usually, this happens when drug therapy and lifestyle changes fail to control its symptoms. In such cases, a heart transplant may be the only treatment option. However, candidates for transplantation often have to wait months or even years before a suitable donor heart is found. Recent studies indicate that some transplant candidates improve during this waiting period through drug treatment and other therapy, and can be removed from the transplant list.

Transplant candidates who do not improve sometimes need mechanical pumps, which are attached to the heart. Called left ventricular assist devices (LVADs), the machines take over part or virtually all of the heart's blood-pumping activity. However, current LVADs are not permanent solutions for heart failure but are considered bridges to transplantation.

An experimental surgical procedure for severe heart failure is available at a few U.S. medical centers. The procedure, called cardiomyoplasty, involves detaching one end of a muscle in the back, wrapping it around the heart, and then suturing the muscle to the heart. An implanted electric stimulator causes the back muscle to contract, pumping blood from the heart.

Heart Diseases and Disorders Sourcebook, Second Edition

Common Heart Failure Medications

Listed below are some of the medications prescribed for heart failure. Not all medications are suitable for all patients, and more than one drug may be needed.

Also, the list provides the full range of possible side effects for these drugs. Not all patients will develop these side effects. If you suspect that you are having a side effect, alert your physician.

ACE Inhibitors. These prevent the production of a chemical that causes blood vessels to narrow. As a result, blood pressure drops, and the heart does not have to work as hard to pump blood.

Side effects may include coughing, skin rashes, fluid retention, excess potassium in the bloodstream, kidney problems, and an altered or lost sense of taste.

Digitalis. Increases the force of the heart's contractions. It also slows certain fast heart rhythms. As a result, the heart beats less frequently but more effectively, and more blood is pumped into the arteries.

Side effects may include nausea, vomiting, loss of appetite, diarrhea, confusion, and new heartbeat irregularities.

Diuretics. These decrease the body's retention of salt and so of water. Diuretics are commonly prescribed to reduce high blood pressure. Diuretics come in many types, with different periods of effectiveness.

Side effects may include loss of too much potassium, weakness, muscle cramps, joint pains, and impotence.

Hydralazine. This drug widens blood vessels, easing blood flow.

Side effects may include headaches, rapid heartbeat, and joint pain.

Nitrates. These drugs are used mostly for chest pain, but may also help diminish heart failure symptoms. They relax smooth muscle and widen blood vessels. They act to lower primarily systolic blood pressure.

Side effects may include headaches.

Making the Most Of Your Doctor Visit

Here are some points you may want to discuss with your doctor. Don't hesitate to ask questions to clarify points. Also, ask your doctor to rephrase a reply you cannot understand. You may want to take a family member or friend to the appointment with you to help you better understand and remember what's said.

- Briefly describe your symptoms, even those you feel may not be important. You may want to keep a list so you will remember them.
- Tell the doctor all of the medications you take—including over-the-counter drugs—and any problems you may be having with them.
- Be sure you understand all of the doctor's instructions—especially for medications. Know what drug to take when, how often, and in what amount.
- Find out what side effects are possible from any drug the doctor prescribes for you.
- Ask the meaning of any medical term you don't understand.
- If, after your appointment, you still have questions or are uncertain about your treatment, call the doctor's office to get the information you need.

Readying a Q & A for Your Doctor Visit

Going to the doctor can be a nervous time. It may be hard to remember everything you want to ask and everything you hear.

It helps to prepare a list of important questions. Then take your list with you to your appointment so you can record the answers.

Before you leave the doctor's office, be sure you understand your condition and its treatment, including any medications.

A Question for Your Pharmacist

Your pharmacist is a good resource for information about medications. Ask if any drug you're taking interacts badly with certain foods or with other drugs, including nonprescription ones. Your pharmacist also can help you understand product package inserts and label instructions.

Can a Person Live with Heart Failure?

Heart failure is one of the most serious symptoms of heart disease. About two-thirds of all patients die within 5 years of diagnosis. However, some live beyond 5 years, even into old age. The outlook for an individual patient depends on the patient's age, severity of heart failure, overall health, and a number of other factors.

As heart failure progresses, the effects can become quite severe, and patients often lose the ability to perform even modest physical activity. Eventually, the heart's reduced pumping capacity may interfere with routine functions, and patients may become unable to care for themselves. The loss in functional ability can occur quickly if the heart is further weakened by heart attacks or the worsening of other conditions that affect heart failure, such as diabetes and coronary heart disease.

Heart failure patients also have an increased risk of sudden death, or cardiac arrest, caused by an irregular heartbeat. To improve the chances of surviving with heart failure, patients must take care of themselves. Patients must:

- See their physician regularly;
- Closely follow all of their physicians instructions;
- Take any medication according to instructions; and
- Immediately inform their physician of any significant change in their condition, such as an intensified shortness of breath or swollen feet.

Patients with heart failure also should:

- Control their weight;
- Watch what they eat;
- Not smoke cigarettes or use other tobacco products; and
- Abstain from or strictly limit alcohol consumption.

Even with the best care, heart failure can worsen, but patients who don't take care of themselves are almost writing themselves a prescription for poor health.

The best defense against heart failure is the prevention of heart disease. Almost all of the major coronary risk factors can be controlled or eliminated: smoking, high cholesterol, high blood pressure, diabetes, and obesity.

What Is the Outlook for Heart Failure?

Within the past decade, knowledge of heart failure has improved dramatically but, clearly, much more remains to be learned. The National

Heart Failure

Heart, Lung, and Blood institute (NHLBI) supports numerous research projects aimed at building on what is already known about heart failure and at uncovering new knowledge about its process, diagnosis, and treatment. NHLBI research priorities for heart failure include:

- Learning more about basic cellular changes that lead to heart failure;
- Developing tests to detect the earliest signs of heart failure;
- Identifying factors that cause heart failure to worsen;
- Determining how heart failure can be reversed once it starts;
- Understanding better the heart's ability to compensate for lost pumping ability; and
- Developing new therapies, especially those based on early signs of heart failure.

Glossary

Angiotensin Converting enzyme (ACE) inhibitor: A drug used to decrease pressure inside blood vessels.

Arrhythmia: An irregular heartbeat.

Cardiomyoplasty: A surgical procedure that involves detaching one end of a back muscle and attaching it to the heart. An electric stimulator causes the muscle to contract to pump blood from the heart.

Congestive heart failure: A heart disease condition that involves loss of pumping ability by the heart, generally accompanied by fluid accumulation in body tissues, especially the lungs.

Diastolic heart failure: Inability of the heart to relax properly and fill with blood as a result of stiffening of the heart muscle.

Dyspnea: Shortness of breath.

Echocardiography: Recording sound waves bounced off the heart to produce images of the heart.

Edema: Abnormal fluid accumulation in body tissues.

Electrocardiogram (EKG or ECG): Measurement of electrical activity associated with heartbeats.

Heart failure: Loss of blood-pumping ability by the heart.

Left ventricular assist device: A mechanical device used to increase the heart's pumping ability.

Pulmonary congestion (or edema): Fluid accumulation in the lungs.

Sudden cardiac death: Cardiac arrest caused by an irregular heartbeat.

Systolic heart failure: Inability of the heart to contract with enough force to pump adequate amounts of blood through the body.

Valves: Flap-like structures that control the direction of blood flow through the heart.

Chapter 34

Cardiomyopathy (Heart Muscle Disease)

Introduction

Cardiomyopathy is a disease of the heart muscle. The heart loses its ability to pump blood and, in some instances, heart rhythm is disturbed, leading to irregular heartbeats, or arrhythmias. Usually, the exact cause of the muscle damage is never found.

Cardiomyopathy differs from many other heart disorders in a couple of ways. First, the types not related to coronary atherosclerosis are fairly uncommon. Cardiomyopathy affects about 50,000 Americans. However, the condition is a leading reason for heart transplantation.

Second, unlike many other forms of heart disease that affect middle-aged and older persons, certain types of cardiomopathies can, and often do, occur in the young. The condition tends to be progressive and sometimes worsens fairly quickly.

Nonischemic Cardiomyopathy

As noted, there are various types of cardiomyopathy. These fall into two major categories: "ischemic" and "nonischemic" cardiomyopathy.

- Ischemic cardiomyopathy typically refers to heart muscle damage that results from coronary artery disease, such as heart attack, and will not be discussed here.

National Heart, Lung, and Blood Institute (NHLBI), NIH Pub. No. 97-3082, July 1997.

- Nonischemic cardiomyopathy includes several types. The three main types are covered in this chapter. They are: dilated, hypertrophic, and restrictive. The name of each describes the nature of its muscle damage.

Dilated (Congestive) Cardiomyopathy

By far the most common type of nonischemic cardiomyopathy, the dilated (stretched) form occurs when disease-affected muscle fibers lead to enlargement, or dilation, of one or more chambers of the heart. This weakens the heart's pumping ability. The heart tries to cope with the pumping limitation by further enlarging and stretching—a process known as "compensation."

Dilated cardiomyopathy occurs most often in middle-aged people and more often in men than women. However, the disease has been diagnosed in people of all ages, including children.

In most cases, the disease is idiopathic—a specific cause for the damage is never identified.

But some factors have been linked to the disease's occurrence. For instance, alcohol has a direct suppressant effect on the heart. Dilated cardiomyopathy can be caused by chronic, excessive consumption of alcohol, particularly in combination with dietary deficiencies. Also, dilated cardiomyopathy occasionally occurs as a complication of pregnancy and childbirth. Other factors are: various infections, mostly viral, which lead to an inflammation of the heart muscle (myocarditis); toxins (such as cobalt, once used in beers, for instance); and, rarely, heredity.

Some drugs, used to treat a different medical condition, also can damage the heart and produce dilated cardiomyopathy. Such drugs include doxorubicin and daunorubicin, both used to treat cancer.

Whatever the cause, the clinical and pathological manifestations of dilated cardiomyopathy are usually the same.

Symptoms

Dilated cardiomyopathy can be present for several years without causing significant symptoms. With time, however, the enlarged heart gradually weakens.

This condition is commonly called "heart failure," and it is the hallmark of dilated cardiomyopathy. Typical signs and symptoms of heart failure include: fatigue; weakness; shortness of breath, sometimes severe and accompanied by a cough, particularly with exertion or when lying down; and swelling of the legs and feet, resulting from fluid

Cardiomyopathy (Heart Muscle Disease)

accumulation that may also affect the lungs (congestion) and other parts of the body. It also produces abnormal weight gain. (The cough and congestion mimic and, therefore, can be misdiagnosed as pneumonia or acute bronchitis. Also, heart failure is often from heart disease other than cardiomyopathy.)

Because of the congestion, some physicians use the older term "congestive cardiomyopathy" to refer to dilated cardiomyopathy. In advanced stages of the disease, the congestion may cause pain in the chest or abdomen.

In advanced stages, some patients develop irregular heartbeats, which can be serious and even life threatening.

Diagnosis

Once symptoms appear, the condition may be tentatively diagnosed based on a physical examination and a patient's medical history. More often, though, further examination is needed to differentiate dilated cardiomyopathy from other causes of heart failure.

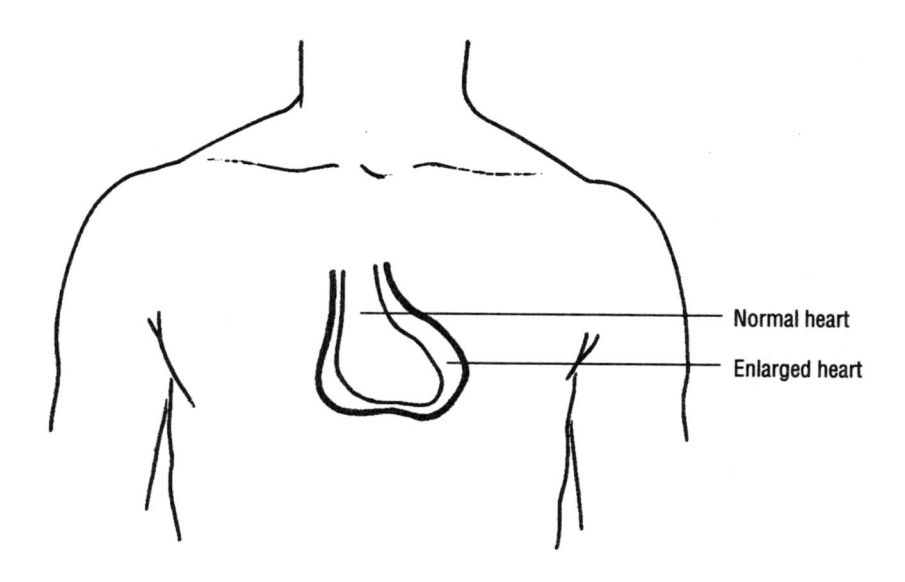

Figure 34.1. The Heart in Cardiamyopathy. In cardiomyopathy, the heart muscle loses its ability to pump effectively. The heart becomes larger as it tries to compensate for its weakened condition. This illustration shows the change in size of the heart muscle.

A firm diagnosis typically requires a chest x-ray to show whether the heart is enlarged, an electrocardiogram to reveal any abnormal electrical activity of the heart, and an echocardiogram, which uses sound waves to produce pictures of the heart.

Other, more specific tests may also be needed. These include:

- *A radionuclide ventriculogram.* This involves injecting low-dose radioactive material (usually equal to that in a set of chest x rays) into a vein, through which it flows to the heart. Pictures are generated by a special camera to show how well the heart is functioning.

- *A cardiac catheterization.* In this procedure, a thin plastic tube is inserted through a blood vessel until it reaches the heart. A dye is injected and x rays taken to assess the heart's structure and function.

Treatment

Since dilated cardiomyopathy is hard to diagnose early, it is rarely treated in its beginning stage.

The goal of treatment is to relieve any complicating factor, if known, control the symptoms, and stop the disease's progression. However, no cure now exists.

Therapy begins with the elimination of obvious risk factors, such as alcohol consumption. Weight loss and dietary changes, especially salt restriction, may also be advised.

Drugs used to treat the condition include:

- Diuretics, which reduce excess fluid in the body;

- Vasodilators, such as angiotensin-converting enzyme (ACE) inhibitors, which relax blood vessels, helping to lower blood pressure and reducing the effort needed by the heart to pump blood through the body;

- Digitalis, which helps to improve pumping action and regulate heartbeat; and,

- Calcium blockers or beta blockers, which may be used in some patients to help regulate heartbeat and to alter the work of the heart muscle.

Also, patients with irregular heartbeats may be put on any of various drugs to control the rhythm.

Cardiomyopathy (Heart Muscle Disease)

In critical cases where the condition is advanced and the patient does not sufficiently respond to other treatments, a heart transplantation may be needed. The patient's heart is replaced with a donor heart. Most heart transplant recipients are under age 60 and in good health other than their diseased heart.

Course of the Disease

As the heart enlarges, it steadily decreases its efficiency in pumping blood and the amount of blood it can pump. As a result, some patients cannot perform even simple physical activities.

However, the disease also may remain fairly stable for years, especially with treatment and regular evaluation by a physician.

Unfortunately, by the time it is diagnosed, the disease often has reached an advanced stage and heart failure has occurred. Consequently, about 50 percent of patients with dilated cardiomyopathy live 5 years once heart failure is diagnosed; about 25 percent live 10 years after such a diagnosis.

Typically, patients die from a continued decline in heart muscle strength, but some die suddenly of irregular heartbeats.

For patients with advanced disease, heart transplantation greatly improves survival: 75 percent of patients live 5 years after a transplantation. However, in the United States, the scarcity of donor hearts

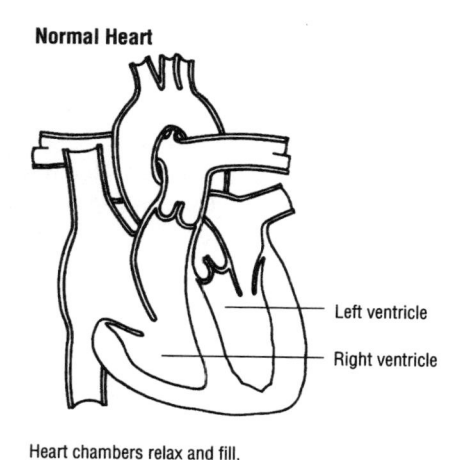

Normal Heart

Left ventricle
Right ventricle

Heart chambers relax and fill, then contract and pump.

Heart with Dilated Cardiomyopathy

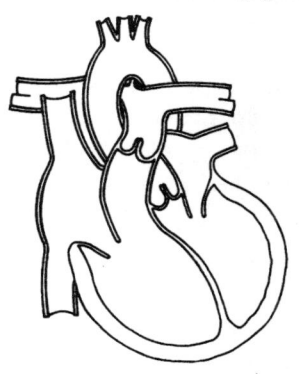

Muscle fibers have stretched. Heart chamber enlarges.

Figure 34.2. *A normal heart compared to a heart with dilated cardiomyopathy.*

limits the number of transplantations to about 2,000 persons a year. Those who qualify for heart transplantation often have to wait months, or even years, for a suitable donor heart. Some patients with dilated cardiomyopathy die awaiting a transplant but, according to recent studies, others improve enough from aggressive medical treatment to be taken off the waiting list.

Also, some critically ill cardiomyopathy patients with declining heart function use a small, implanted mechanical pump as a bridge to transplantation. Called left ventricular assist devices (LVADs), these pumps take over part or virtually all of the heart's blood pumping activity. The devices provide only temporary assistance and are not now used as substitutes for heart transplantation.

Hypertrophic Cardiomyopathy

The second most common form of heart muscle disease is hypertrophic cardiomyopathy. Physicians sometimes call it by other names: idiopathic hypertrophic subaortic stenosis (IHSS), asymmetrical septal hypertrophy (ASH), or hypertrophic obstructive cardiomyopathy (HOCM).

In hypertrophic cardiomyopathy, the growth and arrangement of muscle fibers are abnormal, leading to thickened heart walls. The greatest thickening tends to occur in the left ventricle (the heart's main pumping chamber), especially in the septum, the wall that separates the left and right ventricles. The thickening reduces the size of the pumping chamber and obstructs blood flow. It also prevents the heart from properly relaxing between beats and so filling with blood. Eventually, this limits the pumping action.

Hypertrophic cardiomyopathy is a rare disease, occurring in no more than 0.2 percent of the U.S. population. It can affect men and women of all ages. Symptoms can appear in childhood or adulthood.

Most cases of hypertrophic cardiomyopathy are inherited. Because of this, a patient's family members often are checked for signs of the disease, although the signs may be much less evident or even absent in them. In other cases, there is no clear cause.

Symptoms

Many patients have no symptoms. For those who do, the most common are breathlessness and chest discomfort. Other signs are fainting during physical activity, strong rapid heartbeats that feel like a pounding in the chest, and fatigue, especially with physical exertion.

In some cases, the first and only manifestation of hypertrophic cardiomyopathy is sudden death, caused by a chaotic heartbeat. The

Cardiomyopathy (Heart Muscle Disease)

heart's lower chambers beat so chaotically and fast that no blood is pumped. Instead of beating, the heart quivers.

In advanced stages of the disease, patients may have severe heart failure and its associated symptoms, including fluid accumulation or congestion.

Diagnosis

By listening through a stethoscope, a physician may hear the abnormal heart sounds characteristic of hypertrophic cardiomyopathy. The electrocardiogram (EKG, or ECG) may help diagnose the condition by detecting changes in the electrical activity of the heart as it beats.

Echocardiography is one of the best tools for diagnosing hypertrophic cardiomyopathy. It uses sound waves to detect the extent of muscle-wall thickening and to assess the status of the heart's functioning.

Physicians also may request radionuclide studies to gather added information about the disease's effect on how the heart is pumping blood.

Other tests that also may provide useful information are the chest x ray, cardiac catheterization, and a heart muscle biopsy.

Treatment

Treatments for hypertrophic cardiomyopathy vary but can include the following:

- *Lifestyle changes.* Patients with serious electrical and blood-flow abnormalities must be less physically active.

- *Medications.* Various drugs are used to treat the disease. They include beta blockers (to ease symptoms by slowing the heart's pumping action), calcium channel blockers (to relax the heart and reduce the blood pressure in it), antiarrhythmic medications, and diuretics (to ease heart failure symptoms).

    However, drugs do not work in all cases or may cause adverse side effects, such as fluid in the lungs, very low blood pressure, and sudden death. Then, other treatment, such as a pacemaker or surgery, may be needed.

- *Pacemakers.* These change the pattern and decrease the force of the heart's contractions. The pacemaker can reduce the degree of obstruction and so relieve symptoms. A pacemaker needs to be carefully monitored after its insertion in order to properly adjust the electrical impulse. Some patients who have a pacemaker inserted feel no relief and go on to have heart surgery.

- *Surgery.* This usually calls for removal of part of the thickened septum (the muscle wall separating the chambers) that is blocking the blood flow. Sometimes, surgery also must replace a heart valve—the mitral valve, which connects the left ventricle and the left atrium, the upper chamber that receives oxygen-rich blood from the lungs.

  Surgery to remove the thickening eases symptoms in about 70 percent of patients but results in death in about 1 to 3 percent of patients. Also, about 5 percent of those who have surgery develop a slow heartbeat, which is then corrected with a pacemaker.

Course of the Disease

The course of the disease varies. Many patients remain stable; some improve; some worsen in symptoms and lead severely restricted lives. Patients may need drug treatment and careful medical supervision for the rest of their lives.

Hypertrophic cardiomyopathy patients also are at risk of sudden death. About 2 to 3 percent die each year because the heart suddenly stops beating. This cardiac arrest is brought on by an abnormal heartbeat. Over 10 years, the risk of sudden death can be 20 percent or more.

Restrictive Cardiomyopathy

Restrictive cardiomyopathy is rare in the United States and most other industrial nations. In this disease, the walls of the ventricles stiffen and lose their flexibility due to infiltration by abnormal tissue. As a result, the heart cannot fill adequately with blood and eventually loses its ability to pump properly.

Restrictive cardiomyopathy typically results from another disease, which occurs elsewhere in the body. In the United States, restrictive cardiomyopathy is most commonly related to the following: amyloidosis, in which abnormal protein fibers (amyloid) accumulate in the heart's muscle; sarcoidosis, an inflammatory disease that causes the formation of small lumps in organs; and hemochromatosis, an iron overload of the body, usually due to a genetic disease.

In general, restrictive cardiomyopathy does not appear to be inherited; however, some of the diseases that lead to the condition are genetically transmitted.

Cardiomyopathy (Heart Muscle Disease)

Symptoms

Typical signs of the condition include symptoms of congestive heart failure: weakness, fatigue, and breathlessness. Swelling of the legs, caused by fluid retention, occurs in a significant number of patients. Other symptoms include nausea, bloating, and poor appetite, probably because of the retention of fluid around the liver, stomach, and intestines.

Diagnosis

A physician may suspect restrictive cardiomyopathy based on a patient's symptoms and the presence of another disease. Although symptoms of congestive heart failure may predominate, the size of the heart remains relatively small, unlike other cardiomyopathies.

Diagnostic information comes from an electrocardiogram or any of several imaging studies that provide pictures of the heart. These include echocardiography, magnetic resonance imaging, and computed tomography.

A definite diagnosis usually requires cardiac catheterization studies or a biopsy, in which a tiny piece of tissue—including heart muscle—is removed for laboratory analysis.

Heart with Hypertrophic Cardiomyopathy

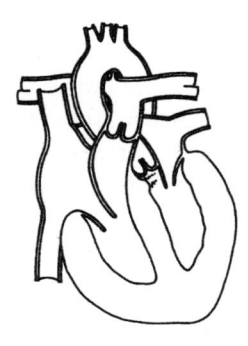

Growth and arrangement of muscle fibers are abnormal. Heart walls thicken, especially in the left ventricle.

Heart with Restrictive Cardiomyopathy

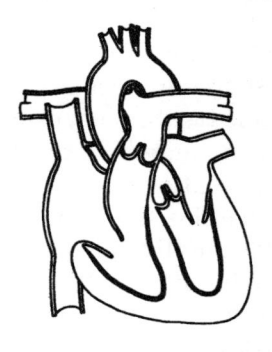

Ventricle walls stiffen and lose flexibility.

Figure 34.3. This diagram shows changes in a heart with hypertrophic cardiomyopathy and a heart with restrictive cardiomyopathy.

Treatment

Restrictive cardiomyopathy has no specific treatment. The underlying disease that leads to the heart problem also may not be treatable.

In general, the use of traditional heart drugs has been limited in this cardiomyopathy, although diuretics may help control fluid accumulation.

In rare cases, surgery is sometimes used to try to improve blood flow into the heart.

Course of the Disease

The condition is similar to dilated cardiomyopathy and tends to worsen with time. Only about 30 percent of patients survive more than 5 years after diagnosis.

Future Directions

Future advances in the diagnosis and treatment of cardiomyopathy depend on a better understanding of the disease process and why heart muscle is damaged. A lot of research is under way to identify these processes and whether they can be halted or even reversed. Much of the research is conducted at or supported by the National Heart, Lung, and Blood Institute (NHLBI).

Promising clues came from investigators at and supported by the NHLBI who discovered some of the genes responsible for hypertrophic cardiomyopathy. Their work represents an important first step in understanding how the disease is transmitted and how it progresses.

Researchers also are trying to determine the best use of currently available treatments, especially drug therapies. Drugs useful for other conditions may help treat cardiomyopathy. For example, drugs effective in treating high blood pressure also help manage heart failure and irregular heartbeats.

Additionally, much work has been—and continues to be—done on identifying factors that increase or decrease the risk of death for persons with cardiomyopathy. Knowing which patients are at the greatest risk is very important in determining the best approach to evaluation and treatment of their condition.

The development of improved treatments for cardiomyopathy, however, awaits still more research and a better understanding of the disease process.

Cardiomyopathy (Heart Muscle Disease)

Glossary

Angiotensin converting enzyme (ACE) inhibitor: A drug used to decrease pressure inside blood vessels.

Arrhythmia: An irregular heartbeat.

Beta blocker: A drug used to slow the heart rate and reduce pressure inside blood vessels. It also can regulate heart rhythm.

Calcium channel blocker (or calcium blocker): A drug used to relax the blood vessel and heart muscle, causing pressure inside blood vessels to drop. It also can regulate heart rhythm.

Cardiac arrest: A sudden stop of heart function. See also "sudden death."

Cardiac catheterization: A procedure in which a thin, hollow tube is inserted into a blood vessel. The tube is then advanced through the vessel into the heart, enabling a physician to study the heart and its pumping activity.

Cardiomyopathy: A disease of the heart muscle (myocardium).

Congestion: Abnormal fluid accumulation in the body, especially the lungs.

Digitalis: A drug used to increase the force of the heart's contraction and to regulate specific irregularities of heart rhythm.

Dilated cardiomyopathy: Heart muscle disease that leads to enlargement of the heart's chambers, robbing the heart of its pumping ability.

Diuretic: A drug that helps eliminate excess body fluid; usually used in the treatment of high blood pressure and heart failure.

Dyspnea: Shortness of breath.

Echocardiography: A test that bounces sound waves off the heart to produce pictures of its internal structures.

Edema: Abnormal fluid accumulation in body tissues.

Electrocardiogram (EKG or ECG): Measurement of electrical activity during heartbeats.

Heart failure: Loss of pumping ability by the heart, often accompanied by fatigue, breathlessness, and excess fluid accumulation in body tissues.

Hypertrophic cardiomyopathy: Heart muscle disease that leads to thickening of the heart walls, interfering with the heart's ability to fill with and pump blood.

Idiopathic: Results from an unknown cause.

Left ventricular assist device (LVAD): A mechanical device used to increase the heart's pumping ability.

Pulmonary congestion (or edema): Fluid accumulation in the lungs.

Restrictive cardiomyopathy: Heart muscle disease in which the muscle walls become stiff and lose their flexibility.

Septum: In the heart, a muscle wall separating the chambers.

Sudden death: Cardiac arrest caused by an irregular heartbeat. The term "death" is somewhat misleading, because some patients survive.

Ventricles: The two lower chambers of the heart. The left ventricle is the main pumping chamber in the heart.

Ventricular fibrillation: Rapid, irregular quivering of the heart's ventricles, with no effective heartbeat.

For More Information

For more information, contact the NHLBI Information Center, a service of the NHLBI and the National institutes of Health. The Information Center provides information to health professionals, patients, and the public about the treatment, diagnosis, and prevention of heart, lung, and blood diseases.

Cardiomyopathy (Heart Muscle Disease)

NHLBI Information Center
P.O. Box 30105
Bethesda, MD 20824-0105
Telephone: (301) 251-1222
Fax: (301) 251-1223

Or check the NHLBI site on the World Wide Web at:
http://www.nhlbi.nih.gov

Chapter 35

Coronary Artery Disease

Blockage of the coronary arteries—or coronary artery disease—is the number one cause of heart attacks. More than 6 million Americans experience symptoms due to coronary artery disease each year, as many as 1.5 million have heart attacks and nearly 500,000 die. Yet, the past decade has seen a dramatic decline in the rates of cardiovascular disease and the age-adjusted death rate from coronary artery disease, which has dropped by approximately 28 percent.

Symptoms of coronary artery disease can take many different forms, but they all have the same cause: The heart muscle doesn't get enough blood and oxygen. The most dramatic symptom of coronary artery disease is sudden death without prior warning, though sudden cardiac death is more commonly caused by a condition known as ventricular fibrillation. Coronary artery disease can also lead to angina (chest pain) or a heart attack. Most coronary artery disease is caused by atherosclerosis, or hardening of the arteries that leads to narrowing of the arteries.

Atherosclerosis

Healthy arteries are flexible, strong and elastic. As you age, your arteries normally become thicker and less elastic, and their calcium content increases. This hardening is believed to occur throughout all the major arteries.

© 1996-1999 Johns Hopkins InteliHealth, updated November 1997; reprinted with permission of InteliHealth.

Atherosclerosis differs from this natural process because it affects mainly the large arteries and the coronary arteries. The inner layers of the artery walls become thick and irregular and certain areas accumulate fats, cholesterol and other materials. This gradual buildup of athersclerotic plaque over a long time reduces the circulation of blood and increases the risk of heart attack, stroke and other serious arterial diseases.

The risk of developing atherosclerosis is increased in people who have inherited certain genes that predispose them to collect fat in their arteries or have high blood cholesterol levels. Smoking cigarettes, diabetes and high blood pressure are additional risk factors.

Cholesterol promotes the development of atherosclerosis. Cholesterol is a naturally occurring fat found in animal products, such as red meat, poultry and dairy products. Low density lipoprotein (LDL) serves as a transport vehicle to carry cholesterol throughout the body, where it is used to mend damaged cells. LDL cholesterol is referred to as "bad cholesterol" because it tends to accumulate in arteries as fatty plaques, thus narrowing the internal opening of the blood vessels, slowing the flow of blood and leading to heart disease.

Because high density lipoprotein (HDL) gathers up excess amounts of cholesterol so it can be excreted from the body, HDL cholesterol is known as the "good cholesterol." There is no "good cholesterol"—it is all bad. HDL cholesterol is call good because HDL can remove cholesterol from the atherosclerotic plaque. Platelets often clump at microscopic sites of injury to the innerwall of arteries at the site of atherosclerotic plaques. Platelet clumps can initiate a blood clot that completely blocks the artery.

Angina

Chest pain, or angina occurs when blockages in the coronary arteries prevent the heart from getting enough blood and oxygen, a condition known as ischemia. The pain may be dull and heavy, but it may also be choking or squeezing and spread to the throat, neck, jaw, teeth and to the left arm. Sweating, nausea, dizziness or breathing difficulties may result.

Angina can be divided into two types: stable angina, which causes chest pain at predictable times, during exercise for example; and unstable angina, which is pain of increasing severity at different, unpredictable times, especially at rest.

The main problem in stable angina is a fixed blockage of blood flow in one or more of the coronary arteries, caused by atherosclerotic plaques. These plaques narrow the internal diameter of the coronary artery so that only a limited amount of blood can reach the heart muscle.

Unstable angina implies that the underlying situation is worsening. Unstable angina often signals a developing heart attack. It's not exactly clear what's happening during unstable angina, though some researchers believe that the blockage in the coronary arteries is getting worse or spasm occurs. It could be that the blockage is so severe that it's significantly pinching off blood flow, or that the blockage is at a point where the artery makes a turn. Blockages at bends in arteries tend to cause platelets to pile up as they come around the turn, and thus can lead to additional clumping of blood.

Congestive Heart Failure

Heart failure doesn't mean that the heart has stopped beating. This disorder varies in degree and the extent it can be reversed or treated. Heart failure can be caused by anything that impairs the heart's ability to pump blood effectively, including congenital heart disease, coronary artery disease, hypertension, damage from a heart attack, valve damage, diabetes or drug or alcohol damage.

Symptoms of heart failure occur when the heart muscle is weakened or when the work load is too great for the heart muscle to accommodate. In either case, two things can happen:

- The heart can't pump enough blood to provide the tissues with vital oxygen and nutrients and to remove wastes.

- Pressure builds up in the veins because the heart isn't pumping blood efficiently through the arteries. In other words, as the heart becomes less and less effective as a pump, it becomes more and more like a dam. The result, a build up of fluid in the lungs (and elsewhere in the body) leading to congestion, is why heart failure is often referred to as congestive heart failure.

Heart failure can lead to a host of symptoms: shortness of breath and fatigue with exertion; shortness of breath at rest, especially when lying down because of fluid buildup in the lungs; swelling or accumulation of fluid in the feet and legs; and general fatigue. With mild heart failure you may not have any symptoms while sitting and resting, but you may be short of breath during physical activity. With severe heart failure, you may experience distress even at rest, including shortness of breath and coolness in the arms and legs; your skin may be pale, and your lips, fingers and toes may turn blue.

Chapter 36

Atherosclerosis

What is atherosclerosis?

Atherosclerosis narrows the arteries (blood vessels that carry blood from the heart to the body tissues). It is the underlying cause of more deaths in the U.S. than any other condition. Atherosclerosis can block the coronary arteries that carry oxygen to the heart muscle, resulting in a heart attack. It can block the carotid arteries that carry oxygen to the brain, resulting in a stroke. It can impede blood flow to the kidneys, legs, and intestines. Atherosclerosis increases with age. Men are affected earlier than women since women aren't usually affected until after menopause.

How does it occur?

In atherosclerosis, arteries are narrowed by fatty deposits called plaques. Plaques interrupt the smooth flow of blood, causing turbulence and leading to clotting. A blood clot or piece of broken off plaque may become stuck in a narrowed area, cutting off the blood supply. Atherosclerosis has been linked with cigarette smoking, high blood pressure, high blood cholesterol, being overweight, lack of exercise, diabetes, an aggressive personality, and a fatty diet. There may be a family history of atherosclerosis.

What are the symptoms?

There are no symptoms of atherosclerosis.

Copyright 1998 Clinical Reference Systems. Reprinted with permission.

How is it diagnosed?

Atherosclerosis is usually diagnosed as a result of clinical investigation of problems it causes, such as pain in the calf muscles with exercise (intermittent claudication), pain due to restriction of blood to the heart muscle (angina), or a mini-stroke or dizziness due to restriction of blood to the brain (transient ischemic attack). The diagnosis is confirmed by special x-rays to outline the arteries (angiography), by ultrasound (sonogram), or by pulse tracing techniques.

How is it treated?

Your doctor will prescribe treatment for condition(s) related to the atherosclerosis and possibly medication to reduce blood clotting or to relax the blood vessels, depending on your symptoms. Surgical treatment may be necessary. Your doctor may advise major lifestyle changes to try to halt or reverse the atherosclerotic process. These may include quitting smoking, losing weight, starting an exercise program, practicing stress reduction, and switching to a low-fat, low-cholesterol diet.

How can I take care of myself?

- Take the medication prescribed and follow your doctor's advice for lifestyle changes.
- Have your blood pressure and blood cholesterol checked regularly.
- If you smoke, quit. Tell your doctor if you need help quitting.
- If you are overweight, talk to your doctor about losing weight.
- Exercise regularly. Walk at least a mile a day.
- Switch to a low-fat, low-cholesterol, high-fiber diet. Your doctor or a dietician can tell you which foods to avoid.

—Developed by Ann Carter, M.D.

Chapter 37

Congenital Heart Disorders

What Is Congenital Cardiovascular Disease or Congenital Heart Disease?

Congenital means inborn or existing at birth. Among the terms you may hear are congenital heart defect, congenital heart disease, and congenital cardiovascular disease. The word "defect" is more accurate than "disease." A congenital cardiovascular defect occurs when the heart or blood vessels near the heart don't develop normally before birth.

What Causes Congenital Cardiovascular Defects?

Congenital cardiovascular defects are present in about one percent of live births and are the most frequent congenital malformations in newborns. In most cases scientists don't know why they occur. Sometimes a viral infection causes serious problems. German measles (also called rubella) is an example. If a mother contracts German measles during pregnancy, it can interfere with the development of the baby's heart or produce other malformations. Other viral diseases also may produce congenital defects.

Heredity sometimes plays a role in congenital cardiovascular disease. More than one child in a family may have a congenital cardiovascular defect, but this rarely occurs. Certain conditions affecting

---

Reproduced with permission of American Heart Association World Wide Web site. Copyright 1999 American Heart Association.

multiple organs, such as Down's syndrome, can involve the heart, too. Some prescription drugs and over-the-counter medicines, as well as alcohol and "street" drugs, may increase the risk of having a baby with a heart defect.

Other factors that affect the heart's development are under study. The fact is that we don't know what causes most congenital cardiovascular defects.

What Are the Types of Congenital Defects?

Most heart defects either 1) obstruct blood flow in the heart or vessels near it or 2) cause blood to flow through the heart in an abnormal pattern. Rarely defects occur in which only one ventricle (single ventricle) is present, or both the pulmonary artery and aorta arise from the same ventricle (double outlet ventricle). A third rare defect occurs when the right or left side of the heart is incompletely formed—hypoplastic heart.

[Visit the American Heart Association's web site at www.amhrt.org for information on congenital heart defects in Spanish.]

Patent Ductus Arteriosus (P.D.A.)

This defect allows blood to mix between the pulmonary artery and the aorta. Before birth there's an open passageway (the ductus arteriosus) between these two blood vessels. Normally this closes within a few hours of birth. When this doesn't happen, however, some blood that should flow through the aorta and on to nourish the body returns to the lungs. A ductus that doesn't close is quite common in premature infants but rather rare in full-term babies.

If the ductus arteriosus is large, a child may tire quickly, grow slowly, catch pneumonia easily and breathe rapidly. In some children symptoms may not occur until after the first weeks or months of life. If the ductus arteriosus is small, the child seems well. If surgery is needed, the surgeon can close the ductus arteriosus by tying it, without opening the heart. If there's no other defect, this restores the circulation to normal.

Obstruction Defects

An obstruction is a narrowing that partly or completely blocks the flow of blood. Obstructions called stenoses can occur in heart valves, arteries or veins.

Congenital Heart Disorders

The three most common forms of obstructed blood flow are pulmonary stenosis, aortic stenosis, and coarctation of the aorta. Related but less common forms include bicuspid aortic valve, subaortic stenosis and Ebstein's anomaly.

Pulmonary stenosis (P.S.): The pulmonary or pulmonic valve is between the right ventricle and the pulmonary artery. It opens to allow blood to flow from the right ventricle to the lungs. A defective pulmonary valve that does not open properly is called stenotic. That means the right ventricle must pump harder than normal to overcome the obstruction.

If the stenosis is severe, especially in babies, some cyanosis (blueness) may occur. Older children usually have no symptoms. Treatment is needed when the pressure in the right ventricle is higher than normal. In most children the obstruction can be relieved by a procedure called balloon valvuloplasty. In other patients, open heart surgery may be needed. During surgery, the valve can usually be opened satisfactorily. The outlook after balloon valvuloplasty or surgery is favorable, but follow-up is required to determine if heart function returns to normal.

People with pulmonary stenosis, before and after treatment, are at risk for getting an infection of the valve (endocarditis). To help prevent this, they'll need to take antibiotics before certain dental and surgical procedures.

Aortic stenosis (A.S.): The aortic valve, between the left ventricle and the aorta, is narrowed. This makes it hard for the heart to pump blood to the body. Aortic stenosis occurs when the aortic valve didn't form properly. A normal valve has three leaflets or cusps, but a stenotic valve may have only one cusp (unicuspid) or two cusps (bicuspid), which are thick and stiff. (See bicuspid aortic valve below.)

Sometimes stenosis is severe and symptoms occur in infancy. Otherwise, most children with aortic stenosis have no symptoms. In some children, chest pain, unusual tiring, dizziness, or fainting may occur. The need for surgery depends on how bad the stenosis is. In children, a surgeon may be able to enlarge the valve opening. Although surgery may improve the stenosis, the valve remains deformed. Eventually, the valve may need to be replaced with an artificial one.

A procedure called balloon valvuloplasty has been used in some children with aortic stenosis. The long-term results of this procedure are still being studied. Children with aortic stenosis need lifelong medical follow-up. Even mild stenosis may worsen over time, and surgical relief of a blockage is sometimes incomplete. Check with your pediatric cardiologist about limiting some kinds of exercise.

People with aortic stenosis, before and after treatment, are at risk for getting an infection of the valve (endocarditis). To help prevent this, they'll need to take antibiotics before certain dental and surgical procedures.

Coarctation of the aorta ("Coarct"): The aorta is pinched or constricted. This obstructs blood flow to the lower part of the body and increases blood pressure above the constriction. Usually there are no symptoms at birth, but they can develop as early as the first week after birth. A baby may develop congestive heart failure or high blood pressure that requires early surgery. Otherwise, surgery usually can be delayed. A child with a severe coarctation should have surgery in early childhood. This prevents problems such as developing high blood pressure as an adult.

The outlook after surgery is favorable, but long-term follow-up is required. Rarely, coarctation of the aorta may recur. Some of these cases can be treated by balloon angioplasty. The long-term results of this procedure are still being studied. Also, blood pressure may stay high even when the aorta's narrowing has been repaired.

People with coarctation of the aorta, before and after treatment, are at risk for getting an infection within the aorta or the heart valves (endocarditis). To help prevent this, they'll need to take antibiotics before certain dental and surgical procedures.

Bicuspid aortic valve: The normal aortic valve has three flaps, or cusps, that open and close. A bicuspid valve has only two flaps, rather than three. There may be no symptoms in childhood, but by adulthood (often middle age or older) the valve can become stenotic (narrowed), making it harder for blood to pass through it, or regurgitant (allowing blood to leak backward through it). Treatment depends on how well the valve functions.

People with bicuspid aortic valve, before and after treatment, are at risk for getting an infection within the aorta or the heart valves (endocarditis). To help prevent this, they'll need to take antibiotics before certain dental and surgical procedures.

Subaortic stenosis: Stenosis means constriction or narrowing. Subaortic means below the aorta. Subaortic stenosis refers to a narrowing of the left ventricle just below the aortic valve, which blood passes through to go into the aorta. This stenosis limits the flow of

Congenital Heart Disorders

blood out of the left ventricle. This condition may be congenital or may be due to a particular form of cardiomyopathy known as "idiopathic hypertrophic subaortic stenosis" (I.H.S.S.). Treatment depends on the cause and the severity of the narrowing. It can include drugs or surgery.

People with subaortic stenosis, before and after treatment, are at risk for getting an infection within the aorta or the heart valves (endocarditis). To help prevent this, they'll need to take antibiotics before certain dental and surgical procedures.

Ebstein's anomaly: Ebstein's anomaly is a congenital downward displacement of the tricuspid valve (located between the upper and lower chambers on the right side of the heart) into the right bottom chamber of the heart (or right ventricle). It is usually associated with an atrial septal defect (see below).

People with Ebstein's anomaly, before and after treatment, are at risk for getting an infection within the heart valve (endocarditis). To help prevent this, they'll need to take antibiotics before certain dental and surgical procedures.

Septal Defects

Some congenital cardiovascular defects allow blood to flow between the right and left chambers of the heart. This happens when a baby is born with an opening between the wall (septum) that separates the right and left sides of the heart. This defect is sometimes called "a hole in the heart."

The two most common types of this defect are atrial septal defect and ventricular septal defect. Two variations are Eisenmenger's complex and atrioventricular canal defect.

Atrial septal defect (A.S.D.): An opening exists between the two upper chambers of the heart. This allows some blood from the left atrium (blood that's already been to the lungs) to return via the hole to the right atrium instead of flowing through the left ventricle, out the aorta and to the body. Many children with ASD have few, if any, symptoms. Closing the atrial defect by open heart surgery in childhood can prevent serious problems later in life.

Ventricular septal defect (V.S.D.): An opening exists between the two lower chambers of the heart. Some blood that has returned from the lungs and has been pumped into the left ventricle flows to the right ventricle through the hole instead of being pumped into the aorta. The heart, which has to pump extra blood, is over-worked and may enlarge.

If the opening is small, it doesn't strain the heart. In that case, the only abnormal finding is a loud murmur. But if the opening is large, open heart surgery is recommended to close the hole and prevent serious problems. Some babies with a large ventricular septal defect don't grow normally and may become undernourished. Babies with VSD may develop severe symptoms or high blood pressure in their lungs. Repairing a ventricular septal defect with surgery usually restores the blood circulation to normal. The long-term outlook is good, but long-term follow-up is required.

People with a ventricular septal defect are at risk for getting an infection of the heart's walls or valves (endocarditis). To help prevent this, they'll need to take antibiotics before certain dental and surgical procedures. After a VSD has been successfully fixed with surgery, antibiotics should no longer be needed.

Eisenmenger's complex: Eisenmenger's complex is a ventricular septal defect coupled with pulmonary high blood pressure, the passage of blood from the right side of the heart to the left (right to left shunt), an enlarged right ventricle and a latent or clearly visible bluish discoloration of the skin called cyanosis. It may also include a malpositioned aorta that receives ejected blood from both the right and left ventricles (an overriding aorta).

People with Eisenmenger's complex, before and after treatment, are at risk for getting an infection within the aorta or the heart valves (endocarditis). To help prevent this, they'll need to take antibiotics before certain dental and surgical procedures.

Atrioventricular (A-V) canal defect (also called **endocardial cushion defect** or **atrioventricular septal defect**): A large hole in the center of the heart exists where the wall between the upper chambers joins the wall between the lower chambers. Also, the tricuspid and mitral valves that normally separate the heart's upper and lower chambers aren't formed as individual valves. Instead, a single large valve forms that crosses the defect.

The large opening in the center of the heart lets oxygen-rich (red) blood from the heart's left side—blood that's just gone through the lungs—pass into the heart's right side. There, the oxygen-rich blood, along with venous (bluish) blood from the body, is sent back to the lungs. The heart must pump an extra amount of blood and may enlarge. Most

Congenital Heart Disorders

babies with an atrioventricular canal don't grow normally and may become undernourished. Because of the large amount of blood flowing to the lungs, high blood pressure may occur there and damage the blood vessels.

In some babies the common valve between the upper and lower chambers doesn't close properly. This lets blood leak backward from the heart's lower chambers to the upper ones. This leak, called regurgitation or insufficiency, can occur on the right side, left side, or both sides of the heart. With a valve leak, the heart pumps an extra amount of blood, becomes overworked and enlarges.

In babies with severe symptoms or high blood pressure in the lungs, surgery must usually be done in infancy. The surgeon closes the large hole with one or two patches and divides the single valve between the heart's upper and lower chambers to make two separate valves. Surgical repair of an atrioventricular canal usually restores the blood circulation to normal. However, the reconstructed valve may not work normally.

Rarely, the defect may be too complex to repair in infancy. In this case, the surgeon may do a procedure called pulmonary artery banding to reduce the blood flow and high pressure in the lungs. When a child is older, the band is removed and corrective surgery is done. More medical or surgical treatment is sometimes needed.

People with atrioventricular canal defect, before and after treatment, are at risk for getting an infection within the heart's walls or valves (endocarditis). To help prevent this, they'll need to take antibiotics before certain dental and surgical procedures.

Cyanotic Defects

Another classification of heart defects is congenital cyanotic heart defects. In these defects, blood pumped to the body contains less-than-normal amounts of oxygen. This results in a condition called cyanosis, a blue discoloration of the skin. The term "blue babies" is often applied to infants with cyanosis.

Examples of cyanotic defects are tetralogy of Fallot, transposition of the great arteries, tricuspid atresia, pulmonary atresia, truncus arteriosus and total anomalous pulmonary venous connection.

Tetralogy of Fallot: Tetralogy of Fallot has four components. The two major ones are: 1) a large hole, or ventricular septal defect, that allows blood to pass from the right ventricle to the left ventricle without going through the lungs, and 2) a narrowing (stenosis) at or just beneath the pulmonary valve. This narrowing partially blocks the flow of blood from the right side of the heart to the lungs. The other two components are: 3) the right ventricle is more muscular than normal, and 4) the aorta lies directly over the ventricular septal defect.

This results in cyanosis (blueness), which may appear soon after birth, in infancy or later in childhood. These "blue babies" may have sudden episodes of severe cyanosis with rapid breathing. They may even become unconscious. During exercise, older children may become short of breath and faint. These symptoms occur because not enough blood flows to the lungs to supply the child's body with oxygen.

Some infants with severe tetralogy of Fallot may need an operation to give temporary relief by increasing blood flow to the lungs with a shunt. This is done by making a connection between the aorta and the pulmonary artery. Then some blood from the aorta flows into the lungs to get more oxygen. This reduces the cyanosis and allows the child to grow and develop until the problem can be fixed when the child is older.

Most children with tetralogy of Fallot have open-heart surgery before school age. The operation involves closing the ventricular septal defect and removing the obstructing muscle. After surgery the long-term outlook varies, depending largely on how severe the defects were before surgery. Lifelong medical follow-up is needed.

People with tetralogy of Fallot, before and after treatment, are at risk for getting an infection within the aorta or the heart valves (endocarditis). To help prevent this, they'll need to take antibiotics before certain dental and surgical procedures.

Transposition of the great arteries: The positions of the pulmonary artery and the aorta are reversed. The aorta is connected to the right ventricle, so most of the blood returning to the heart from the body is pumped back out without first going to the lungs. The pulmonary artery is connected to the left ventricle, so that most of the blood returning from the lungs goes back to the lungs again.

Infants born with transposition survive only if they have one or more connections that let oxygen-rich blood reach the body. One such connection may be a hole between the two atria, called atrial septal defect, or between the two ventricles, called ventricular septal defect. Another may be a vessel connecting the pulmonary artery with the aorta, called patent ductus arteriosus. Most babies with transposition of the great arteries are extremely blue (cyanotic) soon after birth because these connections are inadequate.

To improve the body's oxygen supply, a special procedure called balloon atrial septostomy is used. Two general types of surgery may

Congenital Heart Disorders

be used to help fix the transposition. One is a venous switch or intra-atrial baffle procedure that creates a tunnel inside the atria. Another is an arterial switch. After surgery, the long-term outlook is varies quite a bit. It depends largely on how severe the defects were before surgery. Lifelong follow-up is needed.

People with transposition of the great arteries, before and after treatment, are at risk for getting an infection on the heart's walls or valves (endocarditis). To help prevent this, they'll need to take antibiotics before certain dental and surgical procedures.

Tricuspid atresia. In this condition, there's no tricuspid valve. That means no blood can flow from the right atrium to the right ventricle. As a result, the right ventricle is small and not fully developed. The child's survival depends on there being an opening in the wall between the atria called an atrial septal defect and usually an opening in the wall between the two ventricles called a ventricular septal defect. Because the circulation is abnormal, the blood cannot get enough oxygen, and the child looks blue (cyanotic).

Often in these cases a surgical shunting procedure is needed to increase blood flow to the lungs. This reduces the cyanosis. Some children with tricuspid atresia have too much blood flowing to the lungs. They may need a procedure (pulmonary artery banding) to reduce blood flow to the lungs. Other children with tricuspid atresia may have a more functional repair (Fontan procedure). Children with tricuspid atresia require lifelong follow-up by a pediatric cardiologist.

People with tricuspid atresia, before and after treatment, are at risk for getting an infection of the valves (endocarditis). To help prevent this, they'll need to take antibiotics before certain dental and surgical procedures.

Pulmonary atresia: No pulmonary valve exists, so blood can't flow from the right ventricle into the pulmonary artery and on to the lungs. The right ventricle acts as a blind pouch that may stay small and not well developed. The tricuspid valve is often poorly developed, too.

An opening in the atrial septum lets blood exit the right atrium, so venous (bluish) blood mixes with the oxygen-rich (red) blood in the left atrium. The left ventricle pumps this mixture of oxygen-poor blood into the aorta and out to the body. The baby appears blue (cyanotic) because there's less oxygen in the blood circulating through the arteries. The only source of lung blood flow is the patent ductus arteriosus (PDA), an open passageway between the pulmonary artery and the aorta. If the PDA narrows or closes, the lung blood flow is reduced to critically low levels. This can cause very severe cyanosis.

Early treatment often includes using a drug to keep the PDA from closing. A surgeon can create a shunt between the aorta and the pulmonary artery to help increase blood flow to the lungs. A more complete repair depends on the size of the pulmonary artery and right ventricle. If the pulmonary artery and right ventricle are very small, it may not be possible to correct the defect with surgery. In cases where the pulmonary artery and right ventricle are more normal size, open-heart surgery may produce a good improvement in how the heart works.

If the right ventricle stays too small to be a good pumping chamber, then the surgeon can connect the right atrium directly to the pulmonary artery. The atrial defect also can be closed to relieve the cyanosis. This is called a Fontan procedure. Children with tricuspid atresia require lifelong follow-up by a pediatric cardiologist.

People with pulmonary atresia, before and after treatment, are at risk for getting an infection on the heart's walls or valves (endocarditis). To help prevent this, they'll need to take antibiotics before certain dental and surgical procedures.

Truncus arteriosus: This is a complex malformation where only one artery arises from the heart and forms the aorta and pulmonary artery. Surgery for this condition usually is required early in life. It includes closing a large ventricular septal defect within the heart, detaching the pulmonary arteries from the large common artery, and connecting the pulmonary arteries to the right ventricle with a tube graft. Children with truncus arteriosus need lifelong follow-up to see how well the heart is working.

People with truncus arteriosus, before and after treatment, are at risk for getting an infection on the heart's walls or valves (endocarditis). To help prevent this, they'll need to take antibiotics before certain dental and surgical procedures.

Total anomalous pulmonary venous (P-V) connection: The pulmonary veins that bring oxygen-rich (red) blood from the lungs back to the heart aren't connected to the left atrium. Instead, the pulmonary veins drain through abnormal connections to the right atrium.

In the right atrium, oxygen-rich (red) blood from the pulmonary veins mixes with venous (bluish) blood from the body. Part of this mixture passes through the atrial septum (atrial septal defect) into the left atrium. From there it goes into the left ventricle, to the aorta and out to the body. The rest of the poorly oxygenated mixture flows through the right ventricle, into the pulmonary artery and on to the lungs. The blood passing through the aorta to the body doesn't have enough oxygen, which causes the child to look blue (cyanotic).

This defect must be surgically repaired in early infancy. The pulmonary veins are reconnected to the left atrium and the atrial septal defect is closed. When surgical repair is done in early infancy, the long-term outlook is very good. Still, lifelong follow-up is needed to make certain that any remaining problems, such as an obstruction in the pulmonary veins or irregularities in heart rhythm, are treated properly. Lifelong follow-up is important to make certain that a blockage doesn't develop in the pulmonary veins or where they're attached to the left atrium. Heart rhythm irregularities (arrhythmias) also may occur at any time after surgery.

Hypoplastic Left Heart Syndrome

In hypoplastic left heart syndrome, the left side of the heart—including the aorta, aortic valve, left ventricle and mitral valve—is underdeveloped. Blood returning from the lungs must flow through an opening in the wall between the atria, called an atrial septal defect. The right ventricle pumps the blood into the pulmonary artery, and blood reaches the aorta through a patent ductus arteriosus (see above).

The baby often seems normal at birth, but will come to medical attention within a few days of birth as the ductus closes. Babies with this syndrome become ashen, have rapid and difficult breathing and have difficulty feeding. This heart defect is usually fatal within the first days or months of life without treatment.

Although this defect is not correctable, some babies can be treated with a series of operations, or with a heart transplant. Until an operation is performed, the ductus is kept open by intravenous (IV) medication. Because these operations are complex and different for each patient, you need to discuss all the medical and surgical options with your child's doctor. Your doctor will help you decide which is best for your baby.

If you and your child's doctor elect to undergo surgery, the surgery will be performed in several stages. The first stage, called the Norwood procedure, allows the right ventricle to pump blood to both the lungs and the body. It must be performed soon after birth. The final stage(s) has many names including bi-directional Glenn, Fontan operation, and lateral tunnel. These operations create a connection between the veins returning blue blood to the heart and the pulmonary artery. The overall goal of the operation is to allow the right ventricle to pump only oxygenated blood to the body and to prevent or reduce mixing of the red and blue blood. Some infants require several intermediate operations to achieve the final goal.

Some doctors will recommend a heart transplant to treat this problem. Although it does provide the infant with a heart that has normal structure, the infant will require lifelong medications to prevent rejection. Many other problems related to transplants can develop, and you should discuss these with your doctor.

Children with hypoplastic left heart syndrome require lifelong follow-up by a pediatric cardiologist for repeated checks of how their heart is working. Virtually all the children will require heart medicines.

People with hypoplastic left heart syndrome, before and after treatment, are at risk for getting an infection on the heart's valves (endocarditis). To help prevent this, they'll need to take antibiotics before certain dental and surgical procedures. Good dental hygiene also lowers the risk of endocarditis. For more information about dental hygiene and preventing endocarditis, ask your pediatric cardiologist.

Chapter 38

Endocarditis

Endocarditis is a most serious disease of the heart. It's an infection of the endocardium, the membrane that lines the inside of the four valves of your heart, by bacteria or other organisms. Endocarditis can occur whenever these organisms circulate in the bloodstream. It's more common in people with valve disease because bacteria and other germs tend to settle and multiply on misshapen heart valves where blood flow is turbulent.

Endocarditis may be caused by the bacteria that are often present in the mouth and respiratory system. The organisms may enter your bloodstream during dental or other surgical procedures, such as having your tonsils removed, having a tooth pulled—or even a dental cleaning. Other bacteria that may cause endocarditis are those in your intestinal tract that enter your bloodstream and travel to the heart during an examination or surgical procedure on the prostate, bladder, rectum or female reproductive organs. Risk factors for endocarditis include:

- Being born with a defect in your heart or heart valves;
- Having heart valves that have become scarred from rheumatic fever;
- Having an artificial heart valve;
- Injecting illegal drugs with an unsterile needle.

© 1996-1999 Johns Hopkins InteliHealth, updated November 1997; reprinted with permission of InteliHealth.

Endocarditis is a very dangerous disease that can be fatal unless antibiotics are used to control the infection. The best approach to this disease is prevention. Always tell your dentist or doctor if you are at risk for endocarditis before a dental or surgical procedure. Your dentist or doctor may prescribe preventive antibiotic treatment before the procedure to kill any bacteria before they have a chance of getting into your bloodstream.

Chapter 39

Pericarditis

What is pericarditis?

Pericarditis is a condition in which the pericardium becomes inflamed. The pericardium is the thin membrane that covers the heart. It is made up of tissue that is loose enough to allow the heart to move and change in size. Inflammation of the pericardium can cause chest pain.

How does it occur?

Inflammation of the membrane around the heart can be caused by the following:

- infection
- injury to the heart
- rheumatic fever
- myocardial infarction (heart attack)
- pleurisy
- tuberculosis

The space between the inner and outer layers of the pericardium may fill with excess fluid, causing pressure on the heart and limiting its ability to pump blood properly. If this condition continues for a long time, the pericardium can become scarred. This may result in a drop

---

Copyright 1998 Clinical Reference Systems. Reprinted with permission.

in blood pressure, difficulty breathing, swelling in the neck veins, and edema (swelling in the tissues of the legs).

What are the symptoms?

Symptoms of pericarditis include:

- sharp chest pain becoming worse when a deep breath is taken, the body position changes, or coughing begins
- if the back part of the heart covering is inflamed, pain may be felt with swallowing
- fever
- pain decreases when you sit up or lean forward
- feeling that the heart is beating faster than usual
- tiredness
- shortness of breath

How is it diagnosed?

To diagnose pericarditis, the doctor will examine you, take your medical history, and may order the following tests:

- chest x-ray
- ECG
- cardiac ultrasonography (use of high frequency sound to image the heart)
- blood chemistries
- tuberculin skin tests (when the cause of the pericarditis is not readily defined)

How is it treated?

The treatment is usually aspirin every 3 to 4 hours and/or a nonsteroidal medication. Steroid drugs may be prescribed if pericarditis is a complication of a heart attack, connective tissue disease, or metabolic disorder. These medications calm down the inflammation of the pericardium. You can use nonprescription drugs such as acetaminophen for relief of minor aches and pains. You can also use a heating pad or ice bag on your chest to relieve pain.

Pericarditis

If you have a fever:

- Stay in bed if you have a fever above 100 degrees F (37.8 degrees C). After your temperature has fallen below 100 degrees F (37.8 degrees C), become as active as you comfortably can.
- Ask your doctor if you can take aspirin or acetaminophen to control your fever.
- Keep a record of your daily temperature.

How long will the effects last?

Improvement in these conditions will vary from a few days to several weeks.

In severe cases, a pericardectomy is performed. In this surgery an incision is made between the ribs, and the pericardium is removed. Removal of this membranous bag around the heart does not impair the functioning of the heart.

How can I prevent pericarditis from recurring?

Most of the causes are not easily preventable. You can be aware of the symptoms and contact your doctor immediately if they reappear.

Chapter 40

Valve Disease

Types of Valves

Valves have key roles in regulating blood flow through the heart, opening and closing in sequence with each heartbeat. The valves open their flap-like "doors" (called cusps or leaflets) to allow blood to flow from one area into another and then close to prevent backflow of blood.

There are four types of valves in the heart:

- **Tricuspid:** The tricuspid valve regulates blood flow between the right atrium (upper heart chamber) and right ventricle (lower chamber).

- **Pulmonary:** The pulmonary valve controls flow from the right ventricle into the pulmonary artery, which carries blood to the lungs.

- **Mitral:** The mitral valve allows oxygen-rich blood from the lungs to pass from the left atrium (upper heart chamber) into the left ventricle (lower heart chamber).

- **Aortic:** The aortic valve opens the way for oxygenated blood to pass from the left ventricle into the aorta, the body's largest artery, initiating the supply side of blood circulation.

© 1997 Texas Heart Institute. URL: http://www.tmc.edu/thi/valve.html (Modified 6/19/98); reprinted with permission. If you need information about keeping your heart healthy, e-mail the Heart Information Service (his@heart.thi.tmc.edu) or call 1-800-292-2221. (Outside the U.S., call 713/ 794-6536.)

Types of Valve Disease

Two types of problems can occur in valves to disrupt blood flow. Regurgitation occurs when a valve doesn't close properly and blood leaks backward instead of continuing in the normal forward flow. The second kind of problem is stenosis, which occurs when the leaflets don't open wide enough, reducing the amount of blood that can flow through the valve and making the heart work harder to pump the blood.

Causes

Regurgitation and stenosis can occur for a variety of reasons. In many people, the conditions may be congenital (inherited). Sometimes infections, such as rheumatic fever during childhood, may contribute to valve disorders in many older adults. Other cardiovascular disorders, including high blood pressure and coronary artery disease, may lead to valve problems.

Symptoms

Symptoms of valve disease vary from patient to patient. The most common signs and symptoms are:

- Shortness of breath
- Chest pain
- Fatigue
- Syncope (black out)
- Reduced blood output from the heart

Some people have no symptoms. An initial diagnosis often is made by listening to the heart, as valve diseases tend to be associated with distinct, abnormal sounds. A definite diagnosis requires the use of imaging techniques that provide views of the heart and its valves.

Treatment

People whose valve disorders cause no symptoms or only minimal symptoms may not require treatment. Others do well with drug therapy for specific symptoms. But if a patient's condition worsens and becomes difficult to control or tolerate, the patient may need surgery.

Valve Disease

Repairing the valve can be done by one of the three ways:

- Commissurotomy
- Valvuloplasty, or
- Valve replacement

Commissurotomy and valvuloplasty are repair procedures, whereas valve replacement involves surgical implantation of a new valve. Valve surgery is an open-heart technique, and the procedure requires the use of a heart-lung machine, since the heart must temporarily stop beating.

Commissurotomy. When a patient has a stenosed or narrowed valve, the cusps may thicken and adhere to one another. The surgeon addresses this problem by cutting the commissures, the points where the cusps meet.

Valvuloplasty. Valvuloplasty is a procedure that reinforces the cusps to provide more support and permit proper closure of the valve. The support comes from a ring-like device the surgeon attaches to the outside of the valve. Occasionally, a type of nonsurgical procedure may benefit a specific patient with valvular stenosis. The procedure, called balloon valvuloplasty, involves inserting a balloon-tipped tube through an artery and into the heart. The balloon is then inflated in an effort to make the valve open wider.

Valve Replacement. Valve replacement entails surgical removal of a defective valve and stitching in its place a prosthetic valve. The new valve is made of either synthetic materials (a mechanical valve) or of biological tissue mounted to a synthetic ring (bioprosthesis).

Following uncomplicated valve surgery, a patient will stay in the intensive care unit for about a day, followed by several more days in a hospital room. Before the patient is discharged from the hospital, the physician will prescribe medications that may include an anticoagulant, a drug that prevents clots from forming on the new valve. Patients with mechanical heart valves are required to take an anticoagulant for the rest of their lives.

Patients who are otherwise healthy can expect to resume normal activities after recuperating from valve surgery.

Chapter 41

Heart Murmur

What is heart murmur?

A heart murmur is an extra or abnormal sound produced by the heart and heard with the stethoscope.

How does it occur?

In most cases the abnormal sound is the result of noisy or turbulent blood flow in the heart. The turbulence may be caused by the shape of the heart or by abnormalities of specific heart structures, such as the valves or the heart walls.

Most heart murmurs are caused by congenital abnormalities (that is, abnormalities present at birth). Murmurs can result from heart infections when a person has rheumatic fever from streptococcal infections, such as strep throat; however, this occurs less often now than in the past. Some murmurs do arise from heart muscle damage resulting from coronary artery disease or hypertension.

How are murmurs classified?

The classification of heart murmurs is based on their loudness, where in the heart pumping cycle they occur, and where on the chest they are best heard. From these characteristics the likely cause of a murmur can be predicted.

Copyright 1998 Clinical Reference Systems. Reprinted with permission.

Loudness is on a scale of I (faint) to VI (loud enough to be heard even if the stethoscope is not touching the chest).

Each pump of the heart is a two-phase process. Systole is the name for the pumping phase. Diastole is the name for the resting, filling phase. A murmur heard during systole is systolic; likewise, a murmur heard during diastole is diastolic.

Murmurs are not always significant. A murmur is called functional or benign if no symptoms are associated with it and its sound and location do not indicate a heart problem. Such murmurs are usually found incidentally during a physical exam. They require no further evaluation.

The intensity and timing of a murmur, and sometimes associated symptoms, may suggest that the murmur is significant. Such a murmur needs to be evaluated to determine the underlying structural problem. Many heart abnormalities can be corrected before the heart muscle is permanently damaged.

What are the symptoms?

The symptoms of a significant heart murmur depend on the heart abnormality and its severity. Possible symptoms include:

- shortness of breath
- lightheadedness
- inability to tolerate exertion
- frequent episodes of rapid heart rate
- chest pain

How is it diagnosed?

Technology has made great progress beyond the simple stethoscope in the diagnosis of heart murmurs. For example:

- An electrocardiogram can detect any associated electrical abnormalities.
- A chest x-ray screens for an enlarged heart, signs of heart muscle failure, and certain congenital abnormalities.
- An echocardiogram uses sound waves to create images of the heart structure. The images may show a hole in the wall of the heart or an abnormal valve.

Heart Murmur

- In some cases cardiac catheterization may be necessary to determine the structural problem. This technique also allows measurement of the pressures in the heart chambers and of valve function.

How is it treated?

Some murmurs do not require treatment. The decision for treatment depends on several factors:

- the symptoms
- the risk of heart damage over time if the abnormality is not corrected
- the risk of sudden complications, such as stroke or cardiac arrest

The treatment for correcting a defect causing a heart murmur is open heart surgery.

What can be done to help prevent heart murmurs?

Most heart murmurs are present at birth, and little is known about how to prevent these congenital defects. However, the conditions of coronary artery disease or hypertension, which can cause heart muscle damage, can sometimes be prevented, delayed, or minimized by healthy diet and exercise habits, and by not smoking.

Always get prompt treatment for strep infections to prevent rheumatic heart disease.

—by Dee Ann DeRoin, M.D.

Chapter 42

Heart Palpitations

What are heart palpitations?

Palpitations are a sudden change in the rhythm of your heartbeat. Palpitations are called paroxysmal palpitations when they begin and end suddenly. Palpitations are a symptom, not a disease.

How do they occur?

Normally the heart beats harder or faster after exercise, or when you feel stress or fear. Palpitations occur when your heartbeat changes during normal activity, enough to make you aware of it. They can be caused by:

- anxiety
- insulin reaction in diabetics
- an overactive thyroid gland, which quickens the heartbeat
- certain heart problems

What are the symptoms?

The heart may feel like it is:

- pounding
- racing

Copyright 1998 Clinical Reference Systems. Reprinted with permission.

- skipping
- flopping
- fluttering

How are they diagnosed?

The doctor will ask about your medical history, examine you, and order an ECG (electrocardiogram). He or she may use other lab tests if you show signs of a medical condition that could cause paroxysmal palpitations.

How are they treated?

Treatment depends on the cause. Medication may be prescribed for certain heart disorders.

The doctor may suggest you try the following methods for slowing your heartbeat in certain other cases:

- Briefly pinch your nose and hold your mouth closed against an exhaled breath.
- Splash cool water on your face.
- Slowly drink some water.

If these don't work, you may need to go to an emergency room.

How long will the effects last?

How long you continue to have palpitations depends on the cause, medical conditions, and how you respond to the treatment prescribed by the doctor. Many people have palpitations over a long time without the condition becoming life-threatening. However, you need to seek help immediately if, in addition to palpitations, you:

- have chest pain
- have shortness of breath
- feel lightheaded
- faint

How can I take care of myself?

- Keep a record of episodes of palpitations (how long they last, how fast the heartbeat was (beats/minute), what you were doing when it started, and what you did to make it better).

Heart Palpitations

- Keep your follow-up appointments with the doctor.
- Contact your doctor if you feel chest pain or shortness of breath or if you feel lightheaded or faint.

It is also helpful to:

- Get plenty of rest.
- Avoid smoking.
- Ask your doctor for a diet that helps you lose weight safely if you are overweight.
- Walk or exercise daily.
- Discontinue medications such as decongestants or stimulants.
- Avoid foods and beverages that contain caffeine, such as colas, coffee, chocolate, and tea.
- Balance the work, rest, and recreation in your life.
- Learn to use relaxation techniques.

What can be done to help prevent paroxysmal heart palpitations?

- Avoid alcohol.
- Avoid caffeine.
- Avoid smoking.
- Reduce stress and anxiety.
- Lose weight, if necessary.
- Take medications as prescribed by your doctor.

Chapter 43

Fainting Caused by Cardiac Conditions

What is fainting caused by cardiac conditions?

Fainting is a temporary loss of consciousness when not enough blood reaches the brain. Certain heart conditions may cause you to faint.

The medical term for fainting is syncope.

How does it occur?

Heart conditions that may cause you to faint include arrhythmias, which are disorders of the rhythm and rate of the heartbeat. When the heart pumps at a different rate it makes the heart less efficient. Then, not enough blood reaches the brain and causes you to faint.

One common type of arrhythmia that causes fainting is heart block. This occurs when the contractions of the upper and lower chambers of the heart occur at slightly different times causing blood output to decrease.

Tachycardia, the too-rapid beating of your heart, is another cause of fainting. When this condition begins in the ventricles, it is known as ventricular tachycardia. When it begins above the ventricles, it is called supraventricular tachycardia.

What are the symptoms?

Symptoms may include:

Copyright 1998 Clinical Reference Systems. Reprinted with permission.

- heart palpitations (feeling and hearing your heart pound)
- dizziness
- nausea
- weakness
- loss of consciousness without warning
- loss of consciousness when you are lying down

How is it diagnosed?

To determine the cause of fainting, the doctor will take your medical history and examine you. He or she will take your blood pressure and pulse while you are resting and while you are sitting or standing. The doctor may also order the following lab tests:

- An electrocardiogram (ECG). This is a recording of electrical impulses from the heart. Metal plates called electrodes are attached to the surface of your body and are connected to a recording device. The doctor may also want you to wear a Holter monitor. This is a portable, lightweight device that records your heart impulses all day.

- An electroencephalogram (EEG). This is a recording of the brain's electrical impulses. Metal plates called electrodes are attached to the head and connected to a recording device. Any brain wave abnormalities show up. This procedure is used to make sure the brain is not the cause of the problem.

- An echocardiogram. This is a recording produced during a painless procedure called echocardiography. Ultrasound waves are passed through the chest to examine the structure and function of the heart.

How is it treated?

The doctor may prescribe antiarrhythmic drugs.

If you have heart block and there are no symptoms, no treatment may be necessary. If heart block causes fainting, you need a pacemaker. This device uses electrical impulses to correct the heart's irregular rhythms.

In emergency situations, the doctor may prescribe a drug to stabilize the heartbeat.

Fainting Caused by Cardiac Conditions

How long will the effects last?

After you faint, you will return to consciousness when normal blood flow to your brain returns. You should lie down for 10 to 15 minutes after you return to consciousness.

How can I take care of myself?

Follow the full treatment recommended by the doctor. To avoid fainting you can:

- Treat your constipation; straining can cause you to faint.
- Use a fan or air conditioner during hot spells if hot, humid weather makes you feel faint. Drink plenty of fluids and do not go out or exercise in the heat of the day.

First aid for fainting:

- If a person feels faint they should lie down if possible, or at least sit down and lean forward with their head between their knees.
- If a person has already fainted, but has a good pulse and is breathing normally, raise their legs above the level of their chest. This returns more blood to the brain and will probably return the person to consciousness.
- If a person has already fainted and has no pulse or isn't breathing, call 911 and begin CPR. Call 911 if a person faints and remains unconscious for more than 2 minutes.

How can I prevent fainting caused by cardiac conditions?

- Avoid sudden changes in position and physical activities.
- Ask the doctor if you can adjust the dosage of any prescribed medications if fainting is a side effect.
- Eat small meals 5 or 6 times during the day if you have low blood sugar (hypoglycemia).

Part Five

Medications, Interventions, and Other Treatment Options

Chapter 44

Commonly Prescribed Medications for Heart Patients

Angiotensin-Converting Enzyme (ACE) Inhibitors, Systemic

Commonly used brand names in the U.S.:

- Accupril[7]
- Altace[8]
- Capoten[2]
- Lotensin[1]
- Monopril[5]
- Prinivil[6]
- Vasotec[3,4]
- Zestril[6]

Commonly used brand names in Canada:

- Capoten[2]
- Prinivil[6]
- Vasotec[3,4]
- Zestril[6]

Note: For quick reference, the following angiotensin-converting enzyme (ace) inhibitors are numbered to match the corresponding brand names. This information applies to the following medicines:

1. Benazepril (ben-AY-ze-pril)[†]
2. Captopril (KAP-toe-pril)
3. Enalapril (e-NAL-a-pril)
4. Enalaprilat (e-NAL-a-pril-at)

Excerpted from *Advice for the Patient: Drug Information in Lay Language*, 19th Edition, Prepared by the United States Pharmacopeial Convention, Inc. © 1999 Micromedex; reprinted with permission.

Heart Diseases and Disorders Sourcebook, Second Edition

5. Fosinopril (foe-SIN-oh-pril)†
6. Lisinopril (lyse-IN-oh-pril)
7. Quinapril (KWIN-a-pril)†
8. Ramipril (ra-MI-pril)†

†Not commercially available in Canada.

Description

ACE inhibitors belong to the class of medicines called high blood pressure medicines (antihypertensives). They are used to treat high blood pressure (hypertension).

High blood pressure adds to the work load of the heart and arteries. If it continues for a long time, the heart and arteries may not function properly. This can damage the blood vessels of the brain, heart, and kidneys, resulting in a stroke, heart failure, or kidney failure. High blood pressure may also increase the risk of heart attacks. These problems may be less likely to occur if blood pressure is controlled.

Captopril is used in some patients after a heart attack. After a heart attack, some of the heart muscle is damaged and weakened. The heart muscle may continue to weaken as time goes by. This makes it more difficult for the heart to pump blood. Captopril helps slow down the further weakening of the heart.

Captopril is also used to treat kidney problems in some diabetic patients who use insulin to control their diabetes. Over time, these kidney problems may get worse. Captopril may help slow down the further worsening of kidney problems.

In addition, some ACE inhibitors are used to treat congestive heart failure or may be used for other conditions as determined by your doctor.

The exact way that these medicines work is not known. They block an enzyme in the body that is necessary to produce a substance that causes blood vessels to tighten. As a result, they relax blood vessels. This lowers blood pressure and increases the supply of blood and oxygen to the heart.

These medicines are available only with your doctor's prescription, in the following dosage forms:

Oral

- Benazepril: Tablets (U.S.)
- Captopril: Tablets (U.S. and Canada)
- Enalapril: Tablets (U.S. and Canada)

Commonly Prescribed Medications for Heart Patients

- Fosinopril: Tablets (U.S.)
- Lisinopril: Tablets (U.S. and Canada)
- Quinapril: Tablets (U.S.)
- Ramipril: Capsules (U.S.)

Parenteral

- Enalaprilat: Injection (U.S. and Canada)

Beta-Adrenergic Blocking Agents and Thiazide Diuretics, Systemic

Commonly used brand names in the U.S.:

- Corzide[4]
- Inderide[6]
- Inderide LA[6]
- Lopressor HCT[3]
- Tenoretic[1]
- Timolide[7]
- Ziac[2]

Commonly used brand names in Canada:

- Corzide[4]
- Inderide[6]
- Tenoretic[1]
- Timolide[7]
- Viskazide[5]

Note: For quick reference, the following beta-adrenergic blocking agents and thiazide diuretics are numbered to match the corresponding brand names. This information applies to the following medicines:

1. Atenolol and Chlorthalidone (a-TEN-oh-lole and klor-THAL-i-doan)‡
2. Bisoprolol and Hydrochlorothiazide (bis-OH-proe-lol and hye-droe-klor-oh-THYE-a-zide)†
3. Metoprolol and Hydrochlorothiazide (me-TOE-proe-lole and hye-droe-klor-oh-THYE-a-zide)†
4. Nadolol and Bendroflumethiazide (NAY-doe-lole and ben-droe-floo-meth-EYE-a-zide)
5. Pindolol and Hydrochlorothiazide (PIN-doe-lole and hye-droe-klor-oh-THYE-a-zide)*
6. Propranolol and Hydrochlorothiazide (proe-PRAN-oh-lole and hye-droe-klor-oh-THYE-a-zide)*
7. Timolol and Hydrochlorothiazide (TIM-oh-lole and hye-droe-klor-oh-THYE-a-zide)

Heart Diseases and Disorders Sourcebook, Second Edition

*Not commercially available in the U.S.
†Not commercially available in Canada.
‡Generic name product may be available in the U.S.

Description

Beta-adrenergic blocking agent (more commonly, beta-blockers) and thiazide diuretic combinations belong to the group of medicines known as antihypertensives (high blood pressure medicine). Both ingredients of the combination control high blood pressure, but they work in different ways. Beta-blockers (atenolol, bisoprolol, metoprolol, nadolol, pindolol, propranolol, and timolol) reduce the work load on the heart as well as having other effects. Thiazide diuretics (bendroflumethiazide, chlorthalidone, and hydrochlorothiazide) reduce the amount of fluid pressure in the body by increasing the flow of urine.

High blood pressure adds to the work load of the heart and arteries. If it continues for a long time, the heart and arteries may not function properly. This can damage the blood vessels of the brain, heart, and kidneys, resulting in a stoke, heart failure, or kidney failure. High blood pressure may also increase the risk of heart attacks. These problems may be less likely to occur if blood pressure is controlled.

Beta-blocker and thiazide diuretic combinations are available only with your doctor's prescription, in the following dosage forms:

Oral

- Atenolol and chlorthalidone: Tablets (U.S. and Canada)
- Bisoprolol and hydrochlorothiazide: Tablets (U.S.)
- Metoprolol and hydrochlorothiazide: Tablets (U.S.)
- Nadolol and bendroflumethiazide: Tablets (U.S. and Canada)
- Pindolol and hydrochlorothiazide: Tablets (Canada)
- Propranolol and hydrochlorothiazide: Extended-release capsules (U.S.); Tablets (U.S. and Canada)
- Timolol and hydrochlorothiazide: Tablets (U.S. and Canada)

Calcium Channel Blocking Agents, Systemic

Commonly used brand names in the U.S.:

- Adalat[7]
- Adalat CC[7]
- Calan[9]
- Calan SR[9]

Commonly Prescribed Medications for Heart Patients

- Cardene[6]
- Cardizem[2]
- Cardizem CD[2]
- Cardizem SR[2]
- Dilacor-XR[2]
- DynaCirc[5]
- Isoptin[9]

- Isoptin SR[9]
- Nimotop[8]
- Plendil[3]
- Procardia[7]
- Procardia XL[7]
- Vascor[1]
- Verelan[9]

Commonly used brand names in Canada:

- Adalat[7]
- Adalat PA[7]
- Adalat XL[7]
- Apo-Diltiaz[2]
- Apo-Nifed[7]
- Apo-Verap[9]
- Cardene[6]
- Cardizem[2]
- Cardizem SR[2]
- Isoptin[9]
- Isoptin SR[9]
- Nimotop[8]

- Novo-Diltazem[2]
- Novo-Nifedin[7]
- Novo-Veramil[9]
- Nu-Diltiaz[2]
- Nu-Nifed[7]
- Nu-Verap[9]
- Plendil[3]
- Renedil[3]
- Sibelium[4]
- Syn-Diltiazem[2]
- Verelan[9]

Note: For quick reference, the following calcium channel blocking agents are numbered to match the corresponding brand names. This information applies to the following medicines:

1. Bepridil (BE-pri-dil)†
2. Diltiazem (dil-TYE-a-zem)‡§
3. Felodipine (fe-LOE-di-peen)
4. Flunarizine (floo-NAR-i-zeen)*
5. Isradipine (is-RA-di-peen)†
6. Nicardipine (nye-KAR-de-peen)‡
7. Nifedipine (nye-FED-i-peen)‡
8. Nimodipine (nye-MOE-di-peen)
9. Verapamil (ver-AP-a-mil)‡§

*Not commercially available in the U.S.
†Not commercially available in Canada.
‡Generic name product may be available in the U.S.
§Generic name product may be available in Canada.

Description

Bepridil, diltiazem, felodipine, flunarizine, isradipine, nicardipine, nifedipine, nimodipine, and verapamil belong to the group of medicines called calcium channel blocking agents.

Calcium channel blocking agents affect the movement of calcium into the cells of the heart and blood vessels. As a result, they relax blood vessels and increase the supply of blood and oxygen to the heart while reducing its workload.

Some of the calcium channel blocking agents are used to relieve and control angina pectoris (chest pain). Some are also used to treat high blood pressure (hypertension). High blood pressure adds to the workload of the heart and arteries. If it continues for a long time, the heart and arteries may not function properly. This can damage the blood vessels of the brain, heart, and kidneys, resulting in a stroke, heart failure, or kidney failure. High blood pressure may also increase the risk of heart attacks. These problems may be less likely to occur if blood pressure is controlled.

Flunarizine is used to prevent migraine headaches.

Nimodipine is used to prevent and treat problems caused by a burst blood vessel around the brain (also known as a ruptured aneurysm or subarachnoid hemorrhage).

Other calcium channel blocking agents may also be used for these and other conditions as determined by your doctor.

These medicines are available only with your doctor's prescription, in the following dosage forms:

Oral

- Bepridil: Tablets (U.S.)
- Diltiazem: Extended-release capsules (U.S. and Canada); Tablets (U.S. and Canada)
- Felodipine: Extended-release tablets (U.S. and Canada)
- Flunarizine: Capsules (Canada)
- Isradipine: Capsules (U.S.)
- Nicardipine: Capsules (U.S. and Canada)
- Nifedipine: Capsules (U.S. and Canada); Extended-release tablets (U.S. and Canada)
- Nimodipine: Capsules (U.S. and Canada)
- Verapamil: Extended-release capsules (U.S. and Canada); Tablets (U.S. and Canada); Extended-release tablets (U.S. and Canada)

Commonly Prescribed Medications for Heart Patients

Parenteral

- Diltiazem: Injection (U.S. and Canada)
- Verapamil: Injection (U.S. and Canada)

Digitalis Medicines, Systemic

Commonly used brand names in the U.S.:

- Crystodigin[1]
- Lanoxicaps[2]
- Lanoxin[2]

Commonly used brand names in Canada:

- Digitaline[1]
- Lanoxin[2]
- Novo-Digoxin[2]

Note: For quick reference, the following digitalis medicines are numbered to match the corresponding brand names. This information applies to the following medicines:

1. Digitoxin (di-ji-TOX-in)‡
2. Digoxin (di-JOX-in)‡

‡Generic name product may be available in the U.S.

Description

Digitalis medicines are used to improve the strength and efficiency of the heart, or to control the rate and rhythm of the heartbeat. This leads to better blood circulation and reduced swelling of hands and ankles in patients with heart problems.

Although digitalis has been prescribed to help some patients lose weight, it should never be used in this way. When used improperly, digitalis can cause serious problems.

Digitalis medicines are available only with your doctor's prescription, in the following dosage forms:

Oral

- Digitoxin: Tablets (U.S. and Canada)
- Digoxin: Capsules (U.S.); Elixir (U.S. and Canada); Tablets (U.S. and Canada)

Parenteral

- Digoxin: Injection (U.S. and Canada)

Loop Diuretics, Systemic

Commonly used brand names in the U.S.:

- Bumex[1]
- Edecrin[2]
- Lasix[3]
- Myrosemide[3]

Commonly used brand names in Canada:

- Apo-Furosemide[3]
- Edecrin[2]
- Furoside[3]
- Lasix[3]
- Lasix Special[3]
- Novosemide[3]
- Uritol[3]

Note: For quick reference, the following loop diuretics are numbered to match the corresponding brand names. This information applies to the following medicines:

1. Bumetanide (byoo-MET-a-nide)‡†
2. Ethacrynic Acid (eth-a-KRIN-ik AS-id)
3. Furosemide (fur-OH-se-mide)‡§

†Not commercially available in Canada.
‡Generic name product may be available in the U.S.
§Generic name product may be available in Canada.

Description

Loop diuretics are given to help reduce the amount of water in the body. They work by acting on the kidneys to increase the flow of urine.

Furosemide is also used to treat high blood pressure (hypertension) in those patients who are not helped by other medicines or in those patients who have kidney problems.

High blood pressure adds to the work load of the heart and arteries. If it continues for a long time, the heart and arteries may not function properly. This can damage the blood vessels of the brain, heart, and kidneys, resulting in a stroke, heart failure, or kidney failure. High blood pressure may also increase the risk of heart attacks. These problems may be less likely to occur if blood pressure is controlled.

Commonly Prescribed Medications for Heart Patients

Loop diuretics may also be used for other conditions as determined by your doctor. This medicine is available only with your doctor's prescription, in the following dosage forms:

Oral

- Bumetanide: Tablets (U.S.)
- Ethacrynic Acid: Oral solution (U.S. and Canada); Tablets (U.S. and Canada)
- Furosemide: Oral solution (U.S. and Canada); Tablets (U.S. and Canada)

Parenteral

- Bumetanide: Injection (U.S.)
- Ethacrynic Acid: Injection (U.S. and Canada)
- Furosemide: Injection (U.S. and Canada)

Potassium-Sparing Diuretics, Systemic

Commonly used brand names in the U.S.:

- Aldactone[2]
- Dyrenium[3]
- Midamor[1]

Commonly used brand names in Canada:

- Aldactone[2]
- Dyrenium[2]
- Midamor[1]
- Novospiroton[2]

Note: For quick reference, the following potassium-sparing diuretics are numbered to match the corresponding brand names. This information applies to the following medicines:

1. Amiloride (a-MILL-oh-ride)‡
2. Spironolactone (speer-on-oh-LAK-tone)‡
3. Triamterene (trye-AM-ter-een)

‡Generic name product may be available in the U.S.

Description

Potassium-sparing diuretics are commonly used to help reduce the amount of water in the body. Unlike some other diuretics, these medicines do not cause your body to lose potassium.

Amiloride and spironolactone are also used to treat high blood pressure (hypertension). High blood pressure adds to the workload of the heart and arteries. If the condition continues for a long time, the heart and arteries may not function properly. This can damage the blood vessels of the brain, heart, and kidneys, resulting in a stroke, heart failure, or kidney failure. High blood pressure may also increase the risk of heart attacks. These problems may be less likely to occur if blood pressure is controlled.

Spironolactone is also used to help increase the amount of potassium in the body when it is getting too low.

Potassium-sparing diuretics help to reduce the amount of water in the body by acting on the kidneys to increase the flow of urine. This also helps to lower blood pressure.

These medicines can also be used for other conditions as determined by your doctor.

Potassium-sparing diuretics are available only with your doctor's prescription, in the following dosage forms:

Oral

- Amiloride: Tablets (U.S. and Canada)
- Spironolactone: Tablets (U.S. and Canada)
- Triamterene: Capsules (U.S.); Tablets (Canada)

Potassium-Sparing Diuretics and Hydrochlorothiazide, Systemic

Commonly used brand names in the U.S.:

- Aldactazide[2]
- Dyazide[3]
- Maxzide[3]
- Moduretic[1]
- Spirozide[2]

Commonly used brand names in Canada:

- Aldactazide[2]
- Apo-Triazide[3]
- Dyazide[3]
- Moduret[1]
- Novo-Spirozine[2]
- Novo-Triamzide[3]

Note: For quick reference, the following medicines are numbered to match the corresponding brand names. This information applies to the following medicines:

Commonly Prescribed Medications for Heart Patients

1. Amiloride and Hydrochlorothiazide (a-MILL-oh-ride and hye-droe-klor-oh-THYE-a-zide)‡
2. Spironolactone and Hydrochlorothiazide (speer-on-oh-LAK-tone and hye-droe-klor-oh-THYE-a-zide)‡
3. Triamterene and Hydrochlorothiazide (trye-AM-ter-een and hye-droe-klor-oh-THYE-a-zide)‡

‡Generic name product may be available in the U.S.

Description

This medicine is a combination of two diuretics (water pills). It is commonly used to help reduce the amount of water in the body.

This combination is also used to treat high blood pressure (hypertension). High blood pressure adds to the work load of the heart and arteries. If it continues for a long time, the heart and arteries may not function properly. This can damage the blood vessels of the brain, heart, and kidneys, resulting in a stroke, heart failure, or kidney failure. High blood pressure may also increase the risk of heart attacks. These problems may be less likely to occur if blood pressure is controlled.

Diuretics help to reduce the amount of water in the body by acting on the kidneys to increase the flow of urine. This also helps to lower blood pressure.

This combination is also used to treat problems caused by too little potassium in the body.

This medicine is available only with your doctor's prescription, in the following dosage forms:

Oral

- Amiloride and Hydrochlorothiazide: Tablets (U.S. and Canada)
- Spironolactone and Hydrochlorothiazide: Tablets (U.S. and Canada)
- Triamterene and Hydrochlorothiazide: Capsules (U.S.); Tablets (U.S. and Canada)

Thiazide Diuretics, Systemic

Commonly used brand names in the U.S.:

- Aquatensen[6]
- Diucardin[5]
- Diulo[7]
- Diuril[2]
- Enduron[6]
- Esidrix[4]

- Hydro-chlor[4]
- Hydro-D[4]
- HydroDIURIL[4]
- Hydromox[9]
- Hygroton[3]
- Metahydrin[10]
- Microzide[4]
- Mykrox[7]
- Naqua[10]
- Naturetin[1]
- Oretic[4]
- Renese[8]
- Saluron[5]
- Thalitone[3]
- Trichlorex[10]
- Zaroxolyn[7]

Commonly used brand names in Canada:

- Apo-Chlorthalidone[3]
- Apo-Hydro[4]
- Diuchlor H[4]
- Duretic[6]
- HydroDIURIL[4]
- Hygroton[3]
- Naturetin[1]
- Neo-Codema[4]
- Novo-Hydrazide[4]
- Novo-Thalidone[3]
- Uridon[3]
- Urozide[4]
- Zaroxolyn[7]

Note: For quick reference, the following thiazide diuretics are numbered to match the corresponding brand names. This information applies to the following medicines:

1. Bendroflumethiazide (ben-droe-floo-meth-EYE-a-zide)
2. Chlorothiazide (klor-oh-THYE-a-zide)‡†
3. Chlorthalidone (klor-THAL-i-doan)‡§
4. Hydrochlorothiazide (hye-droe-klor-oh-THYE-a-zide)‡§
5. Hydroflumethiazide (hye-droe-floo-meth-EYE-a-zide)‡†
6. Methyclothiazide (meth-ee-kloe-THYE-a-zide)‡
7. Metolazone (me-TOLE-a-zone)
8. Polythiazide (pol-i-THYE-a-zide)†
9. Quinethazone (kwin-ETH-a-zone)†
10. Trichlormethiazide (trye-klor-meth-EYE-a-zide)‡†

†Not commercially available in Canada.
‡Generic name product may be available in the U.S.
§Generic name product may be available in Canada.

Description

Thiazide or thiazide-like diuretics are commonly used to treat high blood pressure (hypertension). High blood pressure adds to the

Commonly Prescribed Medications for Heart Patients

workload of the heart and arteries. If it continues for a long time, the heart and arteries may not function properly. This can damage the blood vessels of the brain, heart, and kidneys, resulting in a stroke, heart failure, or kidney failure. High blood pressure may also increase the risk of heart attacks. These problems may be less likely to occur if blood pressure is controlled.

Thiazide diuretics are also used to help reduce the amount of water in the body by increasing the flow of urine. They may also be used for other conditions as determined by your doctor.

Thiazide diuretics are available only with your doctor's prescription, in the following dosage forms:

Oral

- Bendroflumethiazide: Tablets (U.S. and Canada)
- Chlorothiazide: Oral suspension (U.S.); Tablets (U.S.)
- Chlorthalidone: Tablets (U.S. and Canada)
- Hydrochlorothiazide: Capsules (U.S.); Oral solution (U.S.); Tablets (U.S. and Canada)
- Hydroflumethiazide: Tablets (U.S.)
- Methyclothiazide: Tablets (U.S. and Canada)
- Metolazone: Tablets (U.S. and Canada)
- Polythiazide: Tablets (U.S.)
- Quinethazone: Tablets (U.S.)
- Trichlormethiazide: Tablets (U.S.)

Parenteral

- Chlorothiazide: Injection (U.S.)

Nitrates—Lingual Aerosol, Systemic

This information applies to nitroglycerin oral spray.

Commonly used brand name in the U.S.:

- Nitrolingual

Commonly used brand name in Canada:

- Nitrolingual

Another commonly used name is glyceryl trinitrate.

Description

Nitrates (NYE-trates) are used to treat the symptoms of angina (chest pain). Depending on the type of dosage form and how it is taken, nitrates are used to treat angina in three ways:

- to relieve an attack that is occurring by using the medicine when the attack begins;
- to prevent attacks from occurring by using the medicine just before an attack is expected to occur; or
- to reduce the number of attacks that occur by using the medicine regularly on a long-term basis.

When used as a lingual (in the mouth) spray, nitroglycerin is used either to relieve the pain of angina attacks or to prevent an expected angina attack.

Nitroglycerin works by relaxing blood vessels and increasing the supply of blood and oxygen to the heart while reducing its work load.

Nitroglycerin as discussed here is available only with your doctor's prescription, in the following dosage form:

Oral

- Lingual aerosol (U.S. and Canada)

Nitrates—Oral, Systemic

Commonly used brand names in the U.S.:

- Cardilate[1]
- Dilatrate-SR[2]
- Duotrate[5]
- IMDUR[3]
- ISMO[3]
- Iso-Bid[2]
- Isonate[2]
- Isorbid[2]
- Isordil[2]
- Isotrate[2]
- Klavikordal[4]
- Monoket[3]
- Niong[4]
- Nitrocap[4]
- Nitrocap T.D.[4]
- Nitroglyn[4]
- Nitrolin[4]
- Nitronet[4]
- Nitrong[4]
- Nitrospan[4]
- Pentylan[5]
- Peritrate[5]
- Peritrate SA[5]
- Sorbitrate[2]
- Sorbitrate SA[2]

Commonly Prescribed Medications for Heart Patients

Commonly used brand names in Canada:

- Apo-ISDN[2]
- Cardilate[1]
- Cedocard-SR[2]
- Coronex[2]
- Isordil[2]
- Nitrong SR[4]
- Novosorbide[2]
- Peritrate[5]
- Peritrate Forte[5]
- Peritrate SA[5]

Other commonly used names are: Eritrityl tetranitrate[1], Erythritol tetranitrate[1], Glyceryl trinitrate[4], Pentaerithrityl tetranitrate[5], and P.E.T.N.[5].

Note: For quick reference, the following nitrates are numbered to match the corresponding brand names. This information applies to the following medicines:

1. Erythrityl Tetranitrate (e-RI-thri-til tet-ra-NYE-trate)
2. Isosorbide Dinitrate (eye-soe-SOR-bide dye-NYE-trate)‡
3. Isosorbide Mononitrate (eye-soe-SOR-bide mon-oh-NYE-trate)†
4. Nitroglycerin (nye-troe-GLI-ser-in)‡
5. Pentaerythritol Tetranitrate (pen-ta-er-ITH-ri-tole tet-ra-NYE-trate)‡

Note: This information does not apply to amyl nitrite or mannitol hexanitrate.

†Not commercially available in Canada.
‡Generic name product may be available in the U.S.

Description

Nitrates (NYE-trates) are used to treat the symptoms of angina (chest pain). Depending on the type of dosage form and how it is taken, nitrates are used to treat angina in three ways:

- to relieve an attack that is occurring by using the medicine when the attack begins;
- to prevent attacks from occurring by using the medicine just before an attack is expected to occur; or
- to reduce the number of attacks that occur by using the medicine regularly on a long-term basis.

When taken orally and swallowed, nitrates are used to reduce the number of angina attacks that occur. They do not act fast enough to relieve the pain of an angina attack.

Nitrates work by relaxing blood vessels and increasing the supply of blood and oxygen to the heart while reducing its work load.

Nitrates may also be used for other conditions as determined by your doctor.

The nitrates discussed here are available only with your doctor's prescription, in the following dosage forms:

Oral

- Erythrityl tetranitrate: Tablets (U.S. and Canada)
- Isosorbide dinitrate: Capsules (U.S.); Extended-release capsules (U.S.); Tablets (U.S. and Canada); Chewable tablets (U.S.); Extended-release tablets (U.S. and Canada)
- Isosorbide mononitrate: Extended-release tablets (U.S.); Tablets (U.S.)
- Nitroglycerin: Extended-release capsules (U.S.); Extended-release tablets (U.S. and Canada)
- Pentaerythritol tetranitrate: Extended-release capsules (U.S.); Tablets (U.S. and Canada); Extended-release tablets (U.S. and Canada)

Nitrates—Sublingual, Chewable, or Buccal, Systemic

Commonly used brand names in the U.S.:

- Cardilate[1]
- Isonate[2]
- Isorbid[2]
- Isordil[2]
- Nitrogard[3]
- Nitrostat[3]
- Sorbitrate[2]

Commonly used brand names in Canada:

- Apo-ISDN[2]
- Cardilate[1]
- Coronex[2]
- Isordil[2]
- Nitrogard SR[3]
- Nitrostat[3]

Other commonly used names are: Eritrityl tetranitrate[1], Erythritol tetranitrate[1], and Glyceryl trinitrate[3].

Commonly Prescribed Medications for Heart Patients

Note: For quick reference, the following nitrates are numbered to match the corresponding brand names. This information applies to the following medicines:

1. Erythrityl Tetranitrate (e-RI-ft-til tet-ra-NYE-trate)
2. Isosorbide Dinitrate (eye-soe-SOR-bide dye-NYE-trate)‡
3. Nitroglycerin (nye-troe-GLI-ser-in)†§

Note: This information doses not apply to amyl nitrite or pentaerythritol tetranitrate.

‡Generic name product may be available in the U.S.
§Generic name product may be available in Canada.

Description

Nitrates (NYE-trates) are used to treat the symptoms of angina (chest pain). Depending on the type of dosage form and how it is taken, nitrates are used to treat angina in three ways:

- to relieve an attack that is occurring by using the medicine when the attack begins;
- to prevent attacks from occurring by using the medicine just before an attack is expected to occur; or
- to reduce the number of attacks that occur by using the medicine regularly on a long-term basis.

Nitrates are available in different forms. Sublingual nitrates are generally placed under the tongue where they dissolve and are absorbed through the lining of the mouth. Some can also be used buccally, being placed under the lip or in the cheek. The chewable dosage forms, after being chewed and held in the mouth before swallowing, are absorbed in the same way. It is important to remember that each dosage form is different and that the specific directions for each type must be followed if the medicine is to work properly.

Nitrates that are used to relieve the pain of an angina attack include:

- sublingual nitroglycerin;
- buccal nitroglycerin;
- sublingual isosorbide dinitrate; and
- chewable isosorbide dinitrate.

Those that can be used to prevent expected attacks of angina include:

- sublingual nitroglycerin;
- buccal nitroglycerin;
- sublingual erythrityl tetranitrate;
- sublingual isosorbide dinitrate; and
- chewable isosorbide dinitrate.

Products that are used regularly on a long-term basis to reduce the number of attacks that occur include:

- buccal nitroglycerin;
- oral/sublingual erythrityl tetranitrate;
- chewable isosorbide dinitrate; and
- sublingual isosorbide dinitrate.

Nitrates work by relaxing blood vessels and increasing the supply of blood and oxygen to the heart while reducing its work load.

Nitrates may also be used for other conditions as determined by your doctor.

The nitrates discussed here are available only with your doctor's prescription, in the following dosage forms:

Buccal

- Nitroglycerin: Extended-release tablets (U.S. and Canada)

Chewable

- Isosorbide dinitrate: Tablets (U.S.)

Sublingual

- Erythrityl tetranitrate: Tablets (U.S. and Canada)
- Isosorbide dinitrate: Tablets (U.S. and Canada)
- Nitroglycerin: Tablets (U.S. and Canada)

Nitrates—Topical, Systemic

Commonly used brand names in the U.S.:

- Deponit[2]
- Minitran[2]
- Nitro-Bid[1]
- Nitrodisc[2]

Commonly Prescribed Medications for Heart Patients

- Nitro-Dur[2]
- Nitrol[1]
- Nitrong[1]
- Nitrostat[1]
- Transderm-Nitro[2]

Commonly used brand names in Canada:

- Minitran[2]
- Nitro-Bid[1]
- Nitro-Dur[2]
- Nitrol[1]
- Nitrong[1]
- Transderm-Nitro[2]

Another commonly used name for nitroglycerin is glyceryl trinitrate.

Note: For quick reference, the following nitrates are numbered to match the corresponding brand names. This information applies to the following medicines:

1. Nitroglycerin Ointment
2. Nitroglycerin Transdermal Patches

Description

Nitrates (NYE-trates) are used to treat the symptoms of angina (chest pain). Depending on the type of dosage form and how it is taken, nitrates are used to treat angina in three ways:

- to relieve an attack that is occurring by using the medicine when the attack begins;
- to prevent attacks from occurring by using the medicine just before an attack is expected to occur; or
- to reduce the number of attacks that occur by using the medicine regularly on a long-term basis.

When applied to the skin, nitrates are used to reduce the number of angina attacks that occur. The only nitrate available for this purpose is topical nitroglycerin (nye-troe-GLI-ser-in).

Topical nitroglycerin is absorbed through the skin. It works by relaxing blood vessels and increasing the supply of blood and oxygen to the heart while reducing its work load. This helps prevent future angina attacks from occurring.

Topical nitroglycerin may also be used for other conditions as determined by your doctor.

Nitroglycerin as discussed here is available only with your doctor's prescription, in the following dosage forms:

Topical

- Ointment (U.S. and Canada)
- Transdermal (stick-on) patch (U.S. and Canada)

Chapter 45

The DIG (Digitalis Investigation Group) Trial

Digitalis, one of the oldest medications in the physician's black bag, has been used in various forms for treatment of heart problems since ancient times. Today, the drug is best known as digoxin (Lanoxin) and is regularly used by people with congestive heart failure (CHF) and heart-rhythm abnormalities (arrhythmias). Most physicians believe that patients with these problems benefit from digoxin, but the drug has not been put through the kind of rigorous testing that new medications must undergo today—in part because it is so old and established.

The question of digoxin's effectiveness is important because it can cause side effects, including nausea, depression, and life-threatening arrhythmias (though side effects are less common than they once were, thanks to monitoring of drug and potassium levels in the blood). Studies have shown that digoxin can increase the pumping ability of the failing heart, minimize breathlessness and other symptoms of CHF, and increase a person's ability to exercise. But the drug has never been shown to improve survival for people with heart failure. Some experts have raised the question about whether the U.S. Food and Drug Administration would approve digoxin today if it were a new medication.

Outdoing the "Competition"

Fortunately, a recent study has addressed some of the questions about digoxin. This study, called the DIG (for Digitalis Investigation

Excerpted from July 1997 issue of *Harvard Heart Letter*, © 1997 President and Fellows of Harvard College; reprinted with permission.

Group) trial, is the first large, randomized, clinical trial to assess digoxin's effect on patients with heart failure and a regular heartbeat (also called normal sinus rhythm). Although the drug is used by many people with atrial fibrillation—a common heart-rhythm abnormality—the trial did not include these types of patients. Experts have generally recognized the value of digoxin in patients with heart failure who have atrial fibrillation, but its effectiveness in people who have a normal heart rhythm has often been questioned.

Ironically, one reason why a large, expensive study of digoxin's impact became important is that there has been so much progress with other medications for heart failure. Heart failure arises because of damage to the heart muscle from various causes, including heart attack, infection, or excessive alcohol intake. If the damage is extensive enough, the remaining heart muscle cannot pump blood effectively in order to clear it from the lungs and supply the body's needs for oxygen and nutrients. When this occurs, the patient experiences the symptoms of heart failure, including breathlessness, weakness, and swelling in the legs from fluid retention.

In the past, heart failure was a grim diagnosis, and it remains a serious problem. However, in the last several years, medications called vasodilators—which dilate, or expand, the body's arteries—have been shown to improve both the survival and the quality of life of those with heart failure. One group of vasodilators, the ACE (angiotensin-converting-enzyme) inhibitors have even helped to prevent heart failure in patients with heart-muscle damage from heart attacks and to stave off a second heart attack (see December 1992 and October 1993 *Harvard Heart Letter*). With the combination of vasodilators and diuretics (water pills) so clearly helpful for most heart-failure patients, researchers have been wondering whether digoxin's potential side effects make this drug less than worthwhile for people with this problem.

Physicians have been reluctant to stop prescribing digoxin for heart failure, however, because this medication works in a different way from the vasodilators and diuretics and therefore might offer an added benefit. Digoxin increases the "squeeze" of the muscle fibers in the heart's ventricles, thereby improving the pumping ability of a weakened heart. In theory, the combination of a drug that helps the heart beat more strongly (digoxin) and a drug that opens up the blood vessels to ease the heart's work (a vasodilator) should be ideal. For patients with atrial fibrillation, digoxin also reduces the flow of electrical signals from the atrial chambers at the top of the heart to the ventricles at the bottom of the heart. This latter effect helps slow the heart

The DIG (Digitalis Investigation Group) Trial

rate and improve the filling of the ventricles in these patients (see February 1993 *Harvard Heart Letter*).

However, in the much larger number of people with CHF and a regular heartbeat, digoxin's benefits are limited to helping the heart muscle beat more strongly. These benefits may be real but may be offset by the risk of arrhythmias caused by digoxin. Since digoxin is used widely in this group of patients, the National Heart, Lung, and Blood Institute and the Veterans Affairs Cooperative Studies Program collaborated in conducting the DIG trial to find out whether digoxin is worthwhile in patients with these characteristics.

The DIG Trial

The DIG trial, which ran from 1991 to 1995, involved more than 7,500 patients from 302 centers in the U.S. and Canada. All participants took ACE inhibitors unless these drugs could not be tolerated. The study subjects were divided into two groups: half were randomly assigned to add digoxin to their regimen, and the other half added a dummy tablet (placebo). The study was double-blind—that is, during the course of the trial, neither the patients nor their physicians knew who was taking digoxin or a placebo.

Patients who had never used digoxin as well as those who were already using it took part in the trial. The study examined digoxin's effect in a wide range of patients with heart failure, tested the medication's impact on survival, and examined whether the addition of digoxin to an ACE inhibitor (or to the patient's usual treatment) provided any additional benefits.

The study, recently published in the *New England Journal of Medicine* (February 20, 1997), found that, overall, digoxin (unlike ACE inhibitors) did not lengthen the lives of patients with heart failure and a normal heartbeat when compared to the placebo; but it did not shorten their lives either. While there were slightly fewer deaths from heart failure and slightly more deaths from other heart causes in people taking digoxin compared to those taking the placebo, the overall effect was no increase in deaths from any cause. However, many people consider quality of life as important as length of life, and in this area the results of the DIG study were encouraging. Patients taking digoxin had fewer hospital admissions for heart failure and fewer deaths from worsening heart failure than those who took the placebo—results that most likely reflect less severe heart failure with digoxin therapy. On balance, the study's results should provide reassurance to people and physicians who currently rely on this medication.

Cautious Optimism

For the first time since its introduction into Western medicine more than 200 years ago, digoxin has been subjected to the same rigorous assessment afforded to all new drugs. The DIG trial demonstrates that digoxin is relatively safe and reduces the severe symptoms that limit activity in those with heart failure and a regular heart rate.

What do these findings mean for people with heart failure? First, modern medical therapy that combines drugs with different effects on the body can help patients with heart failure enjoy more active lives. Second, ACE inhibitors remain the medications of choice for helping patients with weakened heart muscles to increase their life expectancy And, third, digoxin—despite its potential side effects—can be a useful addition to ACE inhibitors for many patients.

All of these medications require close collaboration between the person with heart failure and his or her physician. Symptoms like lightheadedness, breathlessness, or fainting spells might be warnings of medication side effects and warrant prompt evaluation by a physician. Other potential innovations for heart failure may also be added to this mix in the coming years. In the near future, the study group will issue other results, including a more formal assessment of the quality of life of the study participants and an analysis of the effect of various digoxin doses. In the meantime, these findings suggest that complicated drug regimens involving several effective medications win offer true benefits for people with heart failure.

Chapter 46

Anticoagulants

Most people know all too well what it's like to nick themselves with a kitchen knife while slicing and dicing. Fortunately for the clumsy chef, blood usually clots fast enough to stanch the leak.

But what is beneficial in this situation can be fatal in others. Heart attacks, the number-one killer in the developed world, happen when a clot blocks vital arteries supplying the heart muscle with blood. And about three-quarters of all strokes are caused by a clot in the blood vessels leading to the brain. Life-threatening clots can also affect the interior chambers of the heart, the lungs, or the legs.

Anticoagulants, drugs that can halt an incipient clot, are among the most widely used medicines in the world. Physicians have long prescribed them for people who are likely to develop clots because they have a prosthetic heart valve or a type of cardiac arrhythmia called atrial fibrillation. More recently, anticoagulants have emerged as a standard preventive measure for patients who've had a heart attack. Experts are also debating whether they should be given to people who haven't had a damaging blockage as yet, but who seem to be headed that way.

A Delicate Balance

The biological mechanisms that balance the flow and the clotting of blood are so wonderfully complex that Rube Goldberg might have

---

"Clot Prevention: Anticoagulants to the Rescue," by Larry Husten. Excerpted from October 1995 issue of *Harvard Health Letter*, © 1995 President and Fellows of Harvard College; reprinted with permission.

dreamed them up. This system relies on constant chemical chatter among the endothelial cells (lining the circulatory system), soluble coagulation factors, and platelets. Platelets are cell-like structures circulating in the bloodstream. They are disc-shaped and inactive until endothelial cells are damaged, which galvanizes them into action. The platelets become round, and their surface bristles like the deck of a battleship with an assortment of biochemical antennas and weapons. They attach themselves to the injured vessel wall and also to each other.

Circulating coagulation factors interact with the platelets to create a blood clot—which is a fine, Jello-like mesh. Two categories of drugs can interfere with this process: antiplatelet agents, which inhibit the action of the platelets, and anticoagulants, which act on certain clotting factors.

These drugs are often referred to as blood thinners, a popular name that can be misleading. In fact, the blood is just as thick with cells as it ever was; it just can't go through the biochemical steps needed to form a clot.

The Secret Life of Aspirin

Although most people think of aspirin primarily as a pain reliever, in fact the world's most popular drug is also an extremely effective antiplatelet agent. Unfortunately, doctors don't take advantage of its anti-clotting action nearly as much as they could, according to researcher Charles H. Hennekens, a professor of ambulatory care and prevention at Harvard Medical School. In a large study comparing the effectiveness of several treatments within the first 24 hours after a heart attack, aspirin reduced mortality by 23%.

Although aspirin causes far fewer complications and is less expensive than thrombolytic agents (clot-busters), Dr. Hennekens estimated that 30-60% of patients suffering a heart attack are not treated with it. If they were, an additional 5,000-10,000 lives probably could be saved each year in the U.S. alone, said Dr. Hennekens. "Aspirin has the best benefit-to-risk and benefit-to-cost ratio of any heart attack treatment."

In addition to being useful for people who have had heart attacks, strokes, or transient ischemic attacks (warning signs of stroke), there is some evidence that taking one aspirin tablet daily can benefit people with angina (cardiac chest pain) or those with a history of deep venous thrombosis (clots in the legs that can travel to the lungs).

In studies of hospitalized patients, researchers have also found that aspirin prevents postoperative clotting in people who have undergone coronary artery bypass grafting or balloon angioplasty.

Many doctors now advise that people at risk for heart disease take one-half to one aspirin tablet daily to prevent clotting problems. However, aspirin in combination with certain medications can cause problems. No one should take aspirin every day without first consulting a doctor.

More controversial is whether healthy people without any risk for heart disease should take an aspirin tablet daily. Large studies now underway at Harvard and elsewhere will eventually shed light on this question.

Although the side effects of daily aspirin intake are usually limited to stomach upset, a small percentage of people do develop gastrointestinal bleeding.

Warfarin Needs Watching

Most people who are prescribed a so-called blood thinner are probably taking warfarin, sold under the trade name Coumadin. This drug interferes with the activity of vitamin K, which in turn causes depletion of several coagulation factors needed to manufacture clots. It is used to treat a wide variety of disorders.

Taken as a pill, warfarin is often started in the hospital while another anticoagulant called heparin is given intravenously. Heparin provides immediate anticoagulation. Warfarin's full effects generally take 4-6 days to build up, and it is sometimes prescribed as a solo treatment for people who are not considered to be at great danger of a clot complication. In either event, warfarin dosage will probably need to be adjusted every few weeks to produce a stable anticoagulant effect.

The risk that warfarin will inadvertently cause dangerous bleeding is proportional to the dose. In one comparison of high and low doses of the drug, both were about 98% effective in preventing clots but the risk for excess bleeding was 22% for people on the high dose and only 4% for those taking less.

Warfarin can cause other problems as well. The drug is never given to pregnant women, for example, because it can cause birth defects or fatal bleeding in the fetus. In about one in 10,000 cases, warfarin can kill skin, destroying nipples, ears, or the penis. The first sign of trouble is often a smooth, red pinpoint rash, and anyone who develops this within 48 hours of starting warfarin should seek medical attention immediately.

Check the Time

Everyone who takes warfarin needs to have his or her prothrombin time (PT) measured at regular intervals—roughly every three days for the first two weeks, and every 3-4 weeks thereafter. This simple test measures how long it takes for blood to clot. For instance, a normal PT is about 10 seconds; warfarin may prolong it to 15-30 seconds. If the PT is too long, then the risk for dangerous hemorrhage is high; on the other hand, too short a PT means that blood clots could form.

Until about five years ago, PT tests varied so greatly that results differed depending on where the test was done. Now about half of all hospitals report the PT using a standard method known as the International Normalized Ratio (INR). "If patients go on vacation and have a prothrombin test in Mexico, the result should be reported back to their personal doctor in INR units," said David J. Kuter, director of clinical hematology at Massachusetts General Hospital in Boston.

Warfarin doesn't have the same anticoagulation effect in everyone. Some people are stable on the same dose for years, others require frequent adjustment.

Monitoring is so labor intensive that many hospitals have set up special anticoagulation clinics, so that routine testing is not left to busy physicians. "It's best for a patient to be part of a system where he has his prothrombin time routinely tested and then two or three days later gets a postcard telling him to increase or decrease his dose by a specific amount," recommended Dr. Kuter. Although few insurance plans will pay for PT monitoring more than once per month, many people believe that it is worth paying the $9 to $15 that it costs for each additional test.

Food and Drugs

Because warfarin keeps blood from clotting by altering the effects of vitamin K, significant changes in diet can either inhibit or enhance the drug's effects. A person who sets out to lose weight by switching from meat and potatoes to a largely vegetarian regimen, for example, could take in enough vitamin K to keep what had been an adequate dose of warfarin from doing its job. On the other hand, the drug's effects could be magnified in people who haven't been eating much due to serious illness or in those on antibiotics. However, "if you are on a consistent diet and haven't changed your medications, then what you eat is a trivial variable," noted Dr. Kuter.

Anticoagulants

Simultaneous use of other medicines can also wreak havoc with warfarin's effects, which is an important consideration because many people who take warfarin have health problems that require other drugs as well. The most noteworthy of these is aspirin, which can increase the risk for dangerous bleeding by potentiating warfarin's influence. The same is true for other nonsteroidal anti-inflammatory drugs, high doses of penicillin, and certain other antibiotics. The flip side is that warfarin's effectiveness can be diminished by taking such drugs as barbiturates. The wisest course is not to make any major changes in diet or medications without first consulting a physician, Dr. Kuter advised.

Who Needs Anticoagulants?

When people with a history of clotting problems undergo surgery, doctors usually prescribe subcutaneous (delivered under the skin) heparin to guard against the formation of postoperative clots. There is also evidence that patients in intensive care units develop clots at higher rates than previously thought and thus may benefit from prophylactic treatment with heparin.

Warfarin is sometimes prescribed for people who have or have had a heart attack, damaged cardiac valves, valve replacement, atrial fibrillation, deep venous thrombosis, thrombophlebitis, peripheral artery disease, pulmonary embolism, or congestive heart failure.

Chapter 47

Blood Pressure–Lowering Drugs

Potential for Primary Prevention of Hypertension

Before considering the active treatment of established hypertension, the even greater need for prevention of disease should be recognized. Without primary prevention, the hypertension problem would never be solved and would rely solely on detection of existing high blood pressure. Primary prevention provides an attractive opportunity to interrupt and prevent the continuing costly cycle of managing hypertension and its complications. Primary prevention reflects a number of realities:

- A significant portion of cardiovascular disease occurs in people whose blood pressure is above the optimal level (120/80 mm Hg) but not so high as to be diagnosed or treated as hypertension. A population-wide approach to lowering blood pressure can reduce this considerable burden of risk.

- Active treatment of established hypertension, as carefully as can be provided, poses financial costs and potential adverse effects.

Excerpted from *The Sixth Report of the Joint National Committee on Prevention, Detection, Evaluation, and Treatment of High Blood Pressure*, National Heart, Lung, and Blood Institute (NHLBI), NIH Pub. No. 98-4080, November 1997. For a copy of the complete report, including references, please contact the NHLBI Information Center, P.O. Box 30105, Bethesda, MD 20824-0105, (301) 251-1222.

- Most patients with established hypertension do not make sufficient lifestyle changes, do not take medication, or do not take enough medication to achieve control.
- Even if adequately treated according to current standards, patients with hypertension may not lower their risk to that of persons with normal blood pressure.
- Blood pressure rise and high blood pressure are not inevitable consequences of aging.

Therefore, an effective population-wide strategy to prevent blood pressure rise with age and to reduce overall blood pressure levels, even by a little, could affect overall cardiovascular morbidity and mortality as much as or more than that of treating only those with established disease.

Such a population-wide approach has been promulgated. It is based on lifestyle modifications that have been shown to prevent or delay the expected rise in blood pressure in susceptible people. A recent study demonstrated that a diet rich in fruits, vegetables, and low-fat dairy foods, and with reduced saturated and total fats, significantly lowers blood pressure.

Lifestyle modifications could have an even greater impact on disease prevention and should be recommended to the entire population. Modifications that do not require active participation of individuals but that can be provided to the entire population, such as a reduction in the amount of sodium chloride added to processed foods, may be even more effective.

Lifestyle Modifications for Hypertension Prevention and Management

- Lose weight if overweight.
- Limit alcohol intake to no more than 1 oz (30 mL) ethanol (e.g., 24 oz [720 mL] beer, 10 oz [300 mL] wine, or 2 oz [60 mL] 100-proof whiskey) per day or 0.5 oz (15 mL) ethanol per day for women and lighter weight people.
- Increase aerobic physical activity (30 to 45 minutes most days of the week).
- Reduce sodium intake to no more than 100 mmol per day (2.4 g sodium or 6 g sodium chloride).

- Maintain adequate intake of dietary potassium (approximately 90 mmol per day).
- Maintain adequate intake of dietary calcium and magnesium for general health.
- Stop smoking and reduce intake of dietary saturated fat and cholesterol for overall cardiovascular health.

Pharmacologic Treatment

The decision to initiate pharmacologic treatment requires consideration of several factors: the degree of blood pressure elevation, the presence of target organ damage, and the presence of clinical cardiovascular disease or other risk factors.

Efficacy

Reducing blood pressure with drugs clearly decreases cardiovascular morbidity and mortality. Protection has been demonstrated for stroke, coronary events, heart failure, progression of renal disease, progression to more severe hypertension, and all-cause mortality.

Among older persons, treatment of hypertension has been associated with an even more significant reduction in CHD.

These results have been obtained in patients in various countries regardless of sex, age, race, blood pressure level, or socioeconomic status. Therefore, these findings can be generalized with confidence to the entire adult population with high blood pressure.

Drug Therapy Considerations

Most antihypertensive drugs currently available in the United States are listed in Tables 47.1 and 47.2. For most patients, a low dose of the initial drug choice should be used, slowly titrating upward at a schedule dependent on the patient's age, needs, and responses. The optimal formulation should provide 24-hour efficacy with a once-daily dose, with at least 50 percent of the peak effect remaining at the end of the 24 hours. Long-acting formulations that provide 24-hour efficacy are preferred over short-acting agents for many reasons: (1) adherence is better with once-daily dosing; (2) for some agents, fewer tablets incur lower cost; (3) control of hypertension is persistent and smooth rather than intermittent; and (4) protection is provided

Heart Diseases and Disorders Sourcebook, Second Edition

against whatever risk for sudden death, heart attack, and stroke that is due to the abrupt increase of blood pressure after arising from overnight sleep. Agents with a duration of action beyond 24 hours are

Table 47.1. Oral Antihypertensive Drugs* (continued on next page)

Drug	Trade Name	Usual Dose Range, Total mg/day* (Frequency per Day)	Selected Side Effects and Comments*
Diuretics (partial list)			Short-term: increases cholesterol and glucose levels; biochemical abnormalities: decreases potassium, sodium, and magnesium levels, increases uric acid and calcium levels; rare: blood dyscrasias, photosensitivity, pancreatitis, hyponatremia
Chlorthalidone (G)†	Hygroton	12.5-50 (1)	
Hydrochlorothiazide (G)	Hydrodiuril, Microzide, Esidrix	12.5-50 (1)	
Indapamide	Lozol	1.25-5 (1)	(Less or no hypercholesterolemia)
Metolazone	Mykrox	0.5-1.0 (1)	
	Zaroxolyn	2.5-10 (1)	
Loop diuretics			
Bumetanide (G)	Bumex	0.5-4 (2-3)	(Short duration of action, no hypercalcemia)
Ethacrynic acid	Edecrin	25-100 (2-3)	(Only nonsulfonamide diuretic, ototoxicity)
Furosemide (G)	Lasix	40-240 (2-3)	(Short duration of action, no hypercalcemia)
Torsemide	Demadex	5-100 (1-2)	
Potassium-sparing agents			Hyperkalemia
Amiloride hydrochloride (G)	Midamor	5-10 (1)	
Spironolactone (G)	Aldactone	25-100 (1)	(Gynecomastia)
Triamterene (G)	Dyrenium	25-100 (1)	
Adrenergic inhibitors			
Peripheral agents			
Guanadrel	Hylorel	10-75 (2)	(Postural hypotension, diarrhea)
Guanethidine monosulfate	Ismelin	10-150 (1)	(Postural hypotension, diarrhea)
Reserpine (G)**	Serpasil	0.05-0.25 (1)	(Nasal congestion, sedation, depression, activation of peptic ulcer)
Central alpha-agonists			Sedation, dry mouth, bradycardia, withdrawal hypertension
Clonidine hydrochloride (G)	Catapres	0.2-1.2 (2-3)	(More withdrawal)
Guanabenz acetate (G)	Wytensin	8-32 (2)	
Guanfacine hydrochloride (G)	Tenex	1-3 (1)	(Less withdrawal)
Methyldopa (G)	Aldomet	500-3,000 (2)	(Hepatic and "autoimmune" disorders)
Alpha-blockers			Postural hypotension
Doxazosin mesylate	Cardura	1-16 (1)	
Prazosin hydrochloride (G)	Minipress	2-30 (2-3)	
Terazosin hydrochloride	Hytrin	1-20 (1)	
Beta-blockers			Bronchospasm, bradycardia, heart failure, may mask insulin-induced hypoglycemia; less serious: impaired peripheral circulation, insomnia, fatigue, decreased exercise tolerance, hypertriglyceridemia (except agents with intrinsic sympathomimetic activity)
Acebutolol§‡	Sectral	200-800 (1)	
Atenolol (G)§	Tenormin	25-100 (1-2)	
Betaxolol§	Kerlone	5-20 (1)	
Bisoprolol fumarate§	Zebeta	2.5-10 (1)	
Carteolol hydrochloride‡	Cartrol	2.5-10 (1)	
Metoprolol tartrate (G)§	Lopressor	50-300 (2)	
Metoprolol succinate§	Toprol-XL	50-300 (1)	
Nadolol (G)	Corgard	40-320 (1)	
Penbutolol sulfate‡	Levatol	10-20 (1)	
Pindolol (G)‡	Visken	10-60 (2)	
Propranolol hydrochloride (G)	Inderal	40-480 (1)	
	Inderal LA	40-480 (1)	
Timolol maleate (G)	Blocadren	20-60 (2)	

Blood Pressure–Lowering Drugs

attractive because many patients inadvertently miss at least one dose of medication each week. Nonetheless, twice-daily dosing may offer similar control at possibly lower cost.

Table 47.1. Oral Antihypertensive Drugs* (continued)

Drug	Trade Name	Usual Dose Range, Total mg/day* (Frequency per Day)	Selected Side Effects and Comments*
Combined alpha- and beta-blockers			Postural hypotension, bronchospasm
Carvedilol	Coreg	12.5-50 (2)	
Labetalol hydrochloride (G)	Normodyne, Trandate	200-1,200 (2)	
Direct vasodilators			Headaches, fluid retention, tachycardia
Hydralazine hydrochloride (G)	Apresoline	50-300 (2)	(Lupus syndrome)
Minoxidil (G)	Loniten	5-100 (1)	(Hirsutism)
Calcium antagonists			
Nondihydropyridines			Conduction defects, worsening of systolic dysfunction, gingival hyperplasia
Diltiazem hydrochloride	Cardizem SR	120-360 (2)	(Nausea, headache)
	Cardizem CD, Dilacor XR, Tiazac	120-360 (1)	
Mibefradil dihydrochloride (T-channel calcium antagonist)	Posicor	50-100 (1)	(No worsening of systolic dysfunction; contraindicated with terfenadine [Seldane], astemizole [Hismanal], and cisapride [Propulsid])
Verapamil hydrochloride	Isoptin SR, Calan SR	90-480 (2)	(Constipation)
	Verelan, Covera HS	120-480 (1)	
Dihydropyridines			Edema of the ankle, flushing, headache, gingival hypertrophy
Amlodipine besylate	Norvasc	2.5-10 (1)	
Felodipine	Plendil	2.5-20 (1)	
Isradipine	DynaCirc	5-20 (2)	
	DynaCirc CR	5-20 (1)	
Nicardipine	Cardene SR	60-90 (2)	
Nifedipine	Procardia XL, Adalat CC	30-120 (1)	
Nisoldipine	Sular	20-60 (1)	
ACE inhibitors			Common: cough; rare: angioedema, hyperkalemia, rash, loss of taste, leukopenia
Benazepril hydrochloride	Lotensin	5-40 (1-2)	
Captopril (G)	Capoten	25-150 (2-3)	
Enalapril maleate	Vasotec	5-40 (1-2)	
Fosinopril sodium	Monopril	10-40 (1-2)	
Lisinopril	Prinivil, Zestril	5-40 (1)	
Moexipril	Univasc	7.5-15 (2)	
Quinapril hydrochloride	Accupril	5-80 (1-2)	
Ramipril	Altace	1.25-20 (1-2)	
Trandolapril	Mavik	1-4 (1)	
Angiotensin II receptor blockers			Angioedema (very rare), hyperkalemia
Losartan potassium	Cozaar	25-100 (1-2)	
Valsartan	Diovan	80-320 (1)	
Irbesartan	Avapro	150-300 (1)	

* These dosages may vary from those listed in the *Physicians' Desk Reference* (51st edition), which may be consulted for additional information. The listing of side effects is not all-inclusive, and side effects are for the class of drugs except where noted for individual drugs (in parentheses); clinicians are urged to refer to the package insert for a more detailed listing.
† (G) indicates generic available.
‡ Has intrinsic sympathomimetic activity.
§ Cardioselective.
**Also acts centrally.

Special Considerations

Special considerations in the selection of initial therapy include demographic characteristics, concomitant diseases that may be beneficially or adversely affected by the antihypertensive agent chosen

Table 47.2. Combination Drugs for Hypertension

Drug	Trade Name
Beta-adrenergic blockers and diuretics	
Atenolol, 50 or 100 mg/chlorthalidone, 25 mg	Tenoretic
Bisoprolol fumarate, 2.5, 5, or 10 mg/hydrochlorothiazide, 6.25 mg	Ziac*
Metoprolol tartrate, 50 or 100 mg/hydrochlorothiazide, 25 or 50 mg	Lopressor HCT
Nadolol, 40 or 80 mg/bendroflumethiazide, 5 mg	Corzide
Propranolol hydrochloride, 40 or 80 mg/hydrochlorothiazide, 25 mg	Inderide
Propranolol hydrochloride (extended release), 80, 120, or 160 mg/hydrochlorothiazide, 50 mg	Inderide LA
Timolol maleate, 10 mg/hydrochlorothiazide, 25 mg	Timolide
ACE inhibitors and diuretics	
Benazepril hydrochloride, 5, 10, or 20 mg/hydrochlorothiazide, 6.25, 12.5, or 25 mg	Lotensin HCT
Captopril, 25 or 50 mg/hydrochlorothiazide, 15 or 25 mg	Capozide*
Enalapril maleate, 5 or 10 mg/hydrochlorothiazide, 12.5 or 25 mg	Vaseretic
Lisinopril, 10 or 20 mg/hydrochlorothiazide, 12.5 or 25 mg	Prinzide, Zestoretic
Angiotensin II receptor antagonists and diuretics	
Losartan potassium, 50 mg/hydrochlorothiazide, 12.5 mg	Hyzaar
Calcium antagonists and ACE inhibitors	
Amlodipine besylate, 2.5 or 5 mg/benazepril hydrochloride, 10 or 20 mg	Lotrel
Diltiazem hydrochloride, 180 mg/enalapril maleate, 5 mg	Teczem
Verapamil hydrochloride (extended release), 180 or 240 mg/trandolapril, 1, 2, or 4 mg	Tarka
Felodipine, 5 mg/enalapril maleate, 5 mg	Lexxel
Other combinations	
Triamterene, 37.5, 50, or 75 mg/hydrochlorothiazide, 25 or 50 mg	Dyazide, Maxide
Spironolactone, 25 or 50 mg/hydrochlorothiazide, 25 or 50 mg	Aldactazide
Amiloride hydrochloride, 5 mg/hydrochlorothiazide, 50 mg	Moduretic
Guanethidine monosulfate, 10 mg/hydrochlorothiazide, 25 mg	Esimil
Hydralazine hydrochloride, 25, 50, or 100 mg/hydrochlorothiazide, 25 or 50 mg	Apresazide
Methyldopa, 250 or 500 mg/hydrochlorothiazide, 15, 25, 30, or 50 mg	Aldoril
Reserpine, 0.125 mg/hydrochlorothiazide, 25 or 50 mg	Hydropres
Reserpine, 0.10 mg/hydralazine hydrochloride, 25 mg/hydrochlorothiazide, 15 mg	Ser-Ap-Es
Clonidine hydrochloride, 0.1, 0.2, or 0.3 mg/chlorthalidone, 15 mg	Combipres
Methyldopa, 250 mg/chlorothiazide, 150 or 250 mg	Aldochlor
Reserpine, 0.125 or 0.25 mg/chlorthalidone, 25 or 50 mg	Demi-Regroton
Reserpine, 0.125 or 0.25 mg/chlorothiazide, 250 or 500 mg	Diupres
Prazosin hydrochloride, 1, 2, or 5 mg/polythiazide, 0.5 mg	Minizide

*Approved for initial therapy.

Blood Pressure–Lowering Drugs

(Table 47.3), quality of life, cost, and use of other drugs that may lead to drug interactions (Table 47.4). When choosing a certain drug for its favorable effect on comorbidity, clinicians should be aware that reduction of long-term cardiovascular morbidity and mortality may not have been demonstrated.

Table 47.3. Considerations for Individualizing Antihypertensive Drug Therapy*

Indication	Drug Therapy
Compelling Indications Unless Contraindicated	
Diabetes mellitus (type 1) with proteinuria	ACE I
Heart failure	ACE I, diuretics
Isolated systolic hypertension (older patients)	Diuretics (preferred), CA (long-acting DHP)
Myocardial infarction	Beta-blockers (non-ISA), ACE I (with systolic dysfunction)
May Have Favorable Effects on Comorbid Conditions†	
Angina	Beta-blockers, CA
Atrial tachycardia and fibrillation	Beta-blockers, CA (non-DHP)
Cyclosporine-induced hypertension (caution with the dose of cyclosporine)	CA
Diabetes mellitus (types 1 and 2) with proteinuria	ACE I (preferred), CA
Diabetes mellitus (type 2)	Low-dose diuretics
Dyslipidemia	Alpha-blockers
Essential tremor	Beta-blockers (non-CS)
Heart failure	Carvedilol, losartan potassium
Hyperthyroidism	Beta-blockers
Migraine	Beta-blockers (non-CS), CA (non-DHP)
Myocardial infarction	Diltiazem hydrochloride, verapamil hydrochloride
Osteoporosis	Thiazides
Preoperative hypertension	Beta-blockers
Prostatism (BPH)	Alpha-blockers
Renal insufficiency (caution in renovascular hypertension and creatinine ≥265.2 mmol/L [3 mg/dL])	ACE I
May Have Unfavorable Effects on Comorbid Conditions†‡	
Bronchospastic disease	Beta-blockers§
Depression	Beta-blockers, central alpha-agonists, reserpine§
Diabetes mellitus (types 1 and 2)	Beta-blockers, high-dose diuretics
Dyslipidemia	Beta-blockers (non-ISA), diuretics (high-dose)
Gout	Diuretics
2° or 3° heart block	Beta-blockers,§ CA (non-DHP)§
Heart failure	Beta-blockers (except carvedilol), CA (except amlodipine besylate, felodipine)
Liver disease	Labetalol hydrochloride, methyldopa§
Peripheral vascular disease	Beta-blockers
Pregnancy	ACE I,§ angiotensin II receptor blockers§
Renal insufficiency	Potassium-sparing agents
Renovascular disease	ACE I, angiotensin II receptor blockers

* For initial drug therapy recommendations, see figure 8. For references, see chapter 4, *Physicians' Desk Reference* (51st edition), and Kaplan and Gifford.[134] ACE I indicates angiotensin-converting enzyme inhibitors; BPH, benign prostatic hyperplasia; CA, calcium antagonists; DHP, dihydropyridine; ISA, intrinsic sympathomimetic activity; MI, myocardial infarction; and non-CS, noncardioselective.

† Conditions and drugs are listed in alphabetical order.

‡ These drugs may be used with special monitoring unless contraindicated.

§ Contraindicated.

Table 47.4. Selected Drug Interactions with Antihypertensive Therapy*

Class of Agent	Increase Efficacy	Decrease Efficacy	Effect on Other Drugs
Diuretics	• Diuretics that act at different sites in the nephron (e.g., furosemide + thiazides)	• Resin-binding agents • NSAIDs • Steroids	• Diuretics raise serum lithium levels. • Potassium-sparing agents may exacerbate hyperkalemia due to ACE inhibitors.
Beta-blockers	• Cimetidine (hepatically metabolized beta-blockers) • Quinidine (hepatically metabolized beta-blockers) • Food (hepatically metabolized beta-blockers)	• NSAIDs • Withdrawal of clonidine • Agents that induce hepatic enzymes, including rifampin and phenobarbital	• Propranolol hydrochloride induces hepatic enzymes to increase clearance of drugs with similar metabolic pathways. • Beta-blockers may mask and prolong insulin-induced hypoglycemia. • Heart block may occur with nondihydropyridine calcium antagonists. • Sympathomimetics cause unopposed alpha-adrenoceptor-mediated vasoconstriction. • Beta-blockers increase angina-inducing potential of cocaine.
ACE inhibitors	• Chlorpromazine or clozapine	• NSAIDs • Antacids • Food decreases absorption (moexipril)	• ACE inhibitors may raise serum lithium levels. • ACE inhibitors may exacerbate hyperkalemic effect of potassium-sparing diuretics.
Calcium antagonists	• Grapefruit juice (some dihydropyridines) • Cimetidine or ranitidine (hepatically metabolized calcium antagonists)	• Agents that induce hepatic enzymes, including rifampin and phenobarbital	• Cyclosporine levels increase† with diltiazem hydrochloride, verapamil hydrochloride, mibefradil dihydrochloride, or nicardipine hydrochloride (but not felodipine, isradipine, or nifedipine). • Nondihydropyridines increase levels of other drugs metabolized by the same hepatic enzyme system, including digoxin, quinidine, sulfonylureas, and theophylline. • Verapamil hydrochloride may lower serum lithium levels.
Alpha-blockers			• Prazosin may decrease clearance of verapamil hydrochloride.
Central alpha$_2$-agonists and peripheral neuronal blockers		• Tricyclic antidepressants (and probably phenothiazines) • Monoamine oxidase inhibitors • Sympathomimetics or phenothiazines antagonize guanethidine monosulfate or guanadrel sulfate • Iron salts may reduce methyldopa absorption	• Methyldopa may increase serum lithium levels. • Severity of clonidine hydrochloride withdrawal may be increased by beta-blockers. • Many agents used in anesthesia are potentiated by clonidine hydrochloride.

* For initial drug therapy recommendations, see figure 8. See also *Physicians' Desk Reference* (51st edition) and *Cardiovascular Pharmacotherapeutics* (New York: McGraw Hill), 1997. NSAIDs indicate nonsteroidal anti-inflammatory drugs; ACE, angiotensin-converting enzyme.

† This is a clinically and economically beneficial drug-drug interaction because it both retards progression of accelerated atherosclerosis in heart transplant recipients and reduces the required daily dose of cyclosporine.

Blood Pressure–Lowering Drugs

Demographics. Neither sex nor age usually affects responsiveness to various agents. In general, hypertension in African Americans is more responsive to monotherapy with diuretics and calcium antagonists than to beta-blockers or ACE inhibitors. However, if a beta-blocker or ACE inhibitor is needed for other therapeutic benefits, differences in efficacy usually can be overcome with reduction of salt intake, higher doses of the drug, or addition of a diuretic.

Concomitant Diseases and Therapies. Antihypertensive drugs may worsen some diseases and improve others (Table 47.3). Selection of an antihypertensive agent that also treats a coexisting disease will simplify therapeutic regimens and reduce costs.

Quality of Life. Although antihypertensive drugs may cause adverse effects in some patients (Table 47.1), quality of life is maintained and possibly improved by any of the agents recommended for initial therapy.

Physiological and Biochemical Measurements. Some clinicians have found certain physiological and biochemical measurements (e.g., body weight, heart rate, plasma renin activity, hemodynamic measurements) to be helpful in choosing specific therapy.

Economic Considerations. The cost of therapy may be a barrier to controlling high blood pressure and should be an important consideration in selecting antihypertensive medication. Generic formulations are acceptable. Nongeneric newer drugs are usually more expensive than diuretics or beta-blockers. If newer agents eventually prove to be equally effective, then cost should be considered in choosing them for initial therapy; if they prove to be more effective, then cost should be a secondary consideration. Treatment costs include not only the price of drugs but also the expense of routine or special laboratory tests, supplemental therapies, office visits, and time lost from work for visits to physicians' offices. The costs of medications may be reduced by using combination tablets and generic formulations. Patients should be advised to check prices at different sources. Some larger tablets can be divided, saving money when larger doses cost little more than smaller doses. Some sustained-release formulations should not be divided because cutting the tablet eliminates the sustained-release function.

Managed Care. Because high blood pressure is so common, its management requires a major commitment from clinicians and managed care organizations. This commitment will need to expand even further because the majority of patients with hypertension do not have adequately controlled blood pressure and additional demands will develop from the projected increase in numbers of persons with hypertension due to the aging of the population. However, the cost of managing hypertension is lower overall than the sum of direct and indirect costs that may be avoided by reducing hypertension-associated heart disease, stroke, and renal failure, especially because these adverse events often lead to expensive hospitalizations, surgical procedures, and high-cost technologies. Randomized controlled trials have demonstrated that these reductions occur in a relatively short time and are sustained for years.

Managed care programs offer the opportunity for a coordinated approach to care, using various health care professionals and featuring an appropriate frequency of office visits, short waiting times, supportive patient counseling, and controlled formularies. The outcomes of the management of hypertension will need to be monitored, in keeping with the requirements of organizations that monitor quality, such as the Health Plan Employer Data and Information Set (HEDIS). These outcomes may be divided into three categories: immediate (e.g., blood pressure levels, percentage of adherence to therapy), intermediate (e.g., cardiac or renal function, health resource utilization), and long-term (e.g., morbidity and mortality, cost-effectiveness).

Hypertension specialists may play an important role in providing more cost-effective management of high blood pressure by adapting national guidelines for local implementation, providing guidance for new drugs and diagnostic methods, and managing patients with identifiable causes of hypertension, resistance to therapy, or complex concomitant conditions.

Drug Interactions. As shown in Table 47.4, some drug interactions may be helpful. For example, diuretics that act on different sites in the nephron, such as furosemide and thiazides, increase natiuresis and diuresis, and certain calcium antagonists reduce the required amount of cyclosporine. Other interactions are deleterious: nonsteroidal anti-inflammatory drugs (NSAIDs) may blunt the action of diuretics, beta-blockers, and ACE inhibitors.

Dosage and Followup

Therapy for most patients (uncomplicated hypertension, stages 1 and 2) should begin with the lowest dosage listed in Table 47.1 to prevent adverse effects of too great or too abrupt a reduction in blood pressure. If blood pressure remains uncontrolled after 1 to 2 months, the next dosage level should be prescribed. It may take months to control hypertension adequately while avoiding adverse effects of therapy. Most antihypertensive medications can be given once daily, and this should be the goal to improve patient adherence. Home or office blood pressure measurement in the early morning before patients have taken their daily dose is useful to ensure adequate modulation of the surge in blood pressure after arising. Measurements in the late afternoon or evening help monitor control across the day. Treatment goals based on out-of-office measurements should be lower than those based on office recordings.

Initial Drug Therapy

When the decision has been made to begin antihypertensive therapy and if there are no indications for another type of drug, a diuretic or beta-blocker should be chosen because numerous randomized controlled trials have shown a reduction in morbidity and mortality with these agents.

As shown in Table 47.3, there are compelling indications for specific agents in certain clinical conditions, based on outcomes data from randomized controlled trials. In other situations where outcomes data are not yet available, there are indications for other agents and the choice should be individualized, using the agent that most closely fits the patient's needs.

If the response to the initial drug choice is inadequate after reaching the full dose, two options for subsequent therapy should be considered:

- If the patient is tolerating the first choice well, add a second drug from another class.
- If the patient is having significant adverse effects or no response, substitute an agent from another class.

If a diuretic is not chosen as the first drug, it is usually indicated as a second-step agent because its addition will enhance the effects of other agents. If the addition of a second agent controls blood pressure satisfactorily, an attempt to withdraw the first agent may be considered.

Before proceeding to each successive treatment step, clinicians should consider possible reasons for lack of responsiveness to therapy, including the following:

Heart Diseases and Disorders Sourcebook, Second Edition

- Pseudoresistance: "White-coat hypertension" or office elevations; Pseudohypertension in older patients; Use of regular cuff on a very obese arm
- Nonadherence to therapy
- Volume overload: Excess salt intake; Progressive renal damage; Fluid retention from reduction of blood pressure; Inadequate diuretic therapy
- Drug-related causes: Doses too low; Wrong type of diuretic; Inappropriate combinations; Rapid inactiviation; Drug actions and interactions
- Associated conditions: Smoking; Increasing obesity; Sleep apnea; Insulin resistance/hyperinsulinemia; Ethanol intake of more than 1 oz. per day; Anxiety-induced hyperventilation or panic attacks; Chronic pain; Intense vasoconstriction (arteritis); Organic brain syndrome (for example, memory deficit)
- Identifiable causes of hypertension

High-Risk Patients

Although similar general approaches are advocated for all patients with hypertension, modifications may be needed for those with stage 3 hypertension [blood pressure measurements of 180 systolic or 110 diastolic or higher], those in risk group C [patients who have clinically manifest cardiovascular disease, target organ damage, and/or diabetes], or those at especially high risk for a coronary event or stroke. Drug therapy should begin with minimal delay. Although some patients may respond adequately to a single drug, it is often necessary to add a second or third agent after a short interval if control is not achieved. The intervals between changes in the regimen should be decreased, and the maximum dose of some drugs may be increased. In some patients, it may be necessary to start treatment with more than one agent. Patients with average systolic blood pressure of 200 mm Hg or greater and average diastolic blood pressure of 120 mm Hg or greater require more immediate therapy and, if symptomatic target organ damage is present, may require hospitalization.

Step-Down Therapy

An effort to decrease the dosage and number of antihypertensive drugs should be considered after hypertension has been controlled effectively for at least 1 year. The reduction should be made in a deliberate, slow, and progressive manner. Step-down therapy is more often successful in patients who also are making lifestyle modifications. Patients whose drugs have been discontinued should have scheduled followup visits because blood pressure usually rises again to hypertensive levels, sometimes months or years after discontinuance, especially in the absence of sustained improvements in lifestyle.

J-Curve Hypothesis

Concerns have been raised that lowering diastolic blood pressure too much may increase the risk for coronary events by lowering diastolic perfusion pressure in the coronary circulation—the so-called J-curve hypothesis. The J-curve also has been detected in the placebo group of clinical trials of older persons with hypertension. The J-curve concern may be more relevant to patients with both hypertension and preexisting coronary disease and to those with pulse pressure greater than 60 mm Hg. On the other hand, data support a progressive reduction in both cerebrovascular disease and renal disease with even greater reductions in blood pressure. All available evidence supports the value of the reduction of diastolic blood pressure (DBP) and systolic blood pressure (SBP) at all ages to the levels achieved in clinical trials—usually DBP to below 90 mm Hg and SBP to below 140 mm Hg in patients with isolated systolic hypertension. In trials of persons with isolated systolic hypertension, no increase in cardiovascular morbidity and mortality was observed, despite further reductions of DBP.

Considerations for Adherence to Therapy

Poor adherence to antihypertensive therapy remains a major therapeutic challenge contributing to the lack of adequate control in more than two-thirds of patients with hypertension. As attempts to improve adherence are made, patients have the right and responsibility to be active and well-informed participants in their own care and to achieve maximal physical and emotional well-being. Health care professionals have the responsibility to provide patients with complete and accurate information about their health status, allowing patients the opportunity to participate in their care and to achieve goal blood pressure.

Followup Visits

Achieving and maintaining target blood pressure often requires continuing encouragement for lifestyle modification and medication adjustment. Most patients should be seen within 1 to 2 months after the initiation of therapy to determine the adequacy of hypertension control, the degree of patient adherence, and the presence of adverse effects. Associated medical problems—including target organ damage, other major risk factors, and laboratory test abnormalities—also play a part in determining the frequency of patient followup. Visits to other members of the health care team may provide opportunities for more frequent followup. Once blood pressure is stabilized, followup at 3- to 6-month intervals (depending on patient status) is generally appropriate. In some patients, particularly older persons and those with orthostatic symptoms, monitoring should include blood pressure measurement in the seated position and, to recognize postural hypotension, after standing quietly for 2 to 5 minutes.

Strategies for Improving Adherence to Therapy and Control of High Blood Pressure

Various strategies may improve adherence significantly.

- Be aware of signs of patient nonadherence to antihypertensive therapy.
- Establish the goal of therapy: to reduce blood pressure to nonhypertensive levels with minimal or no adverse effects.
- Educate patients about the disease, and involve them and their families in its treatments. Have them measure blood pressure at home.
- Maintain contact with patients; consider telecommunication.
- Keep care inexpensive and simple.
- Encourage lifestyle modifications.
- Integrate pill-taking into routine activities of daily living.
- Prescribe medications according to pharmacologic principles, favoring long-acting formulations.
- Be willing to stop unsuccessful therapy and try a different approach.
- Anticipate adverse effects, and adjust therapy to prevent, minimize, or ameliorate side effects.
- Continue to add effective and tolerated drugs, stepwise, in sufficient doses to achieve the goal or therapy.

Blood Pressure–Lowering Drugs

- Encourage a positive attitude about achieving therapeutic goals.
- Consider using nurse case management.

The choice and application of specific strategies depend on individual patient characteristics, and health care providers are not expected to apply all of them at any one time or to all patients. In particular, pharmacists should be encouraged to monitor patients' use of medications, to provide information about potential adverse effects, and to avoid drug interactions. Nurse-managed clinics offer attractive opportunities to improve adherence and outcomes. The services of other members of the health care team, such as those who provide counseling in nutrition or exercise, should be used.

Resistant Hypertension

Hypertension should be considered resistant if blood pressure cannot be reduced to below 140/90 mm Hg in patients who are adhering to an adequate and appropriate triple-drug regimen that includes a diuretic, with all three drugs prescribed in near maximal doses. For older patients with isolated systolic hypertension, resistance is defined as failure of an adequate triple-drug regimen to reduce SBP to below 160 mm Hg.

Of the various causes of true resistance, one of the most common is volume overload due to inadequate diuretic therapy. Frequently, a cause for resistance can be recognized and overcome. However, if goal blood pressure cannot be achieved without intolerable adverse effects, even suboptimal reduction of blood pressure contributes to decreased morbidity and mortality. Patients who have resistant hypertension or who are unable to tolerate antihypertensive therapy may benefit from referral to a hypertension specialist.

Chapter 48

Cholesterol-Lowering Drugs

How They Work and Who May Need Them

Too much of a good thing. That's what you've got if you have high cholesterol—one of the most common health problems Americans face.

Cholesterol is in every cell of your body, and every cell needs it. But your risk for cardiovascular disease goes up considerably if you have too much of this waxy, fatty substance in your blood.

Weight loss, a low-fat diet, and other lifestyle changes can help bring your cholesterol down. But sometimes, they aren't enough. Your cholesterol level may still put you at risk of heart attack or stroke.

Fortunately, there's now an array of powerful drugs available that can rapidly reduce your cholesterol and, ultimately, the health risks it poses.

Why You Need Cholesterol

Cholesterol is just one kind of fat (lipid) in your blood. It's often talked about as if it were a poison, but you can't live without it. It's essential to your body's cell membranes, to the insulation of your nerves and to the production of certain hormones. It also helps you digest food.

"Cholesterol-Lowering Drugs," in *Mayo Clinic Health Letter*, May 1997. Reprinted with permission of Mayo Foundation for Medical Education and Research, Rochester, MN 55905.

Your liver makes about 80 percent of the cholesterol in your body. You take in the rest when you eat animal products.

Like nutrients from digested food, cholesterol is transported throughout your body by your bloodstream. For this to happen, your body coats cholesterol with a protein. The cholesterol-protein package is called a "lipoprotein" (lip-oh-PRO-teen).

Low-density lipoprotein (LDL) cholesterol is often referred to as "bad" cholesterol. Over time, it can build up in your blood vessels with other substances to form plaque. That can cause a blockage, resulting in heart attack or stroke. In contrast, high-density lipoprotein (HDL) cholesterol is often called "good" cholesterol because it helps "clean" cholesterol from your blood vessels.

Why Do You Have High Cholesterol?

Your genes and your lifestyle choices influence how much and what kind of cholesterol you have.

Your liver may make too much LDL cholesterol or may not "clean" enough of it from your blood. Or, your liver may not make enough HDL cholesterol.

Smoking, a high-fat diet, and inactivity can also raise LDL levels and reduce HDL levels. They also affect levels of other blood lipids.

The best way to find out how much and what kind of cholesterol you have is to go to your doctor and have a blood lipids test. Home tests only give you your total cholesterol. They can't tell you how much "good" or "bad" cholesterol you have.

Table 48.1. Understanding Your Cholesterol Test

Test	Desirable	Borderline	Undesirable
Total cholesterol	Below 200	200-240	Above 240
LDL cholesterol	Below 130	130-160	Above 160
HDL cholesterol	Above 45	35-45	Below 35
Triglycerides	Below 200	200-400	Above 400

Levels given in milligrams per deciliter. Levels are for people, without known cardiovascular disease. If you have established cardiovascular disease, your physician may have different guidelines for you.

Cholesterol-Lowering Drugs

Drug Therapy

If, despite dietary changes and exercise, you still have too much bad cholesterol or not enough good (see Table 48.1), your physician may consider drug therapy. Medications can change your blood levels of cholesterol or triglycerides, another type of lipid in your blood.

By reducing LDL cholesterol or other lipids, the drugs can help prevent plaque build-up or even reduce it. And within a few months of taking them, they can help stabilize plaque already in your blood vessels. This may prevent plaque from cracking or breaking off, which can cause an obstruction or blood clot.

Types of drugs available include:

Resins: Cholestyramine (Questran) and colestipol (Colestid), both known as "resins," have been in use for about 20 years. They lower cholesterol indirectly by binding with bile acids in your intestinal tract. Bile acids are made in your liver from cholesterol and are needed for food digestion. By tying up bile acids, the drugs prompt your liver to make more bile acids. Since your liver uses cholesterol to make the acids, less cholesterol is available to reach your bloodstream.

Triglyceride-lowering drugs: Gemfibrozil (Lopid) or large doses of niacin, a vitamin, can reduce triglyceride production and remove triglycerides from circulation.

Statins: These drugs, introduced in the late 1980s, are fast becoming the most widely prescribed drugs to lower cholesterol. You may have seen them advertised and already know their names: fluvastatin (Lescol), lovastatin (Mevacor), simvastatin (Zocor), pravastatin (Pravachol) and atorvastatin (Lipitor).

Taken in tablet or capsule form, statins work directly in your liver to block a substance your liver needs to manufacture cholesterol. That depletes cholesterol in your liver cells and causes the cells to remove cholesterol from circulating blood.

Depending on the dose, statins can reduce your LDL cholesterol by up to 40 percent. That's usually enough to bring your LDL levels within recommended guidelines. Statins may also help your body reabsorb cholesterol from plaques, slowly unplugging blood vessels.

Statins are the only type of lipid-lowering drug proven to reduce your risk of death from cardiovascular disease. Along with niacin, statins have also been proven to reduce your risk of having a second heart attack.

Do You Need Medication?

If your doctor knows you have cardiovascular disease (you've had a heart attack, for example), he or she will likely prescribe medication and lifestyle changes right away if your LDL cholesterol is more than 100 milligrams per deciliter (mg/dl). The decision isn't as clear if you have high cholesterol without known cardiovascular disease.

At first, your doctor may simply recommend exercise, a low-fat diet, and other changes. But if these aren't effective, drug therapy is an option, particularly if you have other risk factors for cardiovascular disease.

Drug therapy, along with lifestyle changes, is often recommended for people without established cardiovascular disease if:

- Your LDL cholesterol is greater than 190 mg/dl after lifestyle changes, or
- Your LDL cholesterol is greater than 160 mg/dl after lifestyle changes and you have two or more risk factors.

Weighing Your Options

Which lipid-lowering drug your doctor recommends for you depends on many factors. These include how much "good" or "bad" cholesterol you have, and whether other lipids in your blood are high. Your age may also be a factor. Sometimes your doctor may recommend a combination of drugs.

The effectiveness of lipid-lowering drugs varies from person to person. There isn't one drug that's best for everyone. Nor is it necessary to take the newest drug if your current medication is effective.

The bottom line is that all lipid-lowering drugs approved by the Food and Drug Administration can reduce your "bad" cholesterol and slow plaque build-up in your blood vessels. That helps reduce your risk of cardiovascular disease—the goal of taking any of these medications.

A Long-Term Program

The decision to take any kind of lipid-lowering drug is a serious matter. Once you start, you must typically stay on the drug the rest of your life. That can be expensive. Lipid-lowering drugs can cost $200 or more a month.

Cholesterol-Lowering Drugs

You also need to have your liver checked regularly. Rarely, the drugs can cause liver damage, which is why they're not recommended if you have liver disease.

Other side effects for most lipid-lowering drugs usually aren't serious, but may be bothersome enough to keep you from taking the medication. The statins, for example, can cause muscle pain when taken in combination with other drugs, such as gemfibrozil, antifungal medications or the popular antibiotic erythromycin. However, this side effect is rare.

The resins can cause constipation and bloating, or decrease the effectiveness of other medications taken at the same time. Niacin sometimes causes irritating skin flushing and can elevate your blood sugar, aggravate a stomach ulcer or trigger an attack of gout. And gemfibrozil can cause gallstones.

In addition, because lipid-lowering drugs have only been available for about 20 years, physicians haven't been able to study their safety when used over a lifetime.

As with any medication, you should carefully weigh the advantages of taking a drug against not taking it. But if you have cardiovascular disease or are at high risk for it, lipid-lowering drugs are one of the most important treatment options you have.

Chapter 49

Heart Catheterization

What Is Heart Catheterization?

Heart catheterization is a procedure in which the doctor inserts a tube and highlights parts with a special dye and then takes x-rays of your heart.

A heart catheterization can:

- show the different chambers of the heart and major blood vessels and evaluate the anatomy and function of the valves
- record the blood pressure in chambers of the heart and blood vessels
- measure blood flow and oxygen content within the heart and lungs.

When Is It Used?

If your heart is not working normally, this test will provide a description from which the doctor can measure future changes in your heart. In particular, these tests may show if you need heart surgery and when that surgery should occur.

Examples of alternatives include:

- having an echocardiogram

Copyright 1998 Clinical Reference Systems. Reprinted with permission.

- choosing not to have treatment, recognizing the risks of your condition

You should ask your doctor about these choices.

How Do I Prepare for Heart Catheterization?

Follow any instructions your doctor may give you. No special preparation is needed for local anesthesia.

What Happens during the Procedure?

The doctor may give you a sedative to relax you and then put a local anesthetic into your groin. A local anesthetic is a drug that should keep you from feeling pain during the operation. The doctor will put a needle into the vein or artery where a catheter (tube) will be inserted for this test. If the doctor cannot insert the needle into a blood vessel near the skin, he or she may make a cut in your groin to expose an area where the vein or artery is big enough to accept the needle. This may require two or three stitches when the procedure is finished.

The doctor can use the tube to inject dye and measure blood pressure and oxygen levels.

The doctor will put some dye into the heart chambers or blood vessels of the heart and take a high-speed motion picture x-ray to see the position, shape, or function of the parts. Often dye is injected into the vessels of the walls of the heart to display narrowing or blockage of the vessels.

The doctor will remove the catheter and apply pressure over your groin to control any bleeding and assist healing.

What Happens after the Procedure?

You will remain under observation for at least 6 hours to ensure that an adequate sealing occurs on the punctured blood vessel in the groin. You may be quietly active for the rest of the day. You may have nausea and vomiting or a fever. Your leg may be swollen and blue for a day. It may feel cool, even though your circulation is OK. A swollen bruise might appear near the puncture site and be uncomfortable for a number of days.

Ask your doctor what other steps you should take and when you should come back for a checkup.

Heart Catheterization

What Are the Benefits of This Procedure?

This procedure is considered the most accurate means to gather information to help your doctor diagnose and treat heart problems.

What Are the Risks Associated with This Procedure?

- A local anesthesia may not numb the area quite enough and you may feel some minor discomfort.
- Also, in rare cases, you may have an allergic reaction to the drug used in this type of anesthesia.
- Your heart could beat in an unusual way. This could be fixed by moving the catheter or giving you medicine, electric cardioversion, or a temporary pacemaker.
- If the catheter is placed in an artery, some blood may form a clot around it where it entered. The doctor may give you a blood thinner and keep you in the hospital for a few days to help dissolve the clot.
- You may lose your pulse, which may or may not be a threat to circulation. The doctor may give you medicine for this. Rarely, surgery would be needed.
- You could have an allergic reaction to the dye and become nauseated or flushed.
- The catheter may puncture the artery and cause internal bleeding.
- Rarely, you may have a seizure during the procedure.
- While it is extremely rare, any of the above could result in death.

You should ask your doctor how these risks apply to you. Your doctor will take every possible precaution, of course, against the above risks.

When Should I Call the Doctor?

Call the doctor immediately if your groin keeps swelling where the catheter went in.

Call the doctor during office hours if:

Heart Diseases and Disorders Sourcebook, Second Edition

- You have questions about the procedure or its result.
- You want to make another appointment.

—by Informational Medical Systems, Minneapolis, MN.

Chapter 50

Procedures for Opening Blocked Arteries

Invasive Treatments

Revascularization—the re-opening of blocked arteries—is the most common procedure in heart attack patients. But revascularization is not without risks. That's why many doctors may try clot-busting drugs to re-open arteries before resorting to angioplasty or surgery. These procedures become an option if drugs are not effective and the patient continues to have chest pain or ischemia. Surgery also is used to prevent heart attacks in people who perform poorly on exercise tests or have several coronary arteries that are blocked.

The two main types of revascularization for heart disease and heart attacks are percutaneous transluminal coronary angioplasty, or PTCA, and coronary artery bypass grafting.

PTCA

PTCA is the fastest method of opening a blocked artery, provided the hospital has a cardiac catheterization facility to do immediate PTCA and cardiac surgeons available to do a bypass if that becomes necessary. The Food and Drug Administration approved the use of angioplasty in 1983; by 1993, more than 360,000 angioplasties were being done each year in the United States. Today, more patients are treated with PTCA than with coronary artery bypass surgery.

Johns Hopkins InteliHealth (www.intelihealth.com), © 1997 The Johns Hopkins University; reprinted with permission of InteliHealth.

Heart Diseases and Disorders Sourcebook, Second Edition

The purpose of PTCA is to widen coronary arteries blocked by atherosclerosis. Prior to the procedure (done in a cardiac catheterization laboratory), the patient begins to take anticoagulant medications, including aspirin. These drugs help prevent blood clots from forming around the catheter.

In the catheter laboratory, a local anesthetic is administered to deaden the site where the catheter is inserted. The patient otherwise remains awake and alert throughout the procedure. Under x-ray guidance, a tiny plastic catheter with a balloon at its end is inserted into an artery in the thigh and threaded up to the coronary arteries in the heart. A dye, which can be seen on x-ray, is injected into the catheter to aid the doctor in guiding it to the site of the blockage. Once the tip of the catheter is at the site of the blockage the balloon is inflated. The balloon may be inflated up to 10 times during the procedure and remains inflated for about one minute each time. The inflated balloon puts direct pressure on the atherosclerotic plaque in the vessel, cracking and compressing it. The interior space of the vessel widens and the outer wall of the vessel bulges a little to accommodate the plaque. When the procedure is over, the patient is given heparin and aspirin to prevent blood clots from forming.

PTCA can be effective in opening up to 95 percent of arteries, usually within 60 minutes. Within six months of the procedure, however, the opened vessel becomes blocked again in 30 to 40 percent of patients. This process is known as restenosis. One technique to prevent restenosis is to insert a stent during the PTCA procedure to keep the vessel open.

Overall, angioplasty is very safe. As with any invasive procedure, however, complications are possible. The rate of these complications can be reduced by first determining who are the best candidates for PTCA (see below). An accidental cut or tear in the vessel itself is the most serious possible consequence of angioplasty. The catheter may snag on the vessel it passes through. If that happens, the doctors must work quickly. The patient is moved to the operating room for emergency coronary artery bypass surgery. Emergency surgery is required in about 3 percent of angioplasty procedures.

Angioplasty restores blood flow through a vessel narrowed by atherosclerosis. The procedure works best on vessels that are severely narrowed, rather than completely blocked. Heart attack patients with unstable ischemia tend to be the most common candidates. Here are some points to consider before undergoing PTCA:

- Before going ahead with the procedure, the doctor must evaluate whether it is likely to be successful for you. He or she will

Procedures for Opening Blocked Arteries

consider noninvasive alternatives, such as drug therapy. If the same results can be achieved with noninvasive techniques, angioplasty should not be performed.

- The condition of the atherosclerotic plaques in question will be considered. Plaques that are not typical, such as those that are rigid, brittle, very soft, or composed of great amounts of fat, typically do not respond well to angioplasty.

- Your overall condition is also a factor. The doctor will need to consider the severity of your heart attack, your age, strength and other medical problems before deciding to go ahead with angioplasty.

- The hospital's record of success with the procedures is important. In general, hospitals that perform large numbers of angioplasties have better success rates than those that perform fewer procedures. Call the hospital or the American Heart Association at 1-800-AHA-USA1 to find out how well your hospital rates.

Stents

Stents are wire mesh tubes used to prop open an artery that has recently been widened with angioplasty. The stent is collapsed to a small diameter, placed over an angioplasty balloon catheter and maneuvered into the constricted area. When the balloon is inflated, the stent locks in place and forms a rigid support to hold the artery open.

The stent procedure is fairly common, sometimes used as an alternative to coronary artery bypass surgery. It's usually reserved for areas that are likely to re-close after angioplasty. Re-closure (called restenosis) is also a problem with the stent procedure. In recent years doctors have used stents covered with drugs that minimize changes in the blood vessel that encourage re-closure. These new stents have shown considerable promise for improving the long-term success of this procedure.

Coronary Artery Bypass Surgery

Coronary artery bypass surgery creates new pathways between the aorta and major coronary arteries blocked by atherosclerosis. By creating this detour, or bypass, blood is again able to reach parts of the heart muscle that had been blocked off.

Heart Diseases and Disorders Sourcebook, Second Edition

Before a bypass procedure is begun, the patient undergoes angiography to give the surgeon a "map" of the heart. The patient then receives a drug such as heparin to prevent clotting and is given general anesthesia. The first order of business is to connect the patient to a pump oxygenator, or heart-lung machine. That device circulates and oxygenates blood throughout the body while the heart and lungs are stilled during surgery.

During bypass surgery, the doctor uses blood vessels from other places in your body. Typically, a piece from a long vein in your leg, called the saphenous vein, is removed or one in your chest, called the mammary artery is used. A saphenous vein graft is connected to the diseased artery just below the blockage. The other end is connected to the aorta. Blood from the aorta therefore is carried through the new graft, bypassing the blockage. Once the grafts have been completed, an electric shock is delivered to start the heart pumping again. The patient is gradually weaned from the heart-lung machine over a period of a few hours.

After bypass surgery, patients should be advised to modify their diets to reduce their consumption of fat and cholesterol. They should also be advised to walk or perform other physical activity to help them regain their strength. Doctors usually recommend following a home routine of increasing activity; doing light housework, going out, visiting friends, climbing stairs. The goal is to help you return to a normal, active lifestyle.

Most people who have sedentary office jobs can return to work in four to six weeks; those with physically demanding jobs will have to wait longer and in some cases may have to find other employment.

In several new approaches, surgeons are replacing clogged arteries with less drastic alternatives by making tiny keyhole incisions between the ribs, instead of opening the entire rib cage. The new techniques, however, are mainly limited to single artery replacements whereas most bypass surgeries involve several arteries.

Deciding between angioplasty and bypass surgery can be difficult. For patients with stable angina, both procedures are safe. Increasingly, angioplasty is used if drug therapy is not successful in relieving ischemia, or chest pain. Because angioplasty is less invasive than bypass surgery, patients recover from it more quickly. However, bypass surgery usually has slightly better results in the first year. In general, a surgeon will do bypass surgery if you have atherosclerotic plaques in more than one coronary artery, if angioplasty was not successful, or if your atherosclerotic plaque is unusually rigid or soft.

Procedures for Opening Blocked Arteries

Atherectomy

Atherectomy is done in the catheterization laboratory to open coronary arteries blocked by plaque. A rotating shaver, which is a disk or burr device on the end of a catheter, is introduced through an artery in the leg (or arm) and threaded through the blood vessels into the blocked coronary artery. The tip of the catheter has a high-speed rotating device that grinds the plaque up into minute particles. One such device, called the Rotablator, rotates at close to 200,000 rpm, grinding away plaque material that blocks arteries. If necessary, balloon angioplasty may then be used on the artery treated with atherectomy.

Laser Angioplasty

This technique is used in some people to open coronary arteries blocked by plaque. A catheter with a laser at the tip is inserted into an artery and advanced through the blood vessels to the blocked coronary artery. The laser emits pulsating beams of light that vaporize the plaque. This procedure has been used alone and in conjunction with balloon angioplasty. The first laser device (the Excimer laser) for opening coronary arteries was approved by the Food and Drug Administration in 1992. The procedure, which is done under local anesthesia, is available at many major medical centers in the United States.

Chapter 51

Angioplasty

What is angioplasty?

Angioplasty is a procedure in which a cardiologist inserts a balloon catheter into a blocked artery. The blockage may be in an artery in your arm or leg, or in a coronary artery (a blood vessel supplying blood to the heart).

A catheter is a thin tube inserted into a blood vessel either at the elbow or groin. The catheter is pushed through the inside of the blood vessel so that the tip of the catheter is at the point of the blockage in the artery. Inflating a balloon at the tip of the catheter stretches the narrowed artery. The doctor then removes the catheter and balloon. The stretching of the artery allows blood to flow normally through the artery again.

When is angioplasty used?

Angioplasty is used to treat blocked arteries in the heart (coronary artery disease) and in the limbs, especially the legs (peripheral vascular disease).

How do I prepare for angioplasty?

- Plan for your care and transportation after the procedure and during recovery at home.
- Before surgery, the doctor will ask you to sign a consent form for angioplasty, bypass surgery, and angiography. (Angiography

Copyright 1998 Clinical Reference Systems. Reprinted with permission.

is an x-ray study of the blood vessels using dye.) This consent form is needed in case complications arise during the angioplasty and emergency surgery is needed.

- The doctor will ask you not to eat or drink anything after midnight on the night before the procedure.
- The doctor will order blood tests, an electrocardiogram (ECG), and a chest x-ray.
- The area where the catheter is inserted (arm or groin) will be shaved and washed with antibacterial soap to prevent infection.
- You will be given an intravenous line (tube into a vein) and medications to relax you before the procedure is performed.

What happens during the procedure?

Before angioplasty, you will be given a local anesthetic where the catheter will be inserted. Using x-ray imaging, a doctor will insert a thin wire into the blocked artery through a needle he or she has inserted into the blood vessel in your arm or groin.

The doctor will guide a catheter with a balloon at the tip along the wire. When the catheter has reached the narrowed artery or vessel, the balloon will be inflated and deflated several times, widening the blocked passageway. Then the doctor will remove the deflated balloon, catheter, and wire.

What happens after the procedure?

After angioplasty, you will stay in a cardiac care unit or a hospital room for several hours to a day or two, depending on the location of the blockage and your medical condition.

If the catheter was inserted into your groin, you will have to lie flat on your back and not move your leg or groin for about 6 hours. A sandbag may be placed on your groin to apply pressure and prevent excess bleeding.

You will be up and walking in 12 to 24 hours after the procedure.

While in the hospital your heart and circulation will be monitored carefully. When your condition is stable, you will be released to rest at home.

What are the benefits of this procedure?

- It can restore the function of the artery without major surgery.

Angioplasty

- It does not require removing blood vessels from another part of your body (as is often necessary in bypass surgery).
- It can be performed without using general anesthesia.

What are the risks associated with this procedure?

- You may have an allergic reaction to the local anesthetic or x-ray dye.
- There may be excessive bleeding that requires additional medications or transfusion.
- There may be damage to the artery, such as the creation of a hole (perforation) during the procedure. Emergency bypass surgery or repair of the perforation would then be required.
- There is a risk of heart injury during the procedure, including a disturbance of your heart's rhythm or heart attack.
- There is a risk of injury to the arm or leg, including the possibility of amputation, if the blockage worsens or cannot be opened.
- There is a possibility of a stroke.

Ask your doctor how these risks apply to you.

When should I call the doctor?

Call the doctor immediately if:

- You have chest pain or persistent or worsening pain in your arm or leg.
- You develop a fever.
- You develop shortness of breath.
- You develop a blue, cold arm or leg.
- You develop bleeding or large swelling where the catheter was inserted.

Call the doctor during office hours if:

- You have questions about the procedure or its result.
- You want to make another appointment.

Chapter 52

Coronary Artery Bypass Surgery

What Is Coronary Artery Bypass Surgery?

Coronary artery bypass surgery is a procedure in which a blockage in a coronary artery is bypassed to restore normal blood flow through the artery. Coronary arteries are blood vessels that carry oxygen and nutrients to the heart. The blockage can be bypassed with a new vessel made from synthetic material or from part of one of your veins (usually from the leg).

When Is It used?

Coronary artery bypass surgery may be necessary when arteries to your heart become narrowed or blocked. If more than one artery is blocked, you may need more than one bypass.

The location and degree of coronary artery blockages are determined before surgery with a procedure called heart catheterization, or coronary angiogram.

How Do I Prepare for Coronary Bypass Surgery?

The night before surgery you will not be allowed to eat or drink after midnight. In the morning you will be weighed; later you will be weighed again so your doctor can see if you are retaining water. To prevent infection, your legs, groin, and chest (if necessary) are shaved.

Copyright 1998 Clinical Reference Systems. Reprinted with permission.

You should take a shower before going to bed. You may be given a mild sedative to help you relax before the anesthetic is given.

What Happens during the Procedure?

Coronary artery bypass surgery is performed by a team of surgeons and lasts from 2 to 6 hours, depending on how many blood vessels need to be bypassed. One incision is made in the center of the chest at the breastbone to expose the heart. Another incision may be made in the leg to remove a vein for the new blood vessel that will bypass the blockage. (Otherwise, synthetic material or an artery in the chest is used.) You are then connected to a heart-lung machine that supplies oxygen to your blood and circulates it back into your body while the surgery is performed.

The new blood vessel is sewn into the blocked artery above and below the areas of blockage. The blood then uses this new vessel as a detour to bypass the blockage before returning to its normal path.

When the surgery is finished, you are disconnected from the heart-lung machine, your breastbone is closed with wire, and your chest is closed with stitches or staples.

What Happens after the Procedure?

After surgery, you are placed in an intensive care unit (ICU) for several days for observation and monitoring. A constant electrocardiogram (ECG) monitor will record the rhythm of your heart.

You will receive respiratory therapy to prevent any complications in your lungs, such as a collapsed lung, infection, or pneumonia. A nurse or therapist will give you a breathing treatment every few hours. It is extremely important to cooperate and ask for pain medication if you need it.

Therapy may include:

- deep breathing exercises
- coughing while holding a pillow against your chest to protect your breastbone
- chest percussion, which is a gentle slapping on the back to help loosen lung secretions that may have accumulated after surgery
- moving your legs to reduce the chance of blood clots

While in the ICU, you may have the following tubes in your body to help in recovery:

Coronary Artery Bypass Surgery

- a breathing tube in your mouth that goes into your lungs and is connected to a ventilator to help you breathe
- a tube through your nose and down to your stomach to drain out natural fluids that may cause discomfort when you are not eating
- a catheter to empty your bladder
- intravenous (IV) tubes in your arms or possibly near your collarbone for fluids, nutrition, and medications
- chest tubes to drain blood from your chest cavity and to help detect any excessive bleeding in your chest
- an arterial line in your forearm to measure the pressure of the blood flowing through the arteries

Some time during the first 1 to 3 days after surgery, the tubes are removed and you are moved to an intermediate care unit. You will stay in this unit until you are ready to leave the hospital. You will participate in physical therapy that includes walking around the hospital and other strengthening activities. You will be taught how to move your upper arms without hurting your breastbone, and you will receive more respiratory therapy. You will be told about specific foods to avoid when you get home, such as foods high in fat, cholesterol, and sodium. Occupational therapy will help you learn how to take it easy while doing daily activities.

What Are the Risks Associated with This Procedure?

- Depending on your age and the condition of your heart, there is about a 2% to 10% risk of death from this operation.
- There will be some stress to your heart during the anesthesia.
- There is a risk of infection or bleeding from this procedure.
- A bypassed vessel may become blocked again, which might require another heart catheterization and surgery.

How Can I Take Care of Myself?

Follow the full treatment prescribed by your doctor, including all medications. In addition:

- Get plenty of rest.

- Plan at least two rest periods during the day (more if you still are tired).
- Enjoy the support and visits of family and friends, but keep visits short and allow yourself to rest.
- Learn deep breathing and relaxation techniques.
- Talk about your feelings.
- Stop smoking.
- Lose weight slowly if you are overweight.
- Follow a healthy, well-balanced diet that is low in salt, saturated fats, and cholesterol.
- Weigh yourself every morning to help detect a water retention problem.
- Develop a regular exercise program prescribed by your doctor.
- If you feel constipated, ask your doctor for a stool softener or a fiber-based laxative. (Constipation is a common problem after having anesthesia and being physically inactive.)
- Wear support hose to prevent swelling and circulatory problems in your legs. Putting powder on your legs can help you pull hose on more easily. Smooth out any wrinkles to avoid pressure spots.

How Can I Prevent Problems from Occurring during Recovery?

- Follow you doctor's recommended schedule of activity after surgery.
- Have someone help you with your bath or shower if you feel dizzy. Consider using a waterproof chair in the shower for safety.
- Avoid extremely hot water in your shower, bath, or hot tub because it can affect your circulation and cause lightheadedness.
- Initially, avoid lifting anything heavier than 5 to 10 pounds.
- Avoid mowing the lawn, mopping, vacuuming, driving, and any other activities that strain your upper arms and chest until you have recovered.

Coronary Artery Bypass Surgery

- Avoid driving and sexual intercourse until your doctor tells you it's okay to resume these activities.
- Ask your doctor whether you can drink any alcoholic beverages.

When Should I Call the Doctor?

Call the doctor immediately if:

- You develop a fever.
- You become short of breath.
- You have worsening chest pain.

Call the doctor during office hours if:

- You have questions about the procedure or its result.
- You want to make another appointment.

—Developed by Clinical Reference Systems, Ltd.

Chapter 53

A Closer Look at Chelation Therapy: Does It Work?

The claims are dramatic and attention-grabbing:

- Cut your risk of heart attack by 85 percent
- Reduce leg and chest pain
- Improve your cardiovascular function

If you're concerned about heart disease, you may be aware that the source for these claims is chelation (key-LAY-shun) therapy, a controversial alternative medical treatment for atherosclerosis.

The claims sound intriguing. But are they accurate? Is chelation therapy a safe and effective option that can eliminate the need for costly bypass surgery or angioplasty? Or is it yet another case of "if it sounds too good to be true, it probably is"? Only a closer look at the facts about chelation therapy can help you decide.

Getting the Lead Out

Chelation therapy began—and still is approved and widely used—as a treatment for lead poisoning. A chemical called EDTA is injected into the bloodstream where it locates metals and binds to them. In this bound state, the metals pass more easily out of the body through the kidneys and urinary tract.

Mayo Clinic Health Oasis, April 17, 1996. Reprinted with permission of Mayo Foundation for Medical Education for Medical Education and Research, Rochester, MN 55905.

The doctor who pioneered chelation therapy for lead poisoning in the early 1950s, Norman E. Clarke, Sr., M.D., noticed that, in addition to removing the poison, chelation also showed evidence of improving heart health. He speculated that EDTA was helping to remove calcium, a component in the plaque that hardens and constricts arteries. It seemed as if chelation therapy was opening diseased arteries.

Clarke and others continued to use and recommend chelation therapy through the 1950s as a treatment for atherosclerosis. However, rigorous scientific studies were never performed.

Who Do You Trust?

In recent years, interest in chelation therapy has increased along with the attention given alternative medicine. But does chelation and the chemical binding of EDTA with calcium in an arterial plaque have a solid, scientifically proven basis? According to a wide range of authorities, including the U.S. Food and Drug Administration (FDA), the National Institutes of Health and the American College of Cardiology, the answer is no.

The reason? All of these groups agree on an important fact: In the decades since Dr. Clarke's initial work, there have been no properly controlled scientific studies to show that chelation therapy actually works as advertised.

Dr. Morie Gertz, a professor of medicine at Mayo Medical School, Rochester, Minn., sums up the current situation this way: "While the risks from chelation therapy are low, there is still no scientific proof of any benefits to cardiac health. And, while chelation is less expensive than other options, it's not cheap. Costs run in the thousands of dollars and typically are not covered by insurance, including Medicare," according to Dr. Gertz.

Some cardiologists caution that calcium is just one component of the plaque that blocks blood vessels. Atherosclerosis is a complex mixture of cholesterol and other lipids, fibrous tissue and calcium. Removal of calcium alone does not deal with the major obstructive components of the plaque.

Conspiracy Theories?

This view sometimes leads proponents of chelation to suggest a disinterest, if not an outright conspiracy, among "mainline" medical groups to keep chelation therapy from the public. Dr. Gertz discounts those claims. "The fact is that the FDA is required by law to evaluate a new drug regimen if it is submitted with appropriate data. Likewise, all the major medical organizations have study groups and task forces dedicated to exploring and evaluating alternative medical treatments. The problem with chelation therapy is its proponents still have not produced the data to justify further scientific consideration," Dr. Gertz said.

Get Information

If you'd like more information on the controversy over chelation therapy, the American Heart Association (AHA) offers a free, easy-to-read booklet called "Questions and Answers About Chelation Therapy." Contact your local AHA chapter or call 1-800-242-8721 and ask for publication #50-074-A.

Chapter 54

New Treatments for Rhythm Disorders

Two-time Olympic gold-medalist skater Sergei Grinkov shocked the world in fall 1995, when he collapsed on the ice rink and died hours later at the young age of 28. A blood clot that blocked blood flow to his heart triggered it to quiver instead of beat. Medical technicians were unable to restore a normal heart rhythm, and by the time he reached a hospital, Grinkov's heart had stopped beating altogether.

Grinkov suffered what is known as ventricular fibrillation. This inefficient and deadly quivering of the heart is one of several types of irregular heartbeats, or arrhythmias, that afflict the lower chambers, called the ventricles, of the heart. Not all arrhythmias are ventricular; some, for example, arise from the upper chambers of the heart.

Ventricular arrhythmias often occur in people with various forms of heart disease and, according to the American Heart Association, cause most cases of sudden cardiac death. But new drugs and devices show promise in curbing the number of deaths from this condition. These new treatments, approved by the Food and Drug Administration, include a longer-acting form of an antiarrhythmia drug, a wide availability of portable and implantable electrical devices that can spark a return to normal heart rhythm, and techniques for destroying heart tissue that triggers ventricular arrhythmias.

FDA Consumer, April 1997, vol. 31, no. 3, p. 12(4).

Heart of the Matter

Not much bigger than a fist, the human heart beats 100,000 times each day, sending about 2,000 gallons of blood coursing through vessels, which, laid end-to-end, would be long enough to circle the earth more than twice.

To carry out the vital task of pumping blood, the electrical timing of millions of heart cells must be exquisitely coordinated. Their timing sparks the heart to pump in a rhythmic, efficient fashion. When that coordination is disrupted, life-threatening ventricular arrhythmias result.

Each heartbeat normally starts in the upper right chamber of the heart, or right atrium. Here, a specialized bunch of cells called the sinus node, or pacemaker, sends an electrical signal. The signal spreads throughout the right and left atria and then travels along specific pathways to the lower chambers or ventricles. As the signal travels, the heart muscle contracts. First the atria (the upper right and left chambers) contract, pumping blood into the ventricles. A fraction of a second later, the ventricles contract in a squeezing motion, sending blood throughout the body. Each contraction is a heartbeat.

Ventricular arrhythmias occur when a group of heart cells in the ventricles triggers contractions out of sync with the normal rhythm established by the sinus node. A number of factors can prompt a ventricular arrhythmia, including stress, exercise, caffeine, tobacco, alcohol, amphetamines, tricyclic antidepressant drugs, and cough and cold medicines containing pseudoephedrine, as well as several drugs (such as diuretics and digitalis) used to treat various heart conditions.

Many types of heart disease also are associated with ventricular arrhythmias. Atherosclerosis, the buildup of plaque on artery walls, can reduce blood flow to heart tissue. That, in turn, can impede the transmission of electrical signals governing heart contractions. This can prompt groups of ventricle cells to generate their own "back-up" rhythm. In the extreme case of a heart attack, blood flow to specific parts of the heart muscle is completely blocked, and that heart tissue dies. If the affected area includes cells in the electrical pathways of the heart, arrhythmias ensue.

People with enlarged hearts or faulty heart valves also are prone to experiencing ventricular arrhythmias. Ventricular arrhythmias also commonly occur after heart attacks, heart infections, or heart surgery, or when the body is under severe physical stress from, for example, lack of oxygen, very low blood pressure, or major blood loss. They also are triggered by heart failure, surgery, and other conditions that cause abnormal blood and tissue concentrations of potassium, magnesium, sodium, or calcium. These minerals play key roles in triggering and conducting electrical impulses in the heart.

Harmless or Deadly Beats

Ventricular arrhythmias can be either deadly or innocuous, depending on their type and persistence and whether the person's heart function is already compromised. The most common type of ventricular arrhythmia in both healthy and diseased individuals is the ventricular premature beat. The incidence of this condition increases with age.

A premature beat occurs when there is an extra contraction of the ventricles midway between two normal contractions or shortly after a normal contraction. In the latter case, they can delay the next heartbeat prompted by the natural pacemaker.

Ventricular premature beats often do not prompt symptoms, but they may be perceived as skipped beats or fluttering or thumping in the chest known as heart palpitations, and they may cause dizziness or weakness. Probably everyone develops ventricular premature beats at one time or another, according to the American Heart Association. This type of arrhythmia is commonly encountered in cardiac monitoring, even in healthy individuals.

Ventricular premature beats are not by themselves harmful, but they can be a precursor to two more serious types of ventricular arrhythmias: ventricular tachycardia and ventricular fibrillation.

Ventricular tachycardia is rapid heartbeat that arises from the lower chambers of the heart and is usually much faster than the normal heart rate of 60 to 100 times per minute. Ventricular tachycardia is considered "nonsustained" if it lasts only seconds or "sustained" if it lasts for more than 30 seconds. Like ventricular premature beats, ventricular tachycardias commonly occur in healthy people, particularly those who are frightened or excited.

Ventricular tachycardias prevent ventricles from properly filling with blood. This reduces pumping efficiency, which can be made worse if there are underlying heart muscle abnormalities. Nonsustained ventricular tachycardias may cause no noticeable symptoms, or they may be felt as palpitations. When sustained, however, tachycardias often cause palpitations, as well as weakness, dizziness, chest pain, and breathing difficulties. Particularly rapid or long-lasting ventricular tachycardias or sustained tachycardias in people whose heart function is already compromised by disease can cause loss of consciousness or lead to fatal cardiac arrest.

A ventricular tachycardia can degenerate into ventricular fibrillation, which is an extremely rapid, chaotic rhythm that starts in the ventricles and causes the heart to quiver. Such quivering prevents the heart from pumping blood to the rest of the body. The onset of a ventricular fibrillation is dramatic: People suddenly lose consciousness and collapse in a shock-like state. Their pulse, heartbeat and blood pressure cannot be detected, and death occurs in minutes without effective treatment. A common cause of ventricular fibrillation is a heart attack.

Emergency Care

Patients with ventricular fibrillation must be treated immediately with one or more electric shocks to the heart, which are transmitted externally with defibrillator paddles placed on the chest. Severe ventricular tachycardias also must often be treated with defibrillators.

Defibrillators tend to synchronize the heart's electrical system. "By giving a shock you start things from scratch again and organize a disorganized rhythm," said Andrew Epstein, M.D., of the University of Alabama at Birmingham.

Defibrillators may become more readily available as a result of FDA's approval in September 1996 of a smaller portable version that may be particularly beneficial to police officers, firefighters, flight attendants, and others who may be the first to respond to cardiac emergencies and can now equip their vehicles with the compact units.

Once the heartbeat has been restored, patients usually are given lidocaine hydrochloride (Xylocaine) or bretylium tosylate (Bretylol) intravenously to stabilize their heart rhythm.

The Telltale Heart

The safety and effectiveness of long-term arrhythmia treatment depend on accurate diagnosis. Sometimes ventricular arrhythmias can be detected by listening to the heart with a stethoscope. The diagnostic tool of choice, though, is the electrocardiogram (ECG or EKG), which shows the relative timing of atrial and ventricular electrical events. ECG's generate telltale spikes, whose characteristic rhythm and shape identify the specific type of arrhythmia.

To make an ECG, a technician attaches several electrodes to the chest and sometimes the limbs. The electrodes detect electrical activity that is recorded on a moving strip of paper or projected on a computer-like screen. The procedure is harmless and painless.

New Treatments for Rhythm Disorders

Because of the fleeting nature of many arrhythmias, they may not occur while the ECG is running, and so they may go undetected on the ECG. In these cases, doctors may ask patients to wear a small portable ECG recorder, called a Holter monitor, for 24 hours. This device, about the size of a tape recorder, records continuous electrocardiographic signals or selectively records arrhythmias causing symptoms. Holter monitoring requires patients to wear electrodes continuously on their chests during the 24 hours.

ECG's of arrhythmias with symptoms that occur less frequently than daily can be transmitted via the telephone to a doctor's office or a hospital with a hand-held device called an event monitor. This monitor converts ECG signals into tones that travel over a telephone line and are then converted to paper tracings. If a telephone is not available at the time the arrhythmia occurs, the ECG signals can be recorded and stored in the device's memory for transmission later. For such transtelephonic monitoring, patients place electrodes on their chests only when they are experiencing symptoms.

Another diagnostic option for infrequent arrhythmias is to provoke them purposely through exercise or with electrical devices. For example, a patient whose arrhythmias are thought to be prompted by exercise may undergo a treadmill workout while his or her heart activity is being monitored by an ECG device.

An arrhythmia also may be induced with electrophysiologic testing. In this procedure, electrodes are attached to small tubes known as electrode catheters, which are threaded through arm or leg veins until they reach the heart. There, they are placed at strategic positions in the ventricles, atria or both.

These electrodes record electrical signals and allow doctors to "map" the spread of electrical impulses during each heartbeat. The electrodes also can electrically stimulate the heart at programmed rates to trigger latent ventricular tachycardias. These arrhythmias are then stopped by electrical stimuli transmitted via the electrode catheters. An externally applied shock may be required if the patient loses consciousness during the tachycardia.

Being able to "turn on" tachycardias during electrophysiologic testing allows doctors to test anti-arrhythmic drugs quickly for effectiveness. It also can indicate the electrically blocked areas of the heart responsible for triggering a patient's arrhythmia. If these areas are limited in size and number, destruction of them is a treatment option.

Cardiologists usually reserve electrophysiologic testing for patients whose arrhythmias do not occur during ECG monitoring or are not controlled by their current medication. Electrophysiologic testing is considered safe, although rare complications, such as bleeding, infection, perforation of the heart, and fatal arrhythmias, can occur.

Preventive Treatment

Before starting any preventive drug treatment regimen, doctors first try to rule out reversible causes of ventricular arrhythmias: for example, caffeine, alcohol and tobacco consumption, and certain over-the-counter and prescribed medicines.

Also, because treatments pose substantial risks relative to the risk of the arrhythmias themselves, doctors tend not to treat ventricular arrhythmias unless they are tied to significant symptoms or are life-threatening. For this reason, FDA has not approved any treatments for premature ventricular beats.

However, there are several drugs approved for preventing ventricular tachycardia. The main types are beta blockers and sodium or potassium channel blockers. Most drugs to prevent ventricular tachycardias are taken orally up to four times daily and often must be taken for life.

Beta blockers, such as propranolol hydrochloride (Inderal and others), stem the automatic stimulation of heart contractions by the nervous system. Sodium and potassium channel blockers hamper transmission of electrical impulses in heart cells. Some sodium channel blockers are quinidine (Quinidex Extentabs, Quinaglute and others) and procainamide hydrochloride (Procan, Pronestyl and others). FDA approved in February 1996 a long-acting form of procainamide, Procanbid, which is taken only twice a day, compared with other procainamides, which must be taken four times daily.

Potassium channel blockers, such as amiodarone hydrochloride (Cordarone) and sotalol (Betapace), also are used to prevent ventricular tachycardias.

Doctors monitor the effectiveness of antiarrhythmia drug therapy with an ECG, or with electrophysiologic testing. Monitoring is essential not only to ensure effectiveness but safety, as well, because many of these drugs can make arrhythmias worse. Other side effects of antiarrhythmia drugs that can limit their use are low blood pressure, lung damage, nausea, and dizziness.

According to Wilber Aronow, M.D., a cardiologist with Mount Sinai School of Medicine in New York City, studies show that people treated with certain beta blockers following a heart attack have a significantly reduced risk of sudden cardiac death. But many large-scale studies of several different types of sodium channel blockers, as well as studies of certain potassium channel blockers, have shown that treatment with these drugs following heart attacks does not improve survival odds, or reduce them.

Ventricular arrhythmias are common within a month of a heart attack and are associated with an increased risk of sudden cardiac death.

An Internal Jolt

Another treatment option for people at risk for life-threatening arrhythmias is an implanted cardioverter defibrillator. FDA approved the first implantable defibrillators more than 10 years ago.

Today's device typically consists of a generator slightly smaller than the size of a wallet attached to electrode catheters. The generator is surgically placed under or over chest or abdominal muscles. The catheters are threaded through veins to their permanent positions in the heart. Complications of implanting defibrillators are rare but serious and include bleeding, infections, and perforation of the heart.

Implanted defibrillators monitor the heart rhythm and automatically treat, with electrical stimuli or shocks, rhythms recognized as abnormal. Newer devices also can record and store data of the electrical activity of the heart that doctors can later download and evaluate for arrhythmias. The data also can be used to perform electrophysiologic testing.

Implanted defibrillators can often stem ventricular arrhythmias with low-energy shocks. Sometimes, however, high-energy shocks are needed. These shocks, though short-lasting, can be painful—somewhat akin to a kick in the chest.

The generators in implanted defibrillators usually last three to five years and can be replaced with a surgical procedure that usually requires only local anesthesia. The electrode leads tend to last longer, although they can develop cracks or component failures that require their replacement.

A recent study of heart attack survivors by Arthur Moss and colleagues from the University of Rochester (N.Y.) Medical Center found implantable defibrillators cut survivors' risk of death in half.

A National Heart, Lung, and Blood Institute study under way is assessing whether implanted defibrillators or drug therapy is more effective in extending the lives of patients with ventricular arrhythmias.

Opening the Chest

Open-heart surgery to remove heart tissue causing or contributing to arrhythmias may be warranted for patients whose ventricular arrhythmias cannot be controlled by drugs. But, this is feasible only for patients whose arrhythmias can be attributed to heart sites that are limited in size and number. Most patients who undergo this procedure survive.

To avoid the risks and painful recovery of this procedure, a number of clinical investigators have used radiofrequency energy, delivered via catheters threaded through veins to the heart, to destroy heart tissue at the root of ventricular arrhythmias. FDA has not yet fully evaluated the safety and effectiveness of this experimental procedure.

But the availability of other treatment options means that many patients with ventricular arrhythmias can be treated effectively.

That wasn't true a decade ago, cardiologist Epstein points out. "We're a lot further along."

—by Margie Patlak

Margie Patlak is writer in Elkins Park, PA.

Chapter 55

Pacemaker Implantation

What is a pacemaker implantation?

A pacemaker implantation is a procedure in which the doctor places a pacemaker in your chest cavity.

When is it used?

This procedure is done when the rhythm of your heart is not normal. As a result of the abnormal rhythm, your heart beats inefficiently, causing symptoms such as fatigue and shortness of breath.

An alternative to this procedure is to take drugs to control the heart rhythm or to choose not to have treatment, recognizing the risks of your condition. You should ask your doctor about these choices.

How do I prepare for pacemaker implantation?

Plan for your care and recovery after the operation, especially if you are to have general anesthesia. Allow for time to rest and try to find people to help you with your day-to-day duties.

Follow any instructions your doctor may give you. If you are to have general anesthesia, eat a light meal, such as soup or salad, the night before the procedure. Do not eat or drink anything after midnight and the morning before the procedure. Do not even drink coffee, tea, or water.

No special preparation is needed for local anesthesia.

Copyright 1998 Clinical Reference Systems. Reprinted with permission.

What happens during the procedure?

You will be given a local anesthetic or a general anesthetic. A general anesthetic will relax your muscles and make you feel as if you are in a deep sleep. It will prevent you from feeling pain during the operation. A local anesthetic is a drug that should keep you from feeling pain during the operation.

The nurse will wash your upper chest and sometimes shave the area. The doctor will make a cut in the skin over the upper chest and separate the tissues to make a place for the pacemaker generator. The doctor will place a wire into a vein and guide it to the inner surface of the heart cavity. The doctor connects this wire to the pacemaker generator and places this unit beneath the skin.

What happens after the procedure?

You may stay in the hospital for 1 to 3 days, depending on your condition. You will remain in bed and your heart will be monitored. The day after the procedure you will be encouraged to walk in preparation for leaving the hospital. Before you are discharged, the doctor may check the pacemaker with a monitoring device to have a baseline (starting point) with which to compare the follow-up calls. You will learn how to use a telephone transmitter to call the doctor's office and check the function of the pacemaker. The doctor may also explain how having a pacemaker might affect your lifestyle and the expected or average time before the battery in the pacemaker may need to be replaced.

You should ask your doctor what other steps you should take and when you should come back for a checkup.

What are the benefits of this procedure?

Your heart may beat in a healthy rhythm, and you may resume a more normal lifestyle.

What are the risks associated with this procedure?

- There are some risks when you have general anesthesia. Discuss these risks with your doctor.

- A local anesthesia may not numb the area quite enough and you may feel some minor discomfort. Also, in rare cases, you may have an allergic reaction to the drug used in this type of anesthesia. Local anesthesia is considered safer than general anesthesia.

Pacemaker Implantation

- The wire could puncture one of the lungs, the vein, or the heart cavity.
- The pacemaker is implanted because the heart is not working normally. The heart problem may still recur or get worse during or after this procedure.
- Like any electrical/mechanical device, the pacemaker may need a replacement if it stops working properly.
- The pacemaker wire may become dislodged and/or break.
- There is a risk of infection and/or bleeding.

You should ask your doctor how these risks apply to you.

When should I call the doctor?

Call the doctor immediately if your pulse becomes abnormally slow, fast, or irregular, or your original symptoms return.

Call the doctor during office hours if:

- You have questions about the procedure or its result.
- You want to make another appointment.

— by Informational Medical Systems, Minneapolis, MN

Chapter 56

Implantable Defibrillators

Implanted Defibrillators Save More Lives than Drugs

A new study finds that implanted defibrillators—mini cassette-sized devices that continuously monitor heart rhythm and deliver precisely calibrated electrical shocks when needed—are better at saving lives than drug therapy for a select group of heart patients.

So convincing were the findings that the National Institutes of Health (NIH), which sponsored the study, ended it a year early and issued a statement advising certain heart patients on anti-arrhythmic medication to ask their doctors about switching to an implantable cardiac defibrillator (ICD).

This news is important to people with rapid heart rhythms known as ventricular tachycardia and ventricular fibrillation. People with ventricular (versus atrial) heart disturbances carry a greater risk for fainting (syncope) and sudden cardiac arrest.

In the first year of the 1,016-patient study, people at moderate risk of death from a ventricular arrhythmia were 38 percent less likely to die if they had an implanted defibrillator than if they were treated with drugs, the NIH said.

This chapter includes information from two documents: "Implanted Defibrillators Save More Lives than Drugs" (April 29, 1997). Reprinted with permission of Mayo Foundation for Medical Education and Research, Rochester, MN 55905. And, "Implantable Defibrillator Can Aid People with Dangerously Irregular Heartbeats." Copyright 1999 by the Cardiovascular Institute of the South. Reprinted with permission.

"This study makes it clearer how best to treat people who have life-threatening arrhythmias, people who have suffered an episode of sudden cardiac arrest, or who have ventricular tachycardia," notes Dr. Marshall S. Stanton, a cardiovascular specialist at Mayo Clinic, Rochester, MN, "However, ICD therapy may not be right for everyone. People on anti-arrhythmia medication should consult with their physicians to determine whether ICD therapy is right for them," he adds.

Some 350,000 sudden cardiac deaths occur in the United States every year. Most are thought to be caused by ventricular tachycardia or ventricular fibrillation. These ventricular arrhythmias often develop in people with coronary artery disease or disease of the heart muscle (cardiomyopathy).

People with ventricular tachycardia or ventricular fibrillation who survive sudden cardiac arrest are often treated with an implanted defibrillator. If they have survived one episode of sudden cardiac arrest by being resuscitated, there is significant risk they'll have another, and an ICD offers the greatest chance for long-term survival.

Cardiologists have long suspected that defibrillators may play a major role in preventing sudden cardiac arrest. The NIH study follows a multicenter trial coordinated by the University of Rochester, which estimated that, with implantable defibrillators, there would be 50 percent fewer deaths in people who had survived a previous heart attack and were shown to be at high risk for sudden death (although they hadn't yet had an episode of cardiac arrest).

Cardiologists or surgeons can now implant defibrillators using less-invasive techniques because defibrillators are smaller and more technologically advanced. Their increased use may lead to fewer hospitalizations—and reduced mortality. "The initial cost of ICD therapy is more than for long-term drug therapy, but over the long run, the cost per year of life saved is in keeping with other well-accepted chronic drug therapies, such as the treatment of elevated cholesterol," Dr. Stanton adds.

Implantable Defibrillators Can Aid People with Dangerously Irregular Heartbeats

The cardiac defibrillator is a staple of Hollywood and television medical dramas—the device with the paddle electrodes the physician applies to the chest of a dying patient to shock the heart back into action. But it might surprise you to learn that quite a number of people live with a device implanted in their chests that does exactly the same thing.

Implantable Defibrillators

The implantable defibrillator protects patients at risk from severe ventricular tachycardia—a runaway heartbeat that kills 500,000 people a year in this country.

Heartbeat irregularities—arrhythmias—are fairly common, and many are harmless. But anyone experiencing lightheadedness, dizziness, fainting spells, shortness of breath and heart palpitations shouldn't simply assume that's the case. There may be little difference between the symptoms of the merely annoying arrhythmias and those stemming from serious underlying heart conditions that can cause sudden cardiac death.

Medication and pacemakers are the most common treatment for arrhythmias, but, for a small proportion of patients, the implantable defibrillator is a literal life preserver—and an increasingly miniaturized and sophisticated one.

Early models were the size of a pack of cigarettes and had to be implanted beneath the skin of the abdomen. Open heart surgery was required to attach three or four electrodes to the surface of the heart. Newer models are much smaller and can be placed beneath the skin of the chest, which significantly reduces the extent of surgery. In most instances, the newer defibrillators also require only a single electrode, routed into the heart through a vein without a major operation.

Through that electrode the tiny computer aboard the defibrillator constantly monitors the heartbeat. If it detects a minor arrhythmia, it activates a built-in conventional pacemaker to restabilize the heart's rhythm. If that fails, it delivers a small defibrillating electrical jolt to the heart. In an extreme case, it resorts to a far stronger jolt to reset the heart rate. This is a marked advance over the first-generation models, which could only deliver a maximum-level defibrillating charge—perhaps as often as 30 times a day.

The operation of the pacemaker is imperceptible to the patient, and the low-level defibrillator charge is hardly noticeable. While the maximum charge of 30 joules is startling and a bit uncomfortable, it is nothing like the muscle-contracting jolt delivered by the traditional "crash cart" external defibrillator. It doesn't have to be, since the electrode is in direct contact with the heart.

Most patients take the minor annoyance of an occasional defibrillator firing in stride, since they know that it means a potentially life-threatening heartbeat irregularity has been detected and corrected. And the success of the device is truly striking. Untreated, the most severe form of ventricular tachycardia will recur, with deadly effect, within one year of its first appearance. Medication can reduce that mortality rate to 15 to 25 percent, while the implantable defibrillator can reduce it to perhaps two percent. And even more sophisticated versions are currently under development.

—This section by Richard P. Abben, M.D., Director, Arrhythmia Center

Chapter 57

Heart and Heart-Lung Transplants

Introduction

In the three decades since the performance of the first human heart transplant in December 1967, the procedure has changed from an experimental operation to an established treatment for advanced heart disease. Approximately 2,300 heart transplants are performed each year in the United States.

In 1981, combined heart and lung transplants began to be used to treat patients with conditions that severely damage both these organs. As of 1995, about 500 people in the United States and 2,000 worldwide have received heart-lung transplants.

There have been two main barriers to increasing the number of successful operations. In 1983, the first barrier to successful transplantations—rejection of the donor organ by the patient—was overcome. The drug cyclosporine was introduced to suppress rejection of a donor heart or heart-lung by the patient's body. Cyclosporine and other medications to control rejection have significantly improved the survival of transplant patients. About 80 percent of heart transplant patients survive 1 year or more. About 60 percent of heart-lung transplants live at least 1 year after surgery. Research is under way to develop even better ways to control transplant rejection and improve survival.

Organ availability is the second barrier to increasing the number of successful transplantations. Hospitals and organizations nationwide

---

National Heart, Lung, and Blood Institute (NHLBI), NIH Pub. No. 97-2990, August 1997.

are trying to increase public awareness of this problem and improve organ distribution.

Questions and Answers about Transplants

What Happens during a Heart or Heart-Lung Transplant?

A transplant is the replacement of a patient's diseased heart or heart and lungs with a normal organ(s) from someone—called a donor—who has died. The donor's organ(s) is completely removed and quickly transplanted to the patient, who may be located across the country. Organs are cooled and kept in a special solution while being taken to the patient.

During the operation, the patient is placed on a heart-lung machine. This machine allows surgeons to bypass the blood flow to the heart and lungs. The machine pumps the blood throughout the rest of the body, removing carbon dioxide (a waste product) and replacing it with oxygen needed by body tissues. Doctors remove the patient's heart except for the back walls of the atria, the heart's upper chambers. The backs of the atria on the new heart are opened, and the heart is sewn into place. A similar process is followed in heart-lung transplants, except doctors remove the heart and lungs as a unit from the donor; the new lungs are attached first, followed by the heart.

Surgeons then connect the blood vessels and allow blood to flow through the heart and lungs. As the heart warms up, it begins beating. Sometimes, surgeons must start the heart with an electrical shock. Surgeons check all the connected blood vessels and heart chambers for leaks before removing the patient from the heart-lung machine.

Patients are usually up and around a few days after surgery, and if there are no signs of the body immediately rejecting the organ(s), patients are allowed to go home within 2 weeks.

Why Are Transplants Done?

A transplant is considered when the heart is failing and does not respond to all other therapies, but health is otherwise good. The leading reasons why people receive heart transplants are:

- Cardiomyopathy—a weakening of the heart muscle.
- Severe coronary artery disease—in which the heart's blood vessels become blocked, and the heart muscle is damaged.
- Birth defects of the heart.

Heart and Heart-Lung Transplants

Heart-lung transplants are performed on patients who will die from end-stage lung disease that also involves the heart. Alternative therapies for these patients have been tried or considered. Leading reasons people receive heart-lung transplants are:

- Severe pulmonary hypertension—a large increase in blood pressure in the vessels of the lungs that limits blood flow and delivery of oxygen to the rest of the body.
- A birth defect of the heart that results in Eisenmenger's complex—another name for acquired pulmonary hypertension.

Who Can Have a Transplant?

Patients under age 60 are the most likely heart transplant candidates. Patients under age 45 are generally accepted for heart-lung transplants. In both cases, patients must be suffering from end-stage disease and be in good health otherwise. The doctor, patient, and family must address the following four basic questions to determine whether a transplant should be considered:

- Have all other therapies been tried or excluded?
- Is the patient likely to die without the transplant?
- Is the person in generally good health other than the heart or heart and lung disease?
- Can the patient adhere to the lifestyle changes—including complex drug treatments and frequent examinations—required after a transplant?

Patients who do not meet the above considerations or who have additional problems—other severe diseases, active infections, or severe obesity—are not good candidates for a transplant.

How Are Donors Found?

Donors are individuals who are brain dead, meaning that the brain shows no signs of life while the person's body is being kept alive by a machine. Donors have often died as a result of an automobile accident, a stroke, a gunshot wound, suicide, or a severe head injury. Most hearts come from those who die before age 45. Donor organs are located through the United Network for Organ Sharing (UNOS).

Not enough organs are available for transplant. At any given time, almost 3,500 to 4,000 patients are waiting for a heart or heart-lung transplant. A patient may wait months for a transplant. More than 25 percent do not live long enough. Yet, only a fraction of those who could donate organs actually do.

Does a Person Lead a Normal Life after a Transplant?

After a heart or heart-lung transplant, patients must take several medications. The most important are those to keep the body from rejecting the transplant. These medications, which must be taken for life, can cause significant side effects, including hypertension, fluid retention, tremors, excessive hair growth, and possible kidney damage. To combat these problems, additional drugs are often prescribed.

A transplanted heart functions differently from the old one. Because the nerves leading to the heart are cut during the operation, the transplanted heart beats faster (about 100 to 110 beats per minute) than the normal heart (70 beats per minute). The new heart also responds more slowly to exercise and doesn't increase its rate as quickly as before.

A patient's prognosis depends on many factors, including age, general health, and response to the transplant. Recent figures show that 73 percent of heart transplant patients live at least 3 years after surgery. Nearly 85 percent of patients return to work or other activities they like. Many patients enjoy swimming, cycling, running, and other sports.

As noted, 60 percent of patients who receive combined heart-lung transplants survive at least 1 year. Fifty percent live at least 3 years.

What Are the Risks from Transplants?

The most common causes of death following a transplant are infection or rejection of the heart. Patients on drugs to prevent transplant rejection are at risk for developing kidney damage, high blood pressure, osteoporosis (a severe thinning of the bones, which can cause fractures), and lymphoma (a type of cancer that affects cells of the immune system).

Coronary artery disease (atherosclerosis) is a problem that develops in almost half the patients who receive transplants. Normally, patients with this disease experience chest pain and/or other symptoms when their hearts are under stress. This is called angina and is an early warning sign of a blocked heart artery. However, transplant patients may have no early pain symptoms of a blockage building up because they have no sensations in their new hearts.

Heart and Heart-Lung Transplants

Thirty to fifty percent of patients who receive a heart-lung transplant develop bronchiolitis obliterans, in which there are obstructive changes in the airways of the lungs.

What Does Rejection Mean?

The body's immune system protects the body from infection. Cells of the immune system move throughout the body, checking for anything that looks foreign or different from the body's own cells. Immune cells recognize the transplanted organ(s) as different from the rest of the body and attempt to destroy it—this is called rejection. If left alone, the immune system would damage the cells of a new heart and eventually destroy it. In a heart-lung transplant, immune cells may also destroy healthy lung tissue.

To prevent rejection, patients receive immunosuppressants, drugs that suppress the immune system so that the new organ(s) is not damaged. Because rejection can occur anytime after a transplant, immunosuppressive drugs are given to patients the day before their transplant and thereafter for the rest of their lives. To avoid complications, patients must strictly adhere to their drug regimen. The three main drugs now being used are cyclosporine, azathioprine, and prednisone.

Researchers are working on safer, more effective immunosuppressants for future testing. Some of the more promising drugs are FK-506 and mycophenolate mofetil.

Doctors must balance the dose of immunosuppressive drugs so that a patient's transplanted organ(s) is protected, but his or her immune system is not completely shut down. Without an active enough immune system, a patient can easily develop severe infections. For this reason, medications are also prescribed to fight any infections.

To carefully monitor transplant patients for signs of heart rejection, small pieces of the transplanted organ are removed for inspection under a microscope. Called a biopsy, this procedure involves advancing a thin tube called a catheter through a vein to the heart. At the end of the catheter is a bioptome, a tiny instrument used to snip off a piece of tissue. If the biopsy shows damaged cells, the dose and kind of immunosuppressive drug may be changed. Biopsies of the heart muscle are usually performed weekly for the first 3 to 6 weeks after surgery, then every 3 months for the first year, and then yearly thereafter.

How Much Do Transplants Cost?

According to the UNOS, the estimated first year charges for a heart transplant is $209,100, and annual followup charges are $15,000. In most cases these costs are paid by private insurance companies. More than 80 percent of commercial insurers and 97 percent of Blue Cross/Blue Shield plans offer coverage for heart transplants. Medicaid programs in 33 states and the District of Columbia also reimburse for transplants. Heart transplants are covered by Medicare for Medicare-eligible patients if the operation is performed at an approved center.

Approximately 70 percent of commercial insurance companies and 92 percent of Blue Cross/Blue Shield plans cover heart-lung transplants. Medicaid coverage for heart-lung transplants is available in 20 states. According to the UNOS, estimated first year charges for a heart-lung transplant is $246,000, and annual followup charges are $18,400.

What Will Transplants Be Like in 5 to 10 years?

Hospitals nationwide are trying to set up a better system for distributing organs to patients in need. Researchers are looking for easier methods to monitor rejection to replace the regular biopsies that are needed now. Work is progressing to make immunosuppressive drugs with fewer long-term side effects so that coronary artery disease development and lung destruction may be prevented.

Where Can I Get More Information on Transplants?

Information is available 24 hours a day, 7 days a week from the UNOS at 1-800-24-DONOR. This hotline provides general information on transplants, current statistics, and listings of transplant centers. Internet address: http://www.ew3.att.NET/UNOS

Additional information is available from the Division of Transplantation, Health Resources and Services Administration, Room 7-29, 5600 Fishers Lane, Rockville, MD 20857. Telephone: 301-443-7577 Internet address: http://www.hrsa.DHHS.gov/bhrd/dot/dotmain.htm

For More Information on Heart and Lung Diseases

NHLBI Information Center
P.O. Box 30105
Bethesda, MD 20824-0105
Telephone: 301-251-1222
Fax: 301-251-1223
Internet address: http://www.nhlbi.nih.gov/nhlbi/nhibi.htm

Part Six

Cardiac Rehabilitation

Chapter 58

Recovering from Heart Problems

The Keys to Heart Health

Exercise. Regular physical activity that is tailored to your abilities, needs, and interests.

Education. Learning about your heart problem, its causes and treatments, and how you can manage it.

Counseling. Advice on why and how to change your lifestyle to lower your risk of further heart problems.

Behavior change. Learning specific skills to enable you to stop unhealthy behaviors such as smoking or to begin healthy behaviors such as eating a heart-healthy diet.

Purpose of This Chapter

Cardiac rehabilitation (rehab) services are designed to help patients with heart disease recover faster and return to full and productive lives. Cardiac rehab includes exercise, education, counseling, and learning ways to live a healthier life. Together with medical and surgical treatments, cardiac rehab can help you feel better and live a healthier life.

Agency for Health Care Policy and Research (AHCPR), AHCPR Pub. No. 96-0674, October 1995.

You can benefit from cardiac rehab if you:

- Have heart disease, such as angina or heart failure, or have had a heart attack.
- Have had coronary bypass surgery or a balloon catheter (PTCA) procedure on your heart.
- Have had a heart transplant.

Cardiac rehab can make a difference. It is a safe and effective way to help you:

- Feel better faster.
- Get stronger.
- Reduce stress.
- Reduce the risks of future heart problems.
- Live longer.

Almost everyone with heart disease can benefit from some type of cardiac rehab. No one is too old or too young. Women benefit from cardiac rehab as much as men.

This chapter can help you learn how to lower your risk for future heart problems. You will also learn tips for finding a cardiac rehab plan that is right for you.

Most important, you will learn what you can do to be healthier.

When you have heart disease, breaking old habits and learning new ones can be stressful. Wondering about your future health can be stressful, too. But the support of family and friends, as well as health care providers, can make a big difference in how well you adjust to these changes. Share this information with others so they will learn about cardiac rehab and how they can help you.

Risk Factors for Coronary Disease

The controllable risk factors for coronary disease are shown below. There are some risk factors that you cannot change, such as older age or a family history of heart disease. But you can change or control the ones shown below. Cardiac rehab **can** help you do this.

Coronary Disease Risk Factors You Can Control

- Smoking

Recovering from Heart Problems

- High blood pressure
- High blood cholesterol
- Sedentary lifestyle
- Overweight
- Diabetes
- Stress

The Cardiac Rehab Team

Cardiac rehab services can involve many health care providers. Your team may include:

- Doctors (your family doctor, a heart specialist, perhaps a surgeon).
- Nurses.
- Exercise specialists.
- Physical and occupational therapists.
- Dietitians.
- Psychologists or other behavior therapists.

Sometimes a primary care provider, such as your family doctor or nurse practitioner, works alone playing many roles or refers patients to other health care specialists as needed.

But the most important member of your cardiac rehab team is **you**. No one else can make you exercise. Or quit smoking. Or eat a more healthful diet.

To be an active member of the cardiac rehab team:

- Learn about your heart condition.
- Learn what you can do to help your heart.
- Follow the treatment plan.
- Feel free to ask questions.
- Report symptoms or problems.

A support network can help you. Your support network may be family, friends, or a group of other people with heart problems.

Family members and friends can make a difference. They may want to learn more about heart problems so their help can be even more valuable. For example, family members may have to learn to let you do things for yourself. Or they may want to learn about preparing heart-healthy meals. Your family and friends can give you emotional support as you adjust to a new, healthier lifestyle.

You may also want the support of other people who have heart disease. Ask your cardiac rehab team if they know of a support group you can join, or get in touch with one of the organizations listed at the end of this chapter.

How Do I Get Started?

Cardiac rehab often begins in the hospital after a heart attack, heart surgery, or other heart treatment. It continues in an outpatient setting after you leave the hospital. Once you learn the habits of heart-healthy living, stick with them for life.

- **In an outpatient setting.** Outpatient rehab may be located at the hospital, in a medical or professional center, in a community facility such as the YMCA, or at your place of work. You may even have cardiac rehab at home. You will be advised to increase the amount of exercise you do. You will also receive education and encouragement to control your risk factors.

- **For life.** After you have learned the skills of heart-healthy living, you should continue to use them for life.

You need your doctor's approval to get started in cardiac rehab. Tell your doctor or nurse that you're interested in cardiac rehab and ask which rehab services or plans are best for you.

How Does Cardiac Rehab Work?

Cardiac rehab has two major parts:

1. **Exercise training** to help you learn how to exercise safely, strengthen your muscles, and improve your stamina. Your exercise plan will be based on your individual ability, needs, and interests.

2. **Education, counseling, and training** to help you understand your heart condition and find ways to reduce your risk of future heart problems. The cardiac rehab team will help you learn how to cope with the stress of adjusting to a new lifestyle and to deal with your fears about the future.

Recovering from Heart Problems

Cardiac rehab often takes place in groups. However, each patient's plan is based on his or her specific risk factors and special needs.

Cardiac rehab helps you recognize and change unhealthy habits you may have and establish new, more healthy ones. Your rehab may last 6 weeks, 6 months, or even longer. It is important that you complete the recommended rehab plan.

No matter how difficult it seems, your hard work in cardiac rehab will have lifetime benefits.

Is It Safe for Me?

Cardiac rehab is safe. Studies show that serious health problems caused by cardiac rehab exercise are rare. The cardiac rehab team is trained to handle emergencies. Your health care provider can help you choose a plan that is safe for you. Many patients can safely exercise without supervision once they learn their own exercise plan.

Checking how your heart reacts and adapts to exercise is an important part of cardiac rehab. You may be connected to an EKG transmitter while you exercise. If your cardiac rehab is done at home, you may be connected to an EKG machine by telephone, or you may phone the cardiac rehab team to let them know how you are doing. In some settings, you check your own pulse rate or estimate how hard you are exercising.

What's in It for Me?

The goals of cardiac rehab are different for each patient. In helping set your personal goals, your health care team will look at your general health, your personal heart problem, your risks for future heart problems, your doctor's recommendations, and, of course, your own preferences.

Cardiac rehab can reduce your symptoms and your chances of having more heart problems. And it has many other benefits:

- Exercise tones your muscles and improves your energy level and spirits. It helps both your heart and your body get stronger and work better. Exercise also can get you back to work and other activities faster.
- A healthy diet can lower blood cholesterol, control weight, and help prevent or control high blood pressure and other problems such as diabetes. Plus, you will feel better and have more energy.

- Cardiac rehab can help you quit smoking. Kicking the habit means less risk of lung cancer, emphysema, and bronchitis, as well as less risk of heart attack, stroke, and other heart and blood vessel problems. It means more energy, and it means better health for your loved ones.

- You can learn to manage stress instead of letting it manage you. You will feel better and improve your heart health.

Aerobic exercise raises your pulse rate and makes you perspire. It helps improve the flow, of oxygen rich blood throughout your body.

Strength training, such as using weights, improves your muscle strength and your stamina.

Both types of exercise in the right amount are safe and important for your heart health.

Make a habit of the heart-healthy lifestyle you learn in cardiac rehab. Your life depends on it!

How Do I Find a Plan That's Right for Me?

Your doctor or nurse may recommend a cardiac rehab plan or help you to arrange for exercise training, education, counseling, and other services. Many hospitals and outpatient health care centers offer cardiac rehab—so do some local schools and community centers. You can also check the Yellow Pages of your telephone book.

When choosing a cardiac rehab plan, ask about:

- **Time.** Is it offered when you can get there without causing added stress? Cardiac rehab services offered at the workplace are sometimes an option.

- **Place.** Is it easy to get to? Keep in mind that traffic problems can add to your stress. Is there parking? Public transportation?

- **Setting.** Is it an individual or group plan? Is it home-based or in a facility? Think about whether you want to be in a group with professional supervision.

- **Services.** Does it offer a wide range of services? More importantly, does it include the areas you need help with, such as quitting smoking?

- **Cost.** Is it affordable? Is it covered by insurance? Your insurance may cover all or part of the cost of some cardiac rehab services but not others. Find out what will be covered and for how long. Consider what you can afford and for how long.

Cardiac rehab has life-long favorable effects, so choose a plan that will serve your needs. For example, if you smoke, look for a plan that will help you quit. Choose a plan that includes activities you enjoy, such as regular walking in a shopping mall or park. Before you sign up, visit and ask any questions you may have.

How Can I Get the Most out Of Cardiac Rehab?

Studies show that controlling your risk factors for heart disease can help you lead a healthier life. So make sure your cardiac rehab plan works for you. Here's how:

- **Plan.** Work with your health care team to design or change your services to meet your needs.
- **Communicate.** Ask questions. If you don't understand the answers, keep asking until you do. Report changes in your feelings or symptoms.
- **Take charge of your recovery.** No one else can do it for you. Your new lifestyle is healthy for your heart, so stick with it—for life.

To gain more control over your cardiac rehab, remember your goals and keep important information where you can find it. You may want to have a special calendar just for your rehab activities or keep a notebook.

Sometimes people who have big changes in their lives feel depressed. Some people with heart problems feel depressed when they find out about their disease or after surgery. Cardiac rehab may help you feel better, but if you are seriously depressed you will need additional help. When you are depressed, it is hard to do things to do things to help yourself get better, such as going to cardiac rehab or getting back to your usual activities. If you are depressed, tell your doctor. Depression can be treated.

Where Can I Get More Information and Support?

For additional information about heart disease and ways you can help yourself through cardiac rehab, contact:

American Association of Cardiovascular and Pulmonary Rehabilitation
(national program directory)
(608) 831-7561

American Heart Association
(patient education materials)
800-AHA-USA 1 (800-242-8721)

Mended Hearts, Inc.
(patient support group)
(214) 706-1442

National Heart, Lung, and Blood Institute
(patient education materials)
(301) 251-1222

For Further Information

The information in this chapter is based on the *Clinical Practice Guideline on Cardiac Rehabilitation*. The guideline was developed by a non-Federal panel of experts sponsored by the Agency for Health Care Policy and Research (AHCPR), a U.S. Government agency. Additional support came from the National Heart, Lung, and Blood Institute. Other guidelines on common health problems are available from AHCPR, and more are being developed.

Three other patient guides available from AHCPR may be of interest to people participating in cardiac rehab:

- *Managing Unstable Angina* (AHCPR Publication No. 94-0604).

- *Living With Heart Disease: Is It Heart Failure?* (AHCPR Publication No. 94-0614).

- *Depression Is a Treatable Illness* (AHCPR Publication No. 93-0553).

For more information about these and other guidelines, or to get more copies of this booklet, call toll free: 800-358-9295

or write to:

Agency for Health Care Policy and Research
Publications Clearinghouse
P.O. Box 8547
Silver Spring, MD 20907

Recovering from Heart Problems

These and other guidelines are available online through a free electronic service from the National Library of Medicine called STAT.

Copies of this text and other consumer brochures are free through InstantFAX, which operates all day every day. If you have a fax machine equipped with a touchtone telephone, dial (301) 594-2800, push 1, and then press the start button for instructions and a list of publications.

Chapter 59

Lifestyle Changes for Recovering Heart Patients

If you have angina, high cholesterol or have had a heart attack, angioplasty or bypass surgery, you should follow a diet that derives less than 7 percent of calories from saturated fat, (from dairy and animal products) and 200 mg or less of cholesterol per day. (For example, a large egg yolk contains about 215 mg of cholesterol.) And you should concentrate on controlling high blood pressure, quitting smoking, using medications if needed to lower blood cholesterol, maintaining optimum weight, controlling diabetes, managing stress and increasing your physical activity.

High blood cholesterol is one of the major risk factors for coronary heart disease, and the risk increases as blood cholesterol levels rise. Other major risk factors are cigarette smoking, high blood pressure and diabetes. Your cholesterol level is determined both by your genetic makeup and the amount of saturated fat and cholesterol in the foods you eat. The liver also manufactures cholesterol, so even if you never eat cholesterol, your body makes enough for its needs. But if you're an adult with high blood cholesterol, for every 1 percent reduction in total cholesterol levels, you reduce your chance of a heart attack by 2 percent. In other words, if you reduce your cholesterol level 15 percent, your risk of coronary heart disease could drop by 30 percent.

Several factors contribute to high blood cholesterol:

© 1996-1999 Johns Hopkins InteliHealth, updated November 1997; reprinted with permission of InteliHealth.

Diet

To reduce your blood cholesterol level, your diet should be low in fat, particularly saturated fat (dairy products, meat and poultry), and low in cholesterol. Studies have shown that your total and LDL cholesterol levels may begin to drop two to three weeks after you begin your lower fat, lower calorie, lower cholesterol diet. When planning meals:

- Choose poultry, fish, and lean cuts of meat more often, remove the skin from chicken, and trim the fat from meat. Lean cuts of meat include tenderloin, flank, top round, eye of the round, and top sirloin. Better pork cuts include tenderloin, loin, and lean ham.

- Choose low-fat dairy products instead of regular milk, cheese, and yogurt. That means skim milk instead of whole or 1 or 2 percent, and non-fat yogurt and reduced-fat cheeses.

- Use tub margarine or liquid vegetable oils that are high in unsaturated fat (like safflower and corn oils) or monounsaturated fats (olive and canola oils) instead of butter, lard, and hydrogenated vegetable shortenings that are high in saturated fat.

- Choose products that list more unsaturated fats than saturated ones on the label. For instance, soft tub margarine is less saturated (hydrogenated) than harder stick margarine.

- Cut down on commercially prepared and processed foods made with saturated fats or palm or coconut oils. Read labels to choose those low in saturated fats.

- Eat at least one vegetarian meal a week, such as bean chili, a pasta or rice dish with vegetables or a vegetable stir-fry with tofu instead of meat.

- Choose low fat snacks, such as bagels, air-blown popcorn, dry cereal, fruit, flavored rice cakes, pretzels, frozen fruit juice bars, nonfat frozen yogurt, or ice milk.

- Use fat-lowering cooking techniques, such as broiling, boiling, grilling, roasting, poaching, microwaving, steaming, or stir-frying.

Weight

Weight control is another key factor because obesity increases blood cholesterol and triglyceride levels, blood pressure, and the risk of developing diabetes. Obese people tend to eat too many calories and excessive amounts of fat.

Exercise

Although it is not clear whether physical activity can prevent atherosclerosis, regular exercise may help a person control weight, lower blood pressure, and increase the level of "good" HDL cholesterol.

Genetics

Genetic factors play a major role in your overall ability to lower your cholesterol levels through diet alone. A small number of people have an inherited tendency to have a high blood cholesterol level. If one person in a family has a genetic disorder contributing to a high blood cholesterol, a physician may suggest that the entire family have their blood cholesterol levels measured. Many people with a genetic reason for very high cholesterol cannot control their levels through diet alone and often require cholesterol-lowering drugs to get their levels in shape.

Sex/Age

Coronary heart disease is the leading cause of death and disability for both men and women in the United States. Estimates are that one in five men and one in 17 women will have symptoms of heart disease before the age of 60. This means that in this age group, men have three times the risk of developing heart disease as women. The female hormone estrogen is one protector against heart disease. (Estrogen boosts levels of protective HDL cholesterol.) After levels of estrogen decline at menopause, a woman's risk of heart disease increases. About 3,000 women between the ages of 29 and 44 have a heart attack each year; that figure climbs to 136,000 among women aged 45 to 64, and skyrockets to 374,000 among women over age 65, according to the Framingham Heart Study.

Alcohol

You may have heard that modest amounts of alcohol can improve your cholesterol profile by increasing the amount of "good" HDL cholesterol in your blood. Although it is not known whether the higher level produced by alcohol protects against coronary heart disease, there is good evidence that moderate alcohol intake does lower the risk of coronary artery disease, whether or not the protection is due to increasing HDL levels. However, alcohol provides "empty calories" that can add to your weight. Because drinking can have serious adverse effects, present guidelines do not recommend drinking alcohol as a way to prevent heart disease.

Smoking

Smoking damages the heart by raising blood pressure, damaging blood vessels, promoting the buildup of fatty plaque in arteries, lowering levels of "good" HDL cholesterol, making the blood more likely to clot, and depriving your heart of oxygen. Quitting smoking is the best thing you can do to prevent a heart attack.

Stress

Stress has been shown to increase the levels of chemicals within the body that chip away at the heart and blood vessels, perhaps increasing the risk of a heart attack. These fight-or-flight stress hormones, such as cortisol and epinephrine, excite the heart and make it work overtime.

Chapter 60

Emotional Effects of Rehabilitation

If you have suffered a heart attack you are probably worried about two things: The immediate threat to your life and the long-term fear that heart disease will affect the way you live. Many heart attack victims feel angry that the attack happened to them, guilty about not taking better care of themselves, or worried whether they will survive the attack or suffer another one. Result: They become depressed. In fact, one of every two people who has had a heart attack goes through a period of depression during or slightly after their recovery.

Anxiety may develop early, during your first few days in a coronary care unit. Anxiety often eases once you begin to understand that you have survived and can make a complete recovery. Depression, however, is not so easily relieved. Heart attack patients who experience depression after recovery say they are most worried that their attack will limit their lifestyle.

Depression can be very hard to detect and diagnose. Heart attack patients often have a general feeling of weakness or uneasiness. Some find that the tranquilizers or other medications they are taking cause them to feel "blue." But these feelings are different from the full-blown depression many heart attack victims experience.

Signs of depression include:

- Depressed mood (despondent, pessimistic about the future, hopeless, withdrawn)

© 1996-1999 Johns Hopkins InteliHealth, updated November 1997; reprinted with permission of InteliHealth.

- Marked loss of interest or pleasure
- Feelings of worthlessness or guilt
- Change in appetite or weight
- Loss of energy
- Fearfulness of activity
- Insomnia
- Lack of interest in personal hygiene
- Lack of interest in sex
- Anxiety
- Easily distressed
- Agitation or restlessness
- Inability to concentrate, make decisions, remember or comprehend instructions
- Thoughts of death or suicide
- Failure to return to work

Depression may also affect whether you stick with the lifestyle changes recommended by your doctor to reduce the risk of a second heart attack. Many people who are depressed lack the energy and motivation to exercise regularly, and they may feel their situation is too hopeless to change.

The Depression-Disease Connection

While there is increasing appreciation that many people with heart disease go through a period of depression, doctors now believe that the link between these two conditions may be stronger than previously thought. New studies from Johns Hopkins, the Montreal Heart Institute and other medical centers suggest a connection between depression and heart disease; in effect, depression may lead to heart disease. But the experts are unable to agree on how depression may increase your risk of heart disease.

Some researchers hold that hormones released during depression create biochemical changes that stress the heart and circulatory system and lead to heart disease. Others believe that a bout of depression before or after a heart attack may leave people so emotionally

Emotional Effects of Rehabilitation

hollow that they forsake their health, ignore recommendations to alter their lifestyle and forget to take their medications. In a sense, it is a debate over whether the biology of depression or the ensuing behavior is more likely to lead to heart disease.

Regardless of the cause and effect relationship, depression takes its toll on the heart. One study found that depressed patients with heart disease were twice as likely to require surgery within one year as heart disease patients who were not depressed. Another study of people without heart disease found that depressed individuals were four times more likely to suffer a heart attack within the following 14 years than those who were not depressed.

One explanation for the increased risk of heart attacks among depressed people is that, like stress, depression triggers the body's fight-or-flight responses. Depression, it turns out, is a two-faced condition: On the surface, depressed people appear lethargic, tired, and sluggish, yet under the surface their hormones are raging. They often sleep less, wake earlier, lose their appetite and secrete much higher levels of stress hormones—cortisol, norepinephrine and epinephrine—than non-depressed people. In fact, they are in a state of constant chemical arousal. Alone, this chronic state of arousal may be enough to increase the risk of heart disease; combined with the well-known behavioral effects of depression, the effect can be devastating. In a sense, heart disease patients who are depressed are fighting a battle on two fronts. They are more likely to ignore their doctor's recommendations to control their disease, and they must further contend with the biochemical effects of depression on the heart.

One thing that becomes clear is that increased levels of dangerous stress hormones level off in patients undergoing treatment for depression. But the use of drugs to treat depression in people with heart disease is a field still in its infancy. Doctors at the government's National Heart, Lung, and Blood Institute are just beginning a study to determine whether anti-depressant drugs can lower the risk of a second attack in depressed heart-attack patients.

Part of the problem is that many anti-depression drugs either put increased stress on the heart or interact with medications used to treat the heart disease itself. Antidepressants from the tricyclic family and serotonin uptake inhibitors, such as Prozac, Zoloft and Paxil, are used in some heart disease patients with depression. However, they can have side effects, including rapid heart beat, dizziness, and possible heart rhythm problems.

If you are like most heart attack patients suffering from depression, you can benefit from education about your disease. Talk to your doctor and have him or her explain what the future is likely to hold if you follow steps to reduce your risks. Depression usually fades within a few weeks to months after the attack. As people become more confident about their life after a heart attack, they begin to realize that with proper care they can lead a healthy, full life.

Some cases of depression, however, can become very serious. If you or a loved one who has suffered a heart attack cannot seem to come out of a bout of depression, it may be time for professional counseling. Talk to your doctor about getting some long-term help. He or she may recommend a visit to a therapist who can offer a host of depression therapies, from counseling to medications.

What Family Members Can Do

Family members need to adjust to their loved one's new life after a heart attack. The first few weeks after a patient comes home can be particularly trying. You may be afraid that something you do or say can trigger another attack. Or you may mistakenly imagine that it was something you did that precipitated the first attack.

There is no one answer for the feelings you may have after a spouse or parent suffers a heart attack. Open, frank communication of everyone's feelings is the best route. Try to learn as much as you can about heart attacks and recovery. By following your doctor's advice, you can help get through the recovery period and back on track to a normal life.

In addition, family members should be aware of the signs of a heart attack and have a heart attack plan in case your loved one experiences a second attack. It is also a good idea to learn cardiopulmonary resuscitation, in the event it becomes necessary to revive your loved one.

Chapter 61

Lowering Cholesterol for the Person with Heart Disease

Coronary Heart Disease

If you have coronary heart disease (CHD), there are some important things for you to know. They could save your life.

Twelve to thirteen million American adults have CHD, which is a major cause of disability and the number one killer of women and of men in the United States. In 1994, almost 500,000 people died from CHD, equally divided between men and women. About 1.25 million people have heart attacks every year, and about half of these occur in persons who are already known to have CHD. For men and women with CHD, the risk of a heart attack is five to seven times higher than for people of the same age and sex who do not have CHD.

If you have CHD, that's the bad news. But the good news is that by lowering your cholesterol you can reduce your risk of having a heart attack. This text was written to help you make healthy changes in your life that can reduce your risk.

I Already Have Heart Disease. Is It Too Late to Reduce My Risk?

No, it's not too late to help your heart. Most CHD patients will benefit from cholesterol lowering. In fact, if you already have heart disease, you should pay even more attention to your cholesterol level,

---

National Heart, Lung, and Blood Institute (NHLBI), NIH Pub. No. 96-3805, September 1996.

Heart Diseases and Disorders Sourcebook, Second Edition

because you stand to benefit even more. A person with CHD has a much greater risk of having a future heart attack than a person without heart disease. If you lower your blood cholesterol level, you will definitely reduce your risk of a future heart attack and could actually prolong your life.

What Is Coronary Heart Disease?

You probably know that CHD is a type of heart disease caused by narrowing of the coronary arteries that feed the heart. Like any muscle, the heart needs a constant supply of oxygen and nutrients, which are carried to it by the blood in the coronary arteries. When the coronary arteries become narrowed or clogged by fat and cholesterol deposits and cannot supply enough blood to the heart, the result is CHD. If not enough oxygen-carrying blood reaches the heart, the person may experience chest pain called angina. If the blood supply to a portion of the heart is completely cut off by total blockage of a coronary artery, the result is a heart attack. This is usually due to a sudden closure from a blood clot forming on top of a previous narrowing.

How Do You Know if You Have Coronary Heart Disease?

If you answer yes to any of these questions, you most probably have CHD.

- Have you ever had a heart attack?
- Do you suffer from chest pain that has been diagnosed as angina?
- Have you had heart surgery such as a bypass operation or a balloon or angioplasty procedure?
- Have you ever had an angiogram (a special x-ray picture of the heart) that showed a blockage in your coronary arteries?

You should be sure to talk to your doctor about cholesterol if you have answered yes to any of these questions.

Role of Cholesterol in CHD

What is cholesterol and what does it have to do with CHD? Cholesterol is a waxy substance that occurs naturally in all parts of the

Lowering Cholesterol for the Person with Heart Disease

body and that your body needs to function normally. It is present in cell walls or membranes everywhere in the body, including the brain, nerves, muscle, skin, liver, intestines, and heart. Your body uses cholesterol to produce many hormones, vitamin D, and the bile acids that help to digest fat. It takes only a small amount of cholesterol in the blood to meet these needs. However, if you have too much cholesterol in your bloodstream, it can lead to atherosclerosis, a condition in which fat and cholesterol are deposited in the walls of the arteries in many parts of the body, including the coronary arteries feeding the heart. In time, narrowing of the coronary arteries by atherosclerosis can produce the signs and symptoms of CHD, including angina and heart attack.

Lipoproteins

Cholesterol travels in the blood in packages called lipoproteins. Just like oil and water, cholesterol, which is fatty, and blood, which is watery, do not mix. In order to be able to travel in the bloodstream, the cholesterol made in the liver is combined with protein, making a lipoprotein. This lipoprotein then carries the cholesterol through the bloodstream.

There are specific kinds of lipoproteins that contain cholesterol in your blood, and each affects your heart disease risk in a different way.

Low density lipoproteins (LDLs): the "bad" cholesterol. LDLs carry most of the cholesterol in the blood, and the cholesterol from LDLs is the main source of damaging buildup and blockage in the arteries. Thus, the more LDL-cholesterol you have in your blood, the greater your risk of CHD. If you have CHD and your LDL is higher than 100 mg/dL, your cholesterol may well be too high for you.

High density lipoproteins (HDLs): the "good" cholesterol. HDLs carry cholesterol in the blood from other parts of the body back to the liver, which leads to its removal from the body. So HDLs help keep cholesterol from building up in the walls of the arteries. If your level of HDL-cholesterol is below 35 mg/dL, you are at substantially higher risk for CHD. The higher your HDL-cholesterol, the better. The average HDL-cholesterol for men is about 45 mg/dL, and for women it is about 55 mg/dL.

Triglycerides: a form of fat carried through the bloodstream. Most of your body's fat is in the form of triglycerides stored in fat tissue.

Only a small portion of your triglycerides is found in the bloodstream. High blood triglyceride levels alone do not cause atherosclerosis. But lipoproteins that are rich in triglycerides also contain cholesterol, which causes atherosclerosis in some people with high triglycerides. So high triglycerides may be a sign of a lipoprotein problem that contributes to CHD.

What Makes Blood Cholesterol High or Low?

Your blood cholesterol level is affected not only by what you eat but also by how quickly your body makes LDL-cholesterol and disposes of it. In fact, your body makes all the cholesterol it needs, and it is not necessary to take in any additional cholesterol from the foods you eat.

Patients with CHD typically have too much LDL-cholesterol in their blood. Many factors help determine whether your LDL-cholesterol level is high or low. The following factors are the most important:

Heredity. Your genes influence how high your LDL-cholesterol is by affecting how fast LDL is made and removed from the blood. One specific form of inherited high cholesterol that affects 1 in 500 people is familial hypercholesterolemia, which often leads to early CHD. But even if you do not have a specific genetic form of high cholesterol, genes play a role in influencing your LDL-cholesterol level.

What you eat. Two main nutrients in the foods you eat make your LDL-cholesterol level go up: saturated fat, a type of fat found mostly in foods that come from animals; and cholesterol, which comes only from animal products. Saturated fat raises your LDL-cholesterol level more than anything else in the diet. Eating too much saturated fat and cholesterol is the main reason for high levels of cholesterol and a high rate of heart attacks in the United States. Reducing the amount of saturated fat and cholesterol you eat is a very important step in reducing your blood cholesterol levels.

Weight. Excess weight tends to increase your LDL-cholesterol level. If you are overweight and have a high LDL-cholesterol level, losing weight may help you lower it. Weight loss also helps to lower triglycerides and raise HDL.

Physical activity/exercise. Regular physical activity may lower LDL-cholesterol and raise HDL-cholesterol levels.

Lowering Cholesterol for the Person with Heart Disease

Age and sex. Before menopause, women usually have total cholesterol levels that are lower than those of men the same age. As women and men get older, their blood cholesterol levels rise until about 60 to 65 years of age. In women, menopause often causes an increase in their LDL-cholesterol and a decrease in their HDL-cholesterol level, and after the age of 50, women often have higher total cholesterol levels than men of the same age. Some women may benefit from hormone replacement therapy (also called estrogen replacement therapy) after menopause, because estrogen lowers LDL and raises HDL.

Alcohol. Alcohol intake increases HDL-cholesterol but does not lower LDL-cholesterol. Doctors don't know for certain whether alcohol also reduces the risk of CHD. Drinking too much alcohol can damage the liver and heart muscle, lead to high blood pressure, and raise triglycerides. Because of the risks, alcoholic beverages should not be used as a way to prevent CHD.

Stress. Stress over the long term has been shown in several studies to raise blood cholesterol levels. One way that stress may do this is by affecting your habits. For example, when some people are under stress, they console themselves by eating fatty foods. The saturated fat and cholesterol in these foods contribute to higher levels of blood cholesterol.

Unstable Plaque

Cholesterol is a major ingredient of the plaque that builds up in the coronary arteries and causes CHD, so it is important to understand how plaques develop. Excess cholesterol is deposited in the artery walls as it travels through the bloodstream. Then, special cells in the artery wall gobble up this excess cholesterol, creating a "bump" in the artery wall. This cholesterol-rich "bump" then is covered by a scar that produces a hard coat or shell over the cholesterol and cell mixture. It is this collection of cholesterol covered by a scar that is called plaque.

The plaque buildup narrows the space in the coronary arteries through which blood can flow, decreasing the supply of oxygen and nutrients to the heart. If not enough oxygen-carrying blood can pass through the narrowed arteries to reach the heart muscle, the heart may respond with a pain called angina. The pain usually happens with exercise when the heart needs more oxygen. It is typically felt in the chest or sometimes in other places like the left arm and shoulder. However, this same inadequate blood supply may cause no symptoms.

Plaques come in various sizes and shapes. Throughout the coronary arteries many small plaques build themselves into the walls of the arteries, blocking less than half of the artery opening. These small plaques are often invisible on many of the tests doctors use to identify coronary heart disease. It used to be thought that the most dangerous plaques and the ones most likely to cause total blockage of coronary arteries were the largest ones. The largest plaques are in fact the ones most likely to cause angina. However, small plaques that are full of cholesterol but not completely covered by scar are now thought to be very unstable and more likely to rupture or burst, releasing their cholesterol contents into the bloodstream.

When this happens, it triggers blood clotting inside the artery. If the blood clot totally blocks the artery, it stops blood flow and a heart attack occurs. The muscle on the far side of the blood clot does not get enough oxygen and begins to die. The damage can be permanent.

Lowering your blood cholesterol level can slow, stop, or even reverse the buildup of plaque. Cholesterol lowering can reduce your risk of a heart attack by lowering the cholesterol content in unstable plaques to make them more stable and less prone to rupture. This is why lowering your LDL-cholesterol is such an important way to reduce your risk for having a heart attack. Even in people who have had one heart attack, the chances of having future attacks can be substantially reduced by cholesterol lowering.

The Benefits Of Cholesterol Lowering

A 1994 study called the Scandinavian Simvastatin Survival Study (also called 4S) found that lowering cholesterol can prevent heart attacks and reduce death in men and women who already have heart disease and high cholesterol. For over 5 years, more than 4,400 patients with heart disease and total cholesterol levels of 213 mg/dL to 310 mg/dL were given either a cholesterol-lowering drug or a placebo (a dummy pill that looks exactly like the medication). The drug they were given is known as a statin, and it reduced total cholesterol levels by 25 percent and LDL-cholesterol levels by 35 percent. The study found that in those receiving statin, deaths from heart disease were reduced by 42 percent, the chance of having a nonfatal heart attack was reduced by 37 percent, and the need for bypass surgery or angioplasty was reduced by 37 percent. A very important finding is that deaths from causes other than cardiovascular disease were not

Lowering Cholesterol for the Person with Heart Disease

increased, and so the 42 percent reduction in heart disease deaths resulted in a 30 percent drop in overall deaths from all causes.

The 4S researchers say that the following benefits could be expected if doctors were to treat their heart disease patients for the same 5-year period and lower cholesterol to the same extent. For every 1,000 patients:

- 40 people would be saved out of the 90 who would otherwise die from heart disease.
- 70 of the expected 210 nonfatal heart attacks would be avoided.
- Heart procedures such as bypass surgery would be avoided in 60 of the 210 patients who would be expected to need these procedures.

In 1996 the results of the Cholesterol and Recurrent Events (CARE) Study also showed the benefits of cholesterol lowering in CHD patients. This study reported that even in patients with seemingly normal cholesterol levels (average of 209 mg/dL), cholesterol lowering with a statin drug lowered the risk of having another heart attack or dying by 24 percent. These patients were also less likely to need bypass surgery (26 percent reduction) or angioplasty (22 percent reduction) during the study. Women benefitted even more than men, reducing their risk of having another heart attack by 45 percent. The CARE researchers estimate that treatment of 1,000 patients similar to those in CARE would result in 153 fewer heart attacks and deaths from heart disease. If the patients were over 60, there would be 214 fewer, and if they were all women, there would be 248 fewer.

These studies along with many others support the need to lower cholesterol levels in CHD patients. If you lower your cholesterol, you too can see benefits like those in 4S and CARE.

Persons with CHD Have a Lower Goal Cholesterol Level

For the general population, a level of LDL-cholesterol below 130 mg/dL is called desirable. But if you have CHD, your goal is lower: You should reduce your LDL-cholesterol to about 100 mg/dL or less. This is because patients with CHD, even if they have relatively low cholesterol levels (say an LDL-cholesterol of 120 mg/dL), have shown that they are susceptible to developing CHD at that level. A recent study has reaffirmed the benefit of lowering LDL-cholesterol levels in CHD patients to 100 mg/dL or less. So, if you have CHD and your LDL-cholesterol level is more than 100 mg/dL, it may well be too high for you.

Getting to Know Your Risk Factors for Coronary Heart Disease

In addition to a high total and LDL-cholesterol level and a low HDL-cholesterol level, other factors also increase your chance of CHD complications. The text below lists risk factors you can do something about. The more of these modifiable risk factors you have, the higher your chance of having another heart attack or worsening your CHD.

Modifiable Risk Factors for Heart Disease

- High total cholesterol and high LDL-cholesterol
- Low HDL-cholesterol
- Cigarette smoking
- High blood pressure
- Diabetes
- Obesity/overweight
- Physical inactivity

You can reduce your risk of having another heart attack or other CHD problem by doing something about your modifiable risk factors. This means that, in addition to controlling your cholesterol level, you should make a major effort to stop smoking, control your high blood pressure, lose weight if you are overweight, and increase your physical activity. Controlling high blood sugar if you have diabetes is important too.

Smoking. Cigarette smoking is a strong risk factor for CHD. Stopping smoking reduces your risk for CHD and stroke, beginning with the first year after stopping smoking. It also reduces your chances of getting lung cancer and other cancers and chronic lung disease. Changing to low-tar or low-nicotine cigarettes does not reduce the risk for CHD.

High blood pressure. High blood pressure (or hypertension) is associated with increased rates of CHD, as well as stroke and kidney failure. Treatment of hypertension reduces your risk for all these complications.

Diabetes. Diabetes, whether insulin dependent or non-insulin dependent, increases the risk for CHD. In men, diabetes increases risk

Lowering Cholesterol for the Person with Heart Disease

for CHD complications by about three times, and the increase in risk may be even greater for women.

Obesity. Obesity or overweight increases the risk for CHD in men and women. If you are overweight, losing weight can improve other risk factors including diabetes, high blood pressure, and cholesterol, making weight loss very important in the treatment of CHD.

Physical inactivity. Physical inactivity can increase your risk for CHD. Regular physical activity can reduce LDL-cholesterol, triglycerides, high blood pressure, and weight while raising HDL-cholesterol and improving the fitness of your heart and lungs. Regular physical activity is recommended to reduce your risk of future CHD complications.

How Do I Find Out My Cholesterol Level?

Since you have heart disease, finding out your blood cholesterol should be done by a blood test called a lipoprotein profile. This test will determine not only your total and HDL-cholesterol levels, but also your LDL-cholesterol and triglyceride levels. In order to take the test, you must fast, usually overnight. That means you may have nothing to eat or drink but water (or black coffee or tea with no milk, cream, or sugar) for 9 to 12 hours beforehand.

When you get your lipoprotein profile report from your doctor, there are several numbers you should look at: total cholesterol, LDL-cholesterol, HDL-cholesterol, and triglycerides. The important thing to remember is that your doctor will decide on the best treatment for you based primarily on your LDL level. The decision to start treatment should be based on the average of two LDL tests taken 1 to 8 weeks apart. The goal of treatment for CHD patients should be an LDL of about 100 mg/dL or less, which is a lower target level than for people who do not have heart disease.

HDL-cholesterol is important to know too. If your HDL is less than 35 mg/dL, your doctor will try to help you raise it, while lowering LDL-cholesterol.

Treatment Summary

If you have CHD, one of the keys to reducing the risk for future heart attacks or other CHD complications is to lower your LDL-cholesterol. The goal LDL-cholesterol for CHD patients is a level of about 100 mg/dL or less. You can lower LDL-cholesterol through changes in life habits: decreasing saturated fat and cholesterol in the diet, increasing physical activity, and controlling body weight. In addition, medications are available to help you lower your LDL-cholesterol level. For many patients it is necessary to combine medications with changes in life habits to get enough of a reduction in LDL-cholesterol, especially to reach the optimum level of 100 mg/dL or less. Your doctor can help to decide which combination of cholesterol-lowering activities is right for you.

Table 61.1. Four steps you can take to reduce your high blood cholesterol

Follow the Step II diet (low saturated fat, low cholesterol).

Be more physically active.

Lose weight if you are overweight.

Take your cholesterol-lowering medication if prescribed by your doctor.

Even if your doctor starts you on a cholesterol-lowering drug, it is important for you to adopt heart-healthy life habits. These will help to bring about a bigger drop in your LDL-cholesterol, and they will reduce your risk for future CHD in other ways as well. It is not enough just to take a drug. If you do only that, you will fail to get the full amount of risk reduction that is possible. Cholesterol-lowering drugs can significantly decrease your risk for future CHD, but you will do even better by modifying your life habits in addition.

What Your LDL-Cholesterol Means to You (For anyone 20 years of age or older)

If you have heart disease and your LDL-cholesterol is 100 mg/dL or less: You do not need to take specific steps to lower your LDL, but you will need to have your level tested again in 1 year. In the meantime, you should closely follow a diet low in saturated fat and cholesterol, maintain a healthy weight, be physically active, and not smoke. You should also follow the medical regimen prescribed by your doctor.

Lowering Cholesterol for the Person with Heart Disease

If you have heart disease and your LDL-cholesterol level is greater than 100 mg/dL: You need to have a complete physical examination done to see if you have a disease or a health condition that is raising your cholesterol levels. You will need to follow the Step II diet, which is low in saturated fat and cholesterol, and be physically active, lose weight if you are overweight, and not smoke. If your LDL level remains too high, you may need to take medication.

Improve Your Diet

A diet lower in saturated fat and cholesterol than the average American diet is a healthy way for the whole family to eat (except infants under 2 years who need more calories from fat). Since you have heart disease and need to lower your blood cholesterol level more than someone who does not have heart disease, you will probably be advised by your doctor to follow a Step II diet, which is lower in saturated fat and cholesterol than the diet the rest of your family may wish to follow. Because this Step II diet may include many changes to your current eating plan, your doctor may refer you to a registered dietitian who can help you make these changes.

On the Step II Diet, You Should Eat

- Less than 7 percent of the day's total calories from saturated fat.
- 30 percent or less of the day's total calories from fat.
- Less than 200 milligrams of dietary cholesterol a day.
- Just enough calories to achieve and maintain a healthy weight. (Ask your doctor or registered dietitian what is a reasonable calorie level for you.)

The recommendations for saturated fat and total fat are based on a percentage of the total calories you eat; the actual amount you can eat daily will vary depending on how many total calories you eat. See Table 61.2. to get an idea of the number of grams of saturated fat and total fat you should be eating.

Next, here are some general ways to lower blood cholesterol through your diet:

Choose foods low in saturated fat. All foods that contain fat have different mixtures of saturated and unsaturated fats. Saturated fat raises your blood cholesterol level more than anything else that you eat. It is found in greatest amounts in foods from animals, such as fatty cuts of meat, poultry with the skin, whole-milk dairy products, and lard, and in tropical oils like coconut, palm kernel, and palm oils. Most other vegetable oils are low in saturated fats. The best way to reduce your blood cholesterol level is to choose foods low in saturated fat. One way to do this is by choosing foods such as fruit, vegetables, and whole grain foods, which are naturally low in fat and high in starch and fiber. You should read the food labels in the grocery store to help you choose foods that are low in saturated fat.

Choose foods low in total fat. Since many foods high in total fat are also high in saturated fat, eating foods low in total fat will help you eat less saturated fat. Any type of fat is a rich source of calories, so eating foods low in fat should also help you eat fewer calories, which will help you lose weight. If you are overweight, losing weight is an important part of lowering your blood cholesterol. When you do eat fat, you should substitute unsaturated fat for saturated fat. Unsaturated fat can be either monounsaturated or polyunsaturated. Examples of foods high in monounsaturated fat are olive and canola oils. Those high in polyunsaturated fats are safflower, sunflower, corn, and soybean oils. The food label is your best guide to how much total fat, saturated fat, and unsaturated fat and how many calories are in the foods you buy.

Choose foods low in cholesterol. Dietary cholesterol also can raise your blood cholesterol level, although usually not as much as

Table 61.2. Step II Recommendations for Saturated Fat and Total Fat According to Total Calorie Level

Total Calories	1,200	1,500	1,800	2,000	2,500
Saturated fat (grams)*	8	10	12	13	17
Total fat (grams)**	40	50	60	65	80

*One gram of fat equals 9 calories. Amounts are equal to 6 percent of total calories for Step II; your intake should be this much or less.

**Amounts are equal to 30 percent of total calories (rounded down to the nearest 5).

NOTE: On average, women consume about 1,800 calories a day and men consume about 2,500 calories a day.

Lowering Cholesterol for the Person with Heart Disease

saturated fat. So it is important to choose foods low in dietary cholesterol. Dietary cholesterol is found only in foods that come from animals. Many of these foods also are high in saturated fat. Foods from plant sources do not have cholesterol but can contain saturated fat. Use the food label when shopping to choose foods low in cholesterol.

Choose foods high in starch and fiber. Foods high in starch and fiber are excellent substitutes for foods high in saturated fat. These foods—breads, cereals, pasta, grains, fruits, and vegetables—are low in saturated fat and cholesterol, unless fat is added in their preparation. They are also usually lower in calories than foods that are high in fat. Foods high in starch and fiber are also good sources of vitamins and minerals.

A word about sodium. If you have high blood pressure as well as high blood cholesterol (and many people do), your doctor may tell you to cut down on sodium or salt. As long as you are working on getting your blood cholesterol number down, this is a good time to work on your blood pressure, too. Try to limit your sodium intake to 2,400 milligrams a day.

Practical Ways to Change Your Diet

Here are some tips on how to choose foods for the Step II diet. To cut back on saturated fats, choose:

- Poultry, fish, and lean cuts of meat. Remove the skin from chicken and trim the fat from meat before cooking.
- Skim or 1 percent milk instead of 2 percent or whole milk.
- Cheeses with no more than 3 grams of fat per ounce (these include low-fat cottage cheese or other low-fat cheeses). Cut down on full-fat processed, natural, and hard cheeses (like American, brie, and cheddar).
- Low-fat or non-fat yogurt, sour cream, and cream cheese instead of the high-fat varieties.
- Liquid vegetable oils that are high in unsaturated fat (these include canola, corn, olive, and safflower oil).
- Margarine made with unsaturated liquid vegetable oil as the first ingredient rather than hydrogenated or partially hydrogenated oil. Choose tub or liquid margarine or vegetable oil

spreads. The softer the margarine, the more unsaturated it is. If you are watching your sodium intake, try unsalted margarine. Use the food label to choose margarines with the least amount of saturated fat.

- Fewer commercially prepared and processed foods made with saturated or hydrogenated fats or oils (like cakes, cookies, and crackers).
- Foods high in starch and fiber such as whole wheat breads and cereals instead of foods high in saturated fats.

Cutting back on saturated fat helps you to control dietary cholesterol as well, because cholesterol and saturated fat are often, but not always, found together in the same foods. Two additional points to remember when cutting back on dietary cholesterol are:

- Strictly limit organ meat (such as liver, brain, and kidney).
- Eat a total of two or fewer egg yolks a week (as whole eggs or in prepared foods). Try substituting two egg whites for each whole egg in recipes, or using an egg substitute.

To include more foods high in starch and fiber, choose:

- More vegetables and fruits. It is recommended that Americans eat five servings of fruits and vegetables every day. They are low in saturated fat and total fat and have no cholesterol. Fruits and vegetables are good sources of starch, fiber, vitamins, and minerals and are low in sodium. They are also low in calories (which helps with weight control) except for avocados and olives, which are high in both fat and calories. Many fruits and vegetables are also high in vitamin C, vitamin E, and beta-carotene—so-called "antioxidants." A diet high in these fruits and vegetables may also help to lower risk for heart disease. So fruits and vegetables are great substitutes for foods high in saturated fat and cholesterol.
- Whole grain breads and cereals, pasta, rice, and dry peas and beans.

You should also cook the low-fat way:

- Bake, broil, microwave, poach, or roast instead of breading and frying.
- When you roast, place the meat on a rack so the fat can drip away.

Lowering Cholesterol for the Person with Heart Disease

Read Food Labels

We've already mentioned that reading food labels will help you choose foods low in saturated fat, total fat, cholesterol, and calories. Food labels have two important parts: nutrition information and an ingredients list.

Read the nutrition information. Look for the amount of saturated fat, total fat, cholesterol, and calories in a serving of the product. Compare similar products to find the one with the least amounts. If you have high blood pressure, do the same for sodium.

Look at the ingredients. All food labels list the product's ingredients in order by weight. The ingredient in the greatest amount is listed first. The ingredient in the least amount is listed last. So, to

- Serving size
- Number of servings
- Calories
- Total fat in grams
- Saturated fat in grams
- Cholesterol in milligrams

Here, the label gives the amounts for the different nutrients in one serving. Use it to help you keep track of how much fat, saturated fat, cholesterol, and calories you are getting from different foods. Pay attention to the actual amounts (in grams or milligrams). *Don't use the percents shown* (percent daily value) because they are not geared to the Step II diet.

Nutrition Facts

Serving Size 1 cup (228g)
Servings Per Container 2

Amount Per Serving
Calories 250 Calories from Fat 110

	% Daily Value*
Total Fat 12g	18%
Saturated Fat 3g	15%
Cholesterol 30mg	10%
Sodium 470mg	20%
Total Carbohydrate 31g	10%
Dietary Fiber 0g	0%
Sugars 5g	
Protein 5g	

Vitamin A 4% • Vitamin C 2%
Calcium 20% • Iron 4%

* Percent Daily Values are based on a 2,000 calorie diet. Your daily vbalues may be higher or lower depending on your calorie needs:

	Calories:	2,000	2,500
Total Fat	Less than	65g	80g
Sat Fat	Less than	20g	25g
Cholesterol	Less than	300mg	300mg
Sodium	Less than	2,400mg	2,400mg
Total Carbohydrate		300g	375g
Dietary Fiber		25g	30g

Calories per gram:
Fat 9 • Carbohydrates 4 • Protein 4

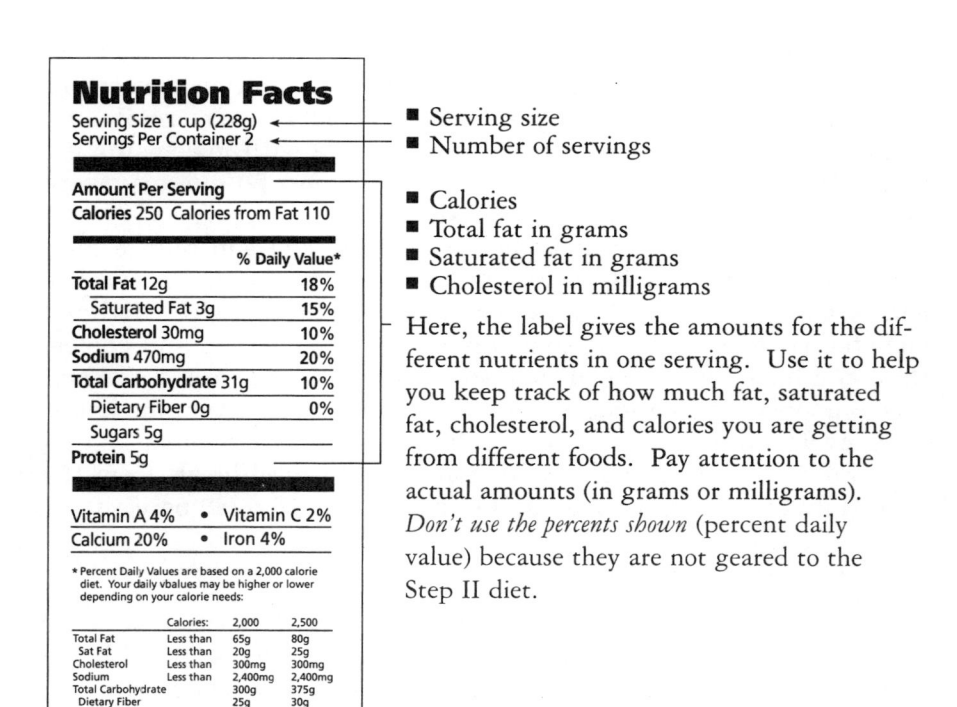

Figure 61.1. Nutrition Fact Food Label

choose foods low in saturated fat or total fat, limit your use of products that list any fat or oil first—or that list many fat and oil ingredients. If you are watching your sodium intake, do the same for sodium or salt.

How Soon Will You See Results?

Generally your blood cholesterol level should show a drop a few weeks after you start on the Step II diet. LDL-cholesterol levels should be measured after being on the diet for 3 to 4 weeks. You should set up a schedule for follow-up cholesterol measurements with your doctor. This schedule will depend on your specific cholesterol level and management program. If your LDL is still too high, your doctor may want you to begin cholesterol-lowering medicine. Once you have reached your goal for LDL-cholesterol, long-term monitoring can begin.

How Much Cholesterol Reduction Can You Expect?

How effective diet is in lowering your LDL-cholesterol level depends on your dietary habits before starting the diet, how well you follow your diet, and how your body responds to your new way of eating. In general, those with higher cholesterol levels have greater reductions in LDL-cholesterol levels than those with lower starting levels. If you are overweight and lose weight, a low-fat diet may work even better to lower your high cholesterol.

Dietary equations predict that the Step II diet can reduce total cholesterol levels in CHD patients who are consuming an average American diet by about 8 to 14 percent. Many people with CHD and elevated cholesterol levels consume more saturated fat and cholesterol and have higher blood cholesterol levels than average and will have an even bigger reduction. Every 1 percent reduction in cholesterol levels lowers your risk for a future heart attack by about 2 percent. So an 8 to 14 percent reduction in cholesterol levels from the Step II diet would lower the CHD risk by about 16 to 28 percent.

Lifetime Changes in Diet

Many people find that advice from a registered dietitian or other qualified nutritionist can help them to be more successful with the Step II diet. Whoever prepares the meals in your house should also participate in these sessions. Your new diet should be maintained for life. You may want to continue diet education sessions with your dietitian quarterly for the first year of long-term monitoring and twice yearly thereafter.

Lowering Cholesterol for the Person with Heart Disease

In addition to making changes in the way you eat, there are other changes you should make.

Become More Physically Active

Regular physical activity by itself may help reduce deaths from heart disease by:

- Lowering LDL levels
- Raising HDL levels
- Lowering high blood pressure
- Lowering triglyceride levels
- Reducing excess weight
- Improving the fitness of your heart and lungs

Since you have heart disease, talk with your doctor before starting an activity to be sure you are following a safe program that works for you.

Your doctor will recommend an activity program to meet your needs. If you have been inactive for a long time, you will be instructed to start with low-to-moderate level activities such as walking, taking the stairs instead of the elevator, gardening, housework, dancing, or exercising at home. Begin by doing the activity for a few minutes most days. Your doctor will then increase your activity level, allowing you to work up to a longer program—your goal is at least 30 minutes per day, 3 or 4 days a week. This can include regular aerobic activities such as brisk walking, jogging, swimming, bicycling, or playing tennis. If you have chest pain, feel faint or light-headed, or become extremely out of breath while exercising, stop the activity at once and tell your doctor as soon as possible.

If you are currently recovering from a heart attack or heart surgery, your doctor may suggest that you begin your new exercise program in a cardiac rehabilitation center. A cardiac rehabilitation center is a place that you can go to exercise under the supervision of a nurse or doctor.

Lose Weight if You Are Overweight

People who are overweight usually have higher blood cholesterol levels than people of desirable weight. When you cut the fat in your diet, you cut down on the richest source of calories. An eating pattern high in starch and fiber instead of fat is a good way to lose weight. Many starchy foods, such as bread, pasta, and rice, have little fat (unless fat is added in preparation) and are lower in calories than high-fat foods. Check the food label to be sure. If you are overweight, losing even a little weight can help to lower LDL-cholesterol and raise HDL-cholesterol. You don't need to reach your desirable weight to see a change in your blood cholesterol levels. But, as a person who has CHD, you should really try to reduce your risk as much as possible by getting your weight down to the desirable level.

Two steps are key to weight loss:

- Eat fewer calories (cutting back on the fat you eat will really help).
- Burn more calories by becoming more physically active.

Cholesterol-Lowering Medicines

To reach an LDL-cholesterol goal of 100 mg/dL or below, you may need to take a cholesterol-lowering medicine in addition to making the life habit changes already mentioned. CHD patients need to lower their LDL more than people without heart disease. As a result, medications are more often used by patients with CHD than by those who do not have CHD.

CHD Patients and Cholesterol-Lowering Medications

CHD patients with LDL levels of 130 mg/dL or greater after diet will generally need to take medicine. If your LDL level is 100 to 129 mg/dL after diet, your doctor will consider all the facts of your case in deciding whether to prescribe medication. If you have been hospitalized for a heart attack, your doctor may choose to start you on a medication at discharge if your LDL-cholesterol is 130 mg/dL or greater. Also, if your LDL-cholesterol is far above the goal level of 100 mg/dL when first measured, your doctor may choose to start a cholesterol-lowering medication together with diet and physical activity right from the beginning of treatment.

If your doctor prescribes medicine, you also will need to:

- Follow your cholesterol-lowering diet.
- Be more physically active.
- Lose weight if overweight.

Lowering Cholesterol for the Person with Heart Disease

- Control all of your other CHD risk factors, including smoking, high blood pressure, and diabetes.

Taking all these steps together may lessen the amount of medicine you need or make the medicine work better—and that reduces your risk for a heart attack. The following is a description of cholesterol-lowering medicines.

Statins

There are currently five statin drugs on the market in the United States: lovastatin, pravastatin, simvastatin, fluvastatin, and atorvastatin. The major effect of the statins is to lower LDL-cholesterol levels, and they lower LDL-cholesterol more than other types of drugs. Statins inhibit an enzyme, HMG-CoA reductase, that controls the rate of cholesterol production in the body. These drugs lower cholesterol by slowing down the production of cholesterol and by increasing the liver's ability to remove the LDL-cholesterol already in the blood. Statins were used to lower cholesterol levels in both the 4S and CARE studies. The large reductions in total and LDL-cholesterol produced by these drugs resulted in large reductions in heart attacks and CHD deaths. Thanks to their track record in these studies and their ability to lower LDL-cholesterol, statins have become the drugs most often prescribed when a person with CHD needs a cholesterol-lowering medicine.

Studies using various statins have reported from 20 to 60 percent lower LDL-cholesterol levels in patients on these drugs. Statin also produce a modest increase in HDL-cholesterol and reduce elevated triglyceride levels.

The statins are usually given in a single dose at the evening meal or at bedtime. It is important that these medications be given in the evening to take advantage of the fact that the body makes more cholesterol at night than during the day.

You should begin to see results from the statins after several weeks, with a maximum effect in 4 to 6 weeks. After about 6 to 8 weeks, your doctor can do the first check of your LDL-cholesterol while on the medication. A second measurement of your LDL-cholesterol level will have to be averaged with the first for your doctor to decide whether your dose of medicine should be changed to help you meet your goal.

The statins are well tolerated by most patients, and serious side effects are rare. A few patients will experience an upset stomach, gas, constipation, and abdominal pain or cramps. These symptoms usually are mild to moderate in severity and generally go away as your body adjusts. Rarely a patient will develop abnormalities in blood tests of the liver. Also rare is the side effect of muscle problems. The symptoms are muscle soreness, pain, and weakness. If this happens, or you have brown urine, contact your doctor right away to get blood tests for possible muscle problems.

Bile Acid Resins

Bile acid resins bind with cholesterol-containing bile acids in the intestines and are then eliminated in the stool. The major effect of bile acid resins is to lower LDL-cholesterol by about 10 to 20 percent. Small doses of resins can produce useful reductions in LDL-cholesterol. Bile acid resins are sometimes prescribed with a statin for patients with CHD to increase cholesterol reduction. When these two drugs are combined, their effects are added together to lower LDL-cholesterol by over 40 percent. Cholestyramine and colestipol are the two main bile acid resins currently available. These two drugs are available as powders or tablets. They are not absorbed from the gastrointestinal tract and 30 years of experience with the resins indicate that their long-term use is safe.

Bile acid resin powders must be mixed with water or fruit juice and taken once or twice (rarely three times) daily with meals. Tablets must be taken with large amounts of fluids to avoid gastrointestinal symptoms. Resin therapy may produce a variety of symptoms including constipation, bloating, nausea, and gas.

The bile acid resins are not prescribed as the sole medicine to lower your cholesterol if you have high triglycerides or a history of severe constipation.

Although resins are not absorbed, they may interfere with the absorption of other medicines if taken at the same time. Other medications therefore should be taken at least 1 hour before or 4 to 6 hours after the resin. Talk to your doctor about the best time to take this medicine, especially if you take other medications.

Nicotinic Acid

Nicotinic acid or niacin, the water-soluble B vitamin, improves all lipoproteins when given in doses well above the vitamin requirement. Nicotinic acid lowers total cholesterol, LDL-cholesterol, and triglyceride levels, while raising HDL-cholesterol levels. There are two types of nicotinic acid: immediate release and timed release. Most experts

Lowering Cholesterol for the Person with Heart Disease

recommend starting with the immediate-release form; discuss with your doctor which type is best for you. Nicotinic acid is inexpensive and widely accessible to patients without a prescription but must not be used for cholesterol lowering without the monitoring of a physician because of the potential side effects. (Nicotinamide, another form of the vitamin niacin, does not lower cholesterol levels and should not be used in the place of nicotinic acid.)

All patients taking nicotinic acid to lower serum cholesterol should be closely monitored by their doctor to avoid complications from this medication. Self-medication with nicotinic acid should definitely be avoided because of the possibility of missing a serious side effect if not under a doctor's care.

Patients on nicotinic acid are usually started on low daily doses and gradually increased to an average daily dose of 1.5 to 3 grams per day.

Nicotinic acid reduces LDL-cholesterol levels by 10 to 20 percent, reduces triglycerides by 20 to 50 percent, and raises HDL-cholesterol by 15 to 35 percent.

A common and troublesome side effect of nicotinic acid is flushing or hot flashes, which are the result of the widening of blood vessels. Most patients develop a tolerance to flushing, and in some patients, it can be decreased by taking the drug during or after meals or by the use of aspirin or other similar medications prescribed by your doctor. The effect of high blood pressure medicines may also be increased while you are on niacin. If you are taking high blood pressure medication, it is important to set up a blood pressure monitoring system while you are getting used to your new niacin regimen.

A variety of gastrointestinal symptoms including nausea, indigestion, gas, vomiting, diarrhea, and the activation of peptic ulcers have been seen with the use of nicotinic acid. Three other major adverse effects include liver problems, gout, and high blood sugar. Risk of the latter three increases as the dose of nicotinic acid is increased. Your doctor will probably not prescribe this medicine for you if you have diabetes, because of the effect on your blood sugar.

Other Drugs

Fibrates

The cholesterol-lowering drugs called fibrates are primarily effective in lowering triglycerides and, to a lesser extent, in increasing HDL-cholesterol levels. Gemfibrozil, the fibrate most widely used in the United States, can be very effective for patients with high triglyceride levels. However, it is not very effective for lowering LDL-cholesterol. As a result, it is used less often than other drugs in patients with CHD for whom LDL-cholesterol lowering is the main goal of treatment. Gemfibrozil therapy by itself is not recommended by the Food and Drug Administration for patients with CHD.

Fibrates are usually given in two daily doses 30 minutes before the morning and evening meals. The reductions in triglycerides generally are in the range of 20 to 50 percent with increases in HDL-cholesterol of 10 to 15 percent.

Fibrates are generally well tolerated by most patients. Gastrointestinal complaints are the most common side effect and fibrates appear to increase the likelihood of developing cholesterol gallstones. Fibrates can increase the effect of medications that thin the blood, and this should be monitored closely by your physician.

Hormone Replacement Therapy

The risk of CHD is increased in postmenopausal women, whether the menopause is natural, surgical, or premature. This increasing risk may be related to the loss of estrogens after menopause. Hormone replacement therapy (HRT) is treatment with estrogen, either alone or with another hormone called progestin. HRT may be prescribed when women experience symptoms from menopause.

HRT can be given in many different forms and amounts. Your doctor will help you select the best form for you.

A recent study called the Postmenopausal Estrogen/Progestin Interventions (PEPI) Trial looked at whether estrogen acts on some of the factors that define a woman's risk of heart disease. Results from the PEPI study showed that:

- Estrogen-only therapy raises the level of HDL-cholesterol.
- Combined estrogen-progestin therapies also increased HDL levels, although less than estrogen alone.
- All of the hormone regimens decreased the level of LDL-cholesterol about equally well.
- None of the hormone regimens caused a significant weight gain.
- All of the hormone regimens caused a rise in triglyceride levels.

In postmenopausal women with CHD, HRT can play a role in improving LDL-and HDL-cholesterol levels.

Lowering Cholesterol for the Person with Heart Disease

Combination Drug Therapy

If your goal LDL level is not reached after 3 months with a single drug, your doctor may consider starting a second medicine to go with it. Combination therapy can increase your cholesterol lowering, reversing or slowing the advance of atherosclerosis and further decreasing the chance of a heart attack or death. The use of low doses of each medicine may help reduce the side effects of the drugs.

Other Medications Commonly Prescribed For CHD

In addition to cholesterol lowering and control of the other risk factors, there are other treatments to help lower your risk from CHD. Aspirin, a drug that has been used for centuries to relieve pain and reduce fever, has been shown to reduce the risk of future heart attacks in patients who have already had one. Aspirin seems to work by reducing the stickiness of the platelets (the cells that cause blood clotting) so that blood clots do not form as readily. After bypass surgery, patients treated with aspirin have fewer early closures of the newly grafted blood vessels in their hearts.

Beta-blockers, another type of drug, have been shown to reduce death rates in patients who have CHD. Beta-blockers slow the heart and make it beat with less contracting force—so blood pressure drops and the heart works less hard.

Many patients with CHD have high blood pressure. Other drugs in addition to beta-blockers may be needed to reach a normal blood pressure.

The amount of risk reduction shown by aspirin and beta-blockers is similar to that of cholesterol lowering, making all three important in the treatment of heart disease.

Next Steps

Talk to Your Doctor—Be Part of Your Health Care Team

There are two key people in your health care team, you and your doctor. You are just as important as your doctor in directing your health care. Only you know how you feel, what you are doing or not doing to improve your health, what you expect from your health, and any difficulties you may be having. It is important for you to tell your doctor these things so he or she can recommend the best treatment.

The first step you should take in becoming an active member of your health care team is to understand what you are being treated for and why. Continue to ask questions until you understand the answer.

It is important for you to understand your coronary heart disease, the special diet you are on, medicines you may be taking, and the tests needed to follow your progress. Ask about the benefits of medications as well as possible side effects. If you are aware of possible side effects of a treatment, you will be able to manage them better. By paying attention to your health and maintaining your own records, you will become an active decision maker in your health care.

Get Support

In addition to your doctor, other health professionals can help you control your blood cholesterol levels. These persons include:

- Registered nurses (RNs) can explain your treatment plan to you, show you how to take your medication, and help you find other sources of information and help. As the health care provider you see the most, nurses are a key resource when you are lowering your cholesterol.

- Registered dietitians (RDs) or qualified nutritionists can explain food plans, show you how to make changes in what you eat, and give you advice on shopping for and preparing foods and eating out. They also can help you set goals for changing the way you eat, so you can successfully lower your high blood cholesterol without making big changes all at once in your eating habits or in your lifestyle.

- Lipid specialists are doctors who are experts in treating high blood cholesterol and similar conditions. You may be referred to a lipid specialist if the treatment your doctor is prescribing does not successfully lower your blood cholesterol levels.

- Pharmacists are aware of the best ways to take medicines to lessen side effects and of the latest research on drugs. They can help you stay on your drug treatment program.

Many people need help while making changes in life habits to reduce their risk; do not be afraid to ask for help from family, friends, and your health care team. Involve your spouse, family members, or significant others in your treatment plan. By sharing your problem and the importance of cholesterol-lowering goals (LDL of 100 mg/dL or less), your current treatment plan, and your medication schedule,

Lowering Cholesterol for the Person with Heart Disease

you can get the help you need to succeed in controlling your cholesterol and lowering your risk.

Long-Term Monitoring

Because you have CHD you will need to monitor your cholesterol and other risk factors for the rest of your life. By discussing your monitoring plan with your health care provider, both you and your physician will be more likely to stick to this plan. Several helpful hints are provided in the text below to help you avoid relapsing to a less healthy lifestyle. If you have a specific problem that is not listed here, discuss it with your doctor, nurse, or dietitian.

Helpful Hints to Monitor Your New Lifestyle

1. Record your test results at each visit.
2. Set realistic short-term goals and write them down.
3. Review your goals during each visit with your health care provider.
4. Share your goals with your family and friends. Support is often the key to success.
5. If you find yourself unable to keep to your plan, write down all of the reasons that you think are responsible. Next, write down what alternatives you have if that situation happens again. If you prepare an alternate strategy in advance, you are more likely to stick to your plan and reach your goals.

When setting your goals with your health care provider, remember the target cholesterol level for persons with CHD:

LDL-cholesterol:100 mg/dL or lower

In addition, since a low HDL-cholesterol level increases CHD risk, patients with CHD should aim to have an HDL-cholesterol higher than 35 mg/dL.

Maintaining Healthy Behaviors and Overcoming Relapse

Question: My last cholesterol level was within my goal. Does that mean I do not have to worry about my cholesterol any more?

Answer: High cholesterol and heart disease are not cured but are only controlled by diet and drug therapy. Stopping your treatment quickly returns your cholesterol to the level that existed before therapy was started.

The goal of diet, physical activity, weight loss, and medicine is to keep your blood cholesterol under control. A slowing in the progression or a regression of atherosclerotic plaque in your coronary arteries is likely to be seen after 1 to 2 years of intensive cholesterol lowering. These observations support the need to continue cholesterol-lowering therapy for years. It seems that maximum benefit is achieved only if therapy is sustained for the rest of your life.

Many people find lifelong changes in diet and activity difficult to manage. It is important to remember that because you may not always stick with your new diet or exercise plan, you are not a failure—just human. The most important part of your new healthy lifestyle is learning how to overcome these challenges and quickly return to your goal.

Eat Right at Social Events

Eating at social events like parties, receptions, family gatherings, and church socials can be a challenge to your heart-healthy eating style. Since you can't control what is served, you may feel pressured to eat foods high in saturated fat and cholesterol.

Here are some tips that will help you eat healthfully at social events:

- At a buffet, look ahead in line to see what low-fat foods are available. Fill up on low-fat items and take only small servings of high-fat foods.

- Bring a low-fat dish to a potluck dinner. That way, you'll have at least one low-fat item from which to choose.

- At parties, focus on activities other than eating. Sit away from the area where the food is being served so you won't be tempted to overeat.

- Ask for help from your family and friends who know you are following a cholesterol-lowering diet. See if they will include some low-fat dishes on the menu.

- Have a few ready answers to politely say no to high-fat foods. For example, "Thank you, but I couldn't eat another bite—everything was delicious."

Lowering Cholesterol for the Person with Heart Disease

- If you do eat too many high-fat foods at a social event, don't feel guilty. Just eat lightly the next day and get back on track.

Eating Out

Are you a smart customer when eating out? You will be if you follow these tips:

- Choose restaurants that have low-fat, low-cholesterol menu choices. And don't be afraid to make special requests—it's your right as a paying customer.
- Control serving sizes by asking for a small serving, sharing a dish with a companion, or taking some home.
- Ask that gravy, butter, rich sauces, and salad dressing be served on the side. That way, you can control the amount you eat.
- Ask to substitute a salad or baked potato for chips, fries, or other extras—or just ask that the extras be left off your plate.
- When ordering pizza, order vegetable toppings like green pepper, onions, and mushrooms instead of meat toppings or extra cheese. To make your pizza even lower in fat and saturated fat, order it with half the cheese or no cheese.
- At fast-food restaurants, go for salads, grilled (not fried or breaded) chicken sandwiches, regular-sized hamburgers, or roast beef sandwiches. Go easy on the regular salad dressings and fatty sauces. Limit jumbo or deluxe burgers or sandwiches.

How to Stay on Your Cholesterol-Lowering Medication

The first step to staying on your medication is understanding what you are taking and why.

- Ask your doctor what you are being treated for and how each medicine helps. For example: If you are taking a statin, you should know that is for lowering your LDL-cholesterol to lower your heart disease risk.
- Know the side effects of any medications you are taking. You can find this out by asking your doctor or pharmacist.
- Ask your doctor how your medicine works with your other medications and the foods you eat. For example: Some medicines

work best if you take them with food, and others work best if you take them at bedtime.

- Ask your doctor what to do if you miss a dose of medicine or have problems with side effects. It is important that you keep your doctor informed of how the medicine is working for you. It may be useful to ask your doctor for help in completing a chart on all of your medicines that includes the name of the medication, what the medication is being taken for, when to take it, what side effects to watch for, and whom to call if you should have a problem.

Remembering to take your medicine is important. Daily reminders are often helpful when scheduling your medication doses. Try to time taking your medicine around activities that you do daily such as setting your alarm clock, brushing your teeth, eating your meals, going to work, or doing other daily activities.

Other ways to help yourself remember to take your medicine could be:

- Setting your watch alarm to go off when it's time to take your medicine.
- Placing a reminder card in a visible place.
- Having a family member or a friend remind you.
- Use a medication box that will hold your entire day's supply of medicine. This will let you know if you missed a dose of medicine.

If you have tried these tricks and still have trouble remembering your medicine, talk to your doctor or pharmacist. It may be possible to simplify your medication schedule or to put your medicine in special containers called blister packs to help you.

Questions You May Be Wondering About

Do I Need to Worry about Lowering My Blood Cholesterol Now That I'm over 70?

A recent study (4S) showed that cholesterol lowering in older patients with CHD significantly reduced the risk for heart attacks and deaths from CHD and prolonged the lives of study participants, just

Lowering Cholesterol for the Person with Heart Disease

as it did in middle-aged patients. Older Americans who have CHD should lower their LDL-cholesterol levels to reduce the risk of having a future heart attack. They should also reduce other cardiovascular risk factors by not smoking and controlling high blood pressure.

Should I Be Concerned about My Child's Blood Cholesterol?

Children from families in which a parent or grandparent has developed heart disease at an early age (before age 55 in father or grandfather, or before age 65 in mother or grandmother) should have their cholesterol levels tested. If a child from such a "high-risk" family has a cholesterol level that is high, it should be lowered under medical supervision, primarily with diet. By following a low-saturated fat and low-cholesterol eating pattern, by being physically active, and by avoiding obesity, even healthy children can lower their risk of developing heart disease as adults.

How Useful Is It to Know My Cholesterol Ratio?

Although the cholesterol ratio can be a useful predictor of heart disease risk, especially in the elderly, it is more important for treatment purposes to know the value for each level separately because both LDL-and HDL-cholesterol separately affect your risk of heart disease and the levels of both may need to be improved by treatment. If you have LDL-cholesterol above 100 mg/dL, lowering your LDL-cholesterol is the main goal of treatment. Your doctor will, however, also consider your HDL when deciding on treatments and goals. The ratio is useful if it helps you and your doctor keep the entire picture of your LDL and HDL levels in mind, but it should not take the place of knowing your separate LDL and HDL levels.

What If I Need Heart Surgery?

Bypass surgery or balloon angioplasty will improve the blood supply to the heart, but it does not mean you can ignore your cholesterol level or the other CHD risk factors. Even though surgery restores blood flow in the heart, poor life habits will clog your new arteries even faster than they clogged your old ones. So pay attention to your risk factors especially after surgery. Trying to lower LDL-cholesterol to about 100 mg/dL or less is an important goal for CH patients. Many patients who have bypass surgery or balloon angioplasty have not actually had a heart attack. Cholesterol-lowering treatment in these patients is very important to lessen the chances of a future heart attack.

What If I Have the Warning Signs of a Heart Attack?

If you have coronary heart disease, you should know the symptoms of a heart attack so that you can get immediate medical help. The most common symptoms are:

- Uncomfortable pressure, fullness, squeezing, or pain in the center of the chest that lasts more than a few minutes, or goes away and comes back.
- Pain that spreads from the chest to the shoulders, jaw, or arms.
- Chest discomfort with lightheadedness, fainting, sweating, nausea, or shortness of breath.

These symptoms may be severe from the start, or they may be mild at first, then gradually worsen. In some people, the warning symptoms come and go.

If you experience any symptoms of a heart attack, get medical help immediately. Be sure you know the phone number so you can get emergency transportation to the hospital. If you are having a heart attack, getting to the hospital fast is very important. Medical treatment, including clot-dissolving medicine, can save lives and reduce damage to the heart muscle, but only if it is started very soon after a heart attack occurs.

Talk with your doctor about the symptoms of a heart attack and what to do if you experience them.

Get More Information

The National Cholesterol Education Program (NCEP), coordinated by the National Heart, Lung, and Blood Institute (NHLBI), has a pamphlet called "Step by Step: Eating To Lower Your High Blood Cholesterol." This pamphlet gives details on how to change your eating habits in order to lower your blood cholesterol levels. The NCEP also has booklets for children with high blood cholesterol levels and their parents. In addition, the NHLBI has a booklet, Exercise and Your Heart: A Guide to Physical Activity. (These publications are available from the government printing office.) The NHLBI can also provide you

Lowering Cholesterol for the Person with Heart Disease

with the names of additional agencies and organizations able to answer questions on cholesterol and the other risk factors for heart disease. To obtain this information please write to:

NHLBI Information Center
P.O. Box 30105
Bethesda, MD 20824-0105

The American Heart Association can also provide you with additional information. Contact your local American Heart Association or call 1-800-AHA-USA1 (1-800-242-8721).

To find a registered dietitian contact:

The National Center for Nutrition and Dietetics' Consumer Nutrition Hotline
1-800-366-1655

Chapter 62

Preventing a Second Heart Attack

If you follow your doctor's advice, take medications as prescribed, and make the necessary lifestyle changes to reduce your risk factors, you may never have another heart attack. However, you and your family members need to be prepared should one occur. Make sure you and family members know the signs of a heart attack and are ready to act quickly if necessary. The sooner you receive treatment, the more likely it is to save heart tissue, and perhaps your life.

You may want to print out and save these warning signs of a heart attack and the heart attack plan so you and your family members can act immediately if trouble develops. It may be reassuring to post the information on the refrigerator or another area where family members can easily find it.

Remember that each heart attack is different and not everyone experiences all the possible warning signs. Also remember that these sensations come and go. Some people feel a lot of pain, others experience very little. Other people experience a feeling of fullness in the chest. Whatever your symptoms, do not delay in getting to an emergency room. The chance of catching a heart attack early is more important than the inconvenience of having doctors check what turns out to be a false alarm.

© 1996-1999 Johns Hopkins InteliHealth, updated November 1997; reprinted with permission of InteliHealth.

Heart Diseases and Disorders Sourcebook, Second Edition

Know the Warning Signs

Not every person experiencing a heart attack has all the signs. In some people, these signs come and go; in others they remain constant and severe. If you experience any of these feelings, get help immediately. Call 911 or get to the nearest emergency room as quickly as possible.

Unless you are suffering from a massive heart attack, which often leads to immediate unconsciousness, you will probably feel at least some of the following warning signs:

- Uncomfortable pressure, fullness, squeezing, or pain in the center of your chest that lasts for a few minutes and then may go away.
- Pain that begins in the chest and spreads to the shoulders, neck and down the arms.
- Lightheadedness, fainting, sweating, nausea, or shortness of breath.

Have a Plan

The key to surviving a heart attack is swift action. After recovering from your first attack, gather the family and talk about what they should do if you experience signs of a repeat attack. You can speed the time between your symptoms and getting care by having a plan ready.

- Get help quickly. Nothing is more important during a heart attack than getting immediate care. The sooner you stop a heart attack, the more heart tissue is saved and the more likely is a full recovery.
- Make a list of hospitals in your area that provide 24-hour emergency cardiac care. Identify which of these hospitals is closest to your home and job. Post a list of the hospitals in your home, where family members can find it, and keep a list with you at all times.
- Don't drive to the hospital alone. Call 911 for emergency rescue if you are alone or if your symptoms are severe.
- Keep two lists of all your medications. Leave one at home where family members can find it and carry the other with you at all

Preventing a Second Heart Attack

times. In the event you do suffer another heart attack, doctors will want to know what medications you are taking so they can prescribe the best treatment for you.

- Have your family trained in cardiopulmonary resuscitation (CPR), a way to help restore heart function and breathing in someone who has collapsed or is unconscious. It is a good idea for family members of heart attack victims to learn CPR in case an emergency ever strikes. Most community centers, hospitals, fire and police organizations and private groups, such as the American Heart Association and the American Red Cross run regular CPR classes. You can reach the American Heart Association at 1-800-AHA-USA1 or the American Red Cross at 1-888-438-2603.

Part Seven

Additional Help and Information

Chapter 63

Glossary of Heart Terms

A

Abdominal aorta: The portion of the aorta in the abdomen (*see also* aorta).

Ablation: Elimination or removal.

ACE (angiotensin-converting enzyme) inhibitor: A drug that lowers blood pressure by interfering with the breakdown of a protein-like substance involved in blood pressure regulation.

Alveoli: Air sacs in the lungs where oxygen and carbon dioxide are exchanged.

Aneurysm: A sac-like protrusion from a blood vessel or the heart, resulting from a weakening of the vessel wall or heart muscle.

Angina or **angina pectoris:** Chest pain that occurs when diseased blood vessels restrict blood flow to the heart.

Angiography: An x-ray technique that makes use of a dye injected into the coronary arteries to study blood circulation through the vessels. The test allows physicians to measure the degrees of obstruction to

"Glossary," © 1997 Texas Heart Institute, URL: http://www.tmc.edu/thi/glossary.html; reprinted with permission. If you need information about keeping your heart healthy, call the Heart Information Service at 1-800-292-2221. (Outside the U.S., call 713/ 794-6536.)

blood flow. Circulation through an artery is not seriously reduced until the inside diameter of the vessel is more than 75% obstructed.

Angioplasty: A nonsurgical technique for treating diseased arteries by temporarily inflating a tiny balloon inside an artery.

Annulus: The ring around a heart valve where the valve leaflet merges with the heart muscle.

Anticoagulant: Any drug that keeps blood from clotting; a blood thinner.

Antihypertensive: Any drug or other therapy that lowers blood pressure.

Aorta: The largest artery in the body and the initial blood-supply vessel from the heart.

Aortic valve: The valve that regulates blood flow from the heart into the aorta.

Arrhythmia (or dysrhythmia): An abnormal heartbeat.

Arterioles: Small, muscular branches of arteries. When they contract, they increase resistance to blood flow, and blood pressure in the arteries increases.

Artery: A vessel that carries oxygen-rich blood to the body.

Arteritis: Inflammation of the arteries.

Arteriosclerosis: A disease process, commonly called hardening of the arteries, which includes a variety of conditions that cause artery walls to thicken and lose elasticity.

Ascending aorta: The first portion of the aorta, emerging from the heart's left ventricle.

Atherectomy: A non-surgical technique for treating diseased arteries with a rotating device that cuts or shaves away obstructing material inside the artery.

Atherosclerosis: A disease process that leads to the accumulation of a waxy substance, called plaque, inside blood vessels.

Glossary of Heart Terms

Atria: The two upper or holding chambers of the heart.

Atrial septal defect: *See* septal defect.

Atrioventricular block: An interruption or disturbance of the electrical signal between the heart's atria (upper two chambers) and the ventricles (lower two chambers).

Atrioventricular (AV) node: A group of cells located between the atria (upper two chambers) and the ventricles (lower two chambers) that regulates the electrical current (heart rhythm) that passes through it to the ventricles.

Atrium: Either one of the heart's two upper chambers.

B

Beta blocker: An antihypertensive drug that limits the activity of epinephrine, a hormone that increases blood pressure.

Biopsy: The process by which a small sample of tissue is taken for examination.

Blalock-Taussig procedure: Palliative shunt between the subclavian and pulmonary arteries used to increase the supply of oxygenated blood in "blue" babies (see below).

Blood clot: A jelly-like mass of blood tissue formed by clotting factors in the blood. Clots stop the flow of blood from an injury; they can also form inside an artery whose walls are damaged by atherosclerotic build-up and can cause a heart attack or stroke.

Blood pressure: The force or pressure exerted by the heart in pumping blood; the pressure of blood in the arteries.

"Blue babies": Babies who have a blue tinge to their skin (cyanosis) resulting from insufficient oxygen in the arterial blood. This condition often indicates a heart defect.

Bradycardia: Abnormally slow heartbeat.

Bundle-branch block: A condition in which portions of the heart's conduction system are defective and unable to conduct the electrical signal normally, causing arrhythmias.

C

Calcium channel blocker (or calcium blocker): A drug that lowers blood pressure by regulating calcium-related electrical activity in the heart.

Capillaries: Microscopically small blood vessels between arteries and veins that distribute oxygenated blood to the body's tissues.

Cardiac: Pertaining to the heart.

Cardiac arrest: The stopping of the heartbeat, usually because of interference with the electrical signal (often associated with coronary heart disease).

Cardiac catheterization: A procedure that involves inserting a fine, hollow tube (catheter) into an artery, usually in the groin area, and passing the tube into the heart. Often used in conjunction with angiography and other procedures, cardiac catheterization has become a prime tool for visualizing the heart and blood vessels and diagnosing and treating heart disease.

Cardiac enzymes: Complex substances capable of speeding up certain biochemical processes in the cardiac muscle. Abnormal levels of these enzymes signal heart attack.

Cardiac output: The amount of blood the heart pumps through the circulatory system in one minute.

Cardiology: The study of the heart and its function in health and disease.

Cardiovascular (CV): Pertaining to the heart and blood vessels. The circulatory system of the heart and blood vessels is the cardiovascular system.

Cardiopulmonary bypass: The process by which a machine is used to do the work of the heart and lungs so the heart can be stopped during surgery.

Cardioversion: A technique of applying an electrical shock to the chest in order to convert an abnormal heartbeat to a normal rhythm.

Cardiomyopathy: A disease of the heart muscle that leads to generalized deterioration of the muscle and its pumping ability.

Glossary of Heart Terms

Carotid artery: A major artery (right and left) in the neck supplying blood to the brain.

Cerebral embolism: A blood clot formed in one part of the body and then carried by the bloodstream to the brain, where it blocks an artery.

Cerebral hemorrhage: Bleeding within the brain resulting from a ruptured blood vessel, aneurysm, or a head injury.

Cerebral thrombosis: Formation of a blood clot in an artery that supplies part of the brain.

Cerebrovascular: Pertaining to the blood vessels of the brain.

Cerebrovascular accident: Also called cerebral vascular accident, apoplexy, or stroke. An impeded blood supply to some part of the brain, resulting in injury to brain tissue.

Cerebrovascular occlusion: The obstruction or closing of a blood vessel in the brain.

Cholesterol: An oily substance that occurs naturally in the body, in animal fats and in dairy products, and that is transported in the blood. Limited quantities are essential to the normal development of cell membranes.

Cineangiography: The technique of taking moving pictures to show the passage of an opaque dye through blood vessels, which allows physicians to diagnose diseases of the heart and blood vessels.

Circulatory system: Pertaining to the heart, blood vessels and the circulation of blood.

Claudication: A tiredness or pain in the arms and legs caused by an inadequate supply of oxygen to the muscles, usually due to narrowed arteries.

Collateral circulation: Blood flow through small, nearby vessels in response to blockage of a main blood vessel.

Computed tomography (CT or CAT scan): An x-ray technique that uses a computer to create cross-sectional images of the body.

Conduction system: Special muscle fibers that conduct electrical impulses throughout the muscle of the heart.

Heart Diseases and Disorders Sourcebook, Second Edition

Congenital: Refers to conditions existing at birth.

Congenital heart defects: Malformation of the heart or of its major blood vessels present at birth.

Congestive heart failure: A condition in which the heart cannot pump all the blood returning to it, leading to a back up of blood in vessels and accumulation of fluid in body tissues, including the lungs.

Coronary arteries: Two arteries arising from the aorta that arch down over the top of the heart and divide into branches. They provide blood to the heart muscle.

Coronary artery bypass (CAB): Surgical rerouting of blood around a diseased vessel that supplies the heart by grafting either a piece of vein from the leg or the artery from under the breastbone.

Coronary artery disease (CAD): A narrowing of the inside diameter of arteries that supply the heart with blood. The condition arises from accumulation of plaque and greatly increases a person's risk of having a heart attack.

Coronary heart disease: Disease of the heart caused by atherosclerotic narrowing of the coronary arteries likely to produce angina pectoris or heart attack; a general term.

Coronary occlusion: An obstruction of one of the coronary arteries that hinders blood flow to some part of the heart muscle.

Coronary thrombosis: Formation of a clot in one of the arteries that carry blood to the heart muscle. Also called coronary occlusion.

Cyanosis: Blueness of skin caused by insufficient oxygen in the blood.

Cyanotic heart disease: A birth defect of the heart that causes oxygen-depleted (blue) blood to circulate to the body without first passing through the lungs.

D

Death rate (age-adjusted): A death rate that has been standardized for age so different populations can be compared or the same population can be compared over time.

Deep vein thrombosis: A blood clot in the deep vein in the calf.

Glossary of Heart Terms

Defibrillator: An electronic device that helps reestablish normal contraction rhythms in a malfunctioning heart.

Diabetes (diabetes mellitus): A disease in which the body doesn't produce or properly use insulin. Insulin is needed to convert sugar and starch into the energy needed in daily life.

Diastolic blood pressure: The lowest blood pressure measured in the arteries, it occurs when the heart muscle is relaxed between beats.

Diuretic: A drug that lowers blood pressure by stimulating fluid loss; promotes urine production.

Doppler ultrasound: A technology that uses sound waves to assess blood flow within the heart and blood vessels and to identify leaking valves.

Dyspnea: A shortness of breath.

E

Echocardiography: A method of studying the heart's structure and function by analyzing sound waves bounced off the heart and recorded by an electronic sensor placed on the chest. A computer processes the information to produce a one-, two- or three-dimensional moving picture that shows how the heart and heart valves are functioning.

Edema: Swelling caused by fluid accumulation in body tissues.

Ejection fraction: A measurement of blood that is pumped out of a filled ventricle. The normal rate is 50 percent or more.

Electrocardiogram (ECG or EKG): A test in which several electronic sensors are placed on the body to monitor electrical activity associated with the heartbeat.

Electroencephalogram (EEG): A graphic record of the electrical impulses produced by the brain.

Electrophysiological study (EPS): A test that uses cardiac catheterization to study patients who have arrhythmias (abnormal heartbeats). An electrical current stimulates the heart in an effort to provoke an arrhythmia, which is immediately treated with medication. EPS is used primarily to identify the origin of arrhythmias and to test the effectiveness of drugs used to treat abnormal heart rhythms.

Embolus: Also called embolism; a blood clot that forms in the blood vessel in one part of the body and travels to another part.

Endarterectomy: Surgical removal of plaque deposits or blood clots in an artery.

Endocardium: The smooth membrane covering the inside surfaces of the heart.

Endothelium: The smooth inner lining of many body structures, including the heart (endocardium) and blood vessels.

Endocarditis: A bacterial infection of the heart's inner lining (endothelium).

Enlarged heart: A state in which the heart is larger than normal due to heredity, long-term heavy exercise, or diseases and disorders such as obesity, high blood pressure, and coronary artery disease.

Enzyme: A complex chemical capable of speeding up specific biochemical processes in the body.

Epicardium: The thin membrane covering the outside surface of the heart muscle.

Estrogen: A female hormone produced by the ovaries that may protect women against heart disease. Estrogen is not produced after menopause.

Exercise stress test: A fairly common test for diagnosing coronary artery disease, especially in patients who have symptoms of heart disease. The test helps physicians assess blood flow through coronary arteries in response to exercise, usually walking, at varied speeds and for various lengths of time on a treadmill. A stress test may include use of electrocardiography, echocardiography, and injected radioactive substances. Also called exercise test, stress test or treadmill test.

F

Familial hypercholesterolemia: A genetic predisposition to dangerously high cholesterol levels.

Glossary of Heart Terms

Fatty acids (fats): Substances that occur in several forms in foods; different fatty acids have different effects on lipid profiles.

Fibrillation: Rapid, uncoordinated contractions of individual heart muscle fibers. The heart chamber involved can't contract all at once and pumps blood ineffectively, if at all.

Flutter: The rapid, ineffective contractions of any heart chamber. A flutter is considered to be more coordinated than fibrillation.

G

Gated blood pool scan: An x-ray analysis of how blood pools in the heart during rest and exercise. The test makes use of a radioactive substance injected into the blood to tag or label red cells. The test provides an estimate of the heart's overall ability to pump and its ability to compensate for one or more blocked arteries. Also called MUGA, for multi-unit gated analysis.

H

Heart attack: Death of, or damage to, part of the heart muscle due to an insufficient blood supply.

Heart block: General term for conditions in which the electrical impulse that activates the heart muscle cells is delayed or interrupted somewhere along its path.

Heart failure: *See* congestive heart failure.

Heart-lung machine: An apparatus that oxygenates and pumps blood to the body during open heart surgery.

Heredity: The genetic transmission of a particular quality or trait from parent to offspring.

High blood pressure: A chronic increase in blood pressure above its normal range.

High density lipoprotein (HDL): A component of cholesterol, HDL helps protect against heart disease by promoting cholesterol breakdown and removal from the blood; hence, its nickname "good cholesterol."

Holter monitor: A portable device for recording heartbeats over a period of 24 hours or more.

Heart Diseases and Disorders Sourcebook, Second Edition

Hypertension: High blood pressure.

Hypertrophic obstructive cardiomyopathy (HOCM): An overgrown heart muscle that creates a bulge into the ventricle and impedes blood flow.

Hypoglycemia: Low levels of glucose in the blood.

Hypotension: Abnormally low blood pressure.

Hypoxia: Less than normal content of oxygen in the organs and tissues of the body.

I

Immunosuppressive medications: Any drug that suppresses the body's immune system. These medications are used to minimize the chances that the body will reject a newly transplanted organ such as a heart.

Impedance plethysmography: A noninvasive diagnostic test used to evaluate blood flow through the leg.

Infarct: The area of heart tissue permanently damaged by an inadequate supply of oxygen.

Inferior vena cava: The large vein returning blood from the legs and abdomen to the heart.

Inotropic medications: Any drug that increases the strength of the heart's contraction.

Intravascular echocardiography: A marriage of echocardiography and cardiac catheterization. A miniature echo device on the tip of a catheter is used to generate images inside the heart and blood vessels.

Ischemia: Decreased blood flow to an organ, usually due to constriction or obstruction of an artery.

Ischemic heart disease: Also called coronary artery disease and coronary heart disease, this term is applied to heart ailments caused by narrowing of the coronary arteries, and therefore characterized by a decreased blood supply to the heart.

Glossary of Heart Terms

J

Jugular veins: The veins that carry blood back from the head to the heart.

L

Lesion: An injury or wound. An atherosclerotic lesion is an injury to an artery due to hardening of the arteries.

Lipid: A fatty substance insoluble in blood.

Lipoprotein: A lipid surrounded by a protein; the protein makes the lipid soluble in blood.

Low density lipoprotein (LDL): The body's primary cholesterol-carrying molecule. High blood levels of LDL increase a person's risk of heart disease by promoting cholesterol attachment and accumulation in blood vessels; hence, the popular nickname "bad cholesterol."

Lumen: The hollow area within a tube, such as a blood vessel.

M

Magnetic resonance imaging (MRI): A technique that produces images of the heart and other body structures by measuring the response of certain elements (such as hydrogen) in the body to a magnetic field. When stimulated by radio waves, the elements emit distinctive signals in a magnetic field. MRI can produce detailed pictures of the heart and its various structures without the need to inject a dye.

Mitral valve: The structure that controls blood flow between the heart's left atrium (upper chamber) and left ventricle (lower chamber).

Mitral valve prolapse: A condition that occurs when the leaflets of the mitral valve between the left atrium (upper chamber) and left ventricle (lower chamber) bulge into the ventricle and permit backflow of blood into the atrium. The condition is often associated with progressive mitral regurgitation.

Monounsaturated fats: A type of fat found in many foods but predominantly in avocados and canola, olive and peanut oil. Monounsaturated fat tends to lower LDL cholesterol levels, and some studies suggest that it may do so without also lowering HDL cholesterol levels.

Mortality: The total number of deaths from a given disease in a population during an interval of time, usually a year.

Murmur: Noises superimposed on normal heart sounds. They are caused by congenital defects or damaged heart valves that do not close properly and allow blood to leak back into the chamber from which it has come.

Myocardial infarction: The damage or death of an area of the heart muscle (myocardium) resulting from a blocked blood supply to the area. The affected tissue dies, injuring the heart. Symptoms include prolonged, intensive chest pain and a decrease in blood pressure that often causes shock.

Myocardial ischemia: Deficient blood flow to part of the heart muscle.

Myocardium: The muscular wall of the heart. It contracts to pump blood out of the heart and then relaxes as the heart refills with returning blood.

N

Nitroglycerin: A drug that helps relax and dilate arteries, often used to treat cardiac chest pain (angina).

Necrosis: Referring to the death of tissue within a certain area.

Noninvasive procedures: Any diagnostic or treatment procedure in which no instrument enters the body.

O

Obesity: The condition of being significantly overweight. It is usually applied to a condition of 30 percent or more over ideal body weight. Obesity puts a strain on the heart and can increase the chance of developing high blood pressure and diabetes.

Occluded artery: An artery in which the blood flow has been impaired by a blockage.

Glossary of Heart Terms

Open heart surgery: An operation in which the chest and heart are opened surgically while the bloodstream is diverted through a heart-lung (cardiopulmonary perfusion) machine.

P

Pacemaker: A surgically implanted electronic device that helps regulate the heartbeat.

Palpitation: An uncomfortable sensation within the chest caused by an irregular heartbeat.

Patent ductus arteriosus: A congenital defect in which the opening between the aorta and the pulmonary artery does not close after birth.

Percutaneous transluminal coronary angioplasty (PTCA): *See* angioplasty.

Pericarditis: Inflammation of the outer membrane surrounding the heart. Rheumatic fever, tuberculosis, and many other agents are its possible causes.

Pericardiocentesis: A diagnostic procedure using a needle to withdraw fluid from the sac or membrane surrounding the heart (pericardium).

Pericardium: The outer fibrous sac that surrounds the heart.

Plaque: A deposit of fatty (and other) substances in the inner lining of the artery wall; it is characteristic of atherosclerosis.

Platelets: One of the three types of cells found in blood; they aid in the clotting of the blood.

Polyunsaturated fat: The major fat constituent in most vegetable oils including corn, safflower, sunflower, and soybean. These oils are liquid at room temperature. Polyunsaturated fat actually tends to lower LDL cholesterol levels but may also reduce HDL cholesterol levels as well.

Positron emission tomography (PET): A test that uses positron emitting substances to assess information about the metabolism of elements that can be used to indicate whether heart muscle is alive and functioning. A ring of radiosensitive detectors positioned around the chest reconstructs a two- or three-dimensional image of the heart.

Prevalence: The total number of cases of a given disease that exist in a population at a specific time.

Pulmonary: Referring to the lungs and respiratory system.

Pulmonary valve: The heart valve between the right ventricle and the pulmonary artery. It controls blood flow from the heart into the lungs.

Pulmonary vein: The blood vessel that carries newly oxygenated blood from the lungs back to the left atrium of the heart.

R

Radionuclide ventriculography: A diagnostic test used to determine the size and shape of the heart's pumping chambers (the ventricles).

Regurgitation: Backward flow of blood through a defective heart valve.

Renal: Pertaining to the kidneys.

Rheumatic fever: A disease, usually occurring in childhood, that may follow a streptococcal infection. Symptoms may include fever, sore or swollen joints, skin rash, involuntary muscle twitching, and development of nodules under the skin. If the infection involves the heart, scars may form on heart valves, and the heart's outer lining may be damaged.

Risk factor: An element or condition involving a certain hazard or danger. When referring to heart and blood vessels, a risk factor is associated with an increased chance of developing cardiovascular disease, including stroke.

Rubella: Commonly known as German measles.

S

Saturated fat: Type of fat found in foods of animal origin and a few of vegetable origin; they are usually solid at room temperature. Abundant

Glossary of Heart Terms

in meat and dairy products, saturated fat tends to increase LDL cholesterol levels, and it may raise the risk of certain types of cancer.

Septal defect: A hole in the wall of the heart separating the atria or in the wall of the heart separating the ventricles.

Septum: The muscular wall dividing a chamber on the left side of the heart from the chamber on the right.

Shock: A condition in which body function is impaired because the volume of fluid circulating through the body is insufficient to maintain normal metabolism. This may be caused by blood loss or by a disturbance in the function of the circulatory system.

Shunt: A connector that allows blood to flow between two locations.

Sick sinus syndrome: The failure of the sinus node to regulate the heart's rhythm.

Silent ischemia: Episodes of cardiac ischemia that are not accompanied by chest pain.

Sinus (SA) node: The "natural" pacemaker of the heart. The node is a group of specialized cells in the top of the right atrium which produces the electrical impulses that travel down to eventually reach the ventricular muscle, causing the heart to contract.

Sodium: A mineral essential to life found in nearly all plant and animal tissue. Table salt (sodium chloride) is nearly half sodium.

Sphygmomanometer: An instrument used to measure blood pressure.

Stent: A device made of expandable, metal mesh that is placed (by using a balloon catheter) at the site of a narrowing artery. The stent is then expanded and left in place to keep the artery open.

Stenosis: The narrowing or constriction of an opening, such as a blood vessel or heart valve.

Stethoscope: An instrument for listening to sounds within the body.

Streptococcal infection ("strep" infection): An infection, usually in the throat, resulting from the presence of streptococcus bacteria.

Streptokinase: A clot-dissolving drug used to treat heart attack patients.

Sternum: The breastbone.

Stress: Bodily or mental tension resulting from physical, chemical or emotional factors. Stress can refer to physical exertion as well as mental anxiety.

Stroke: A sudden disruption of blood flow to the brain, either by a clot or a leak in a blood vessel.

Subarachnoid hemorrhage: Bleeding from a blood vessel on the surface of the brain into the space between the brain and the skull.

Sudden death: Death that occurs unexpectedly and instantaneously or shortly after the onset of symptoms. The most common underlying reason for patients dying suddenly is cardiovascular disease, in particular coronary heart disease.

Superior vena cava: The large vein that returns blood from the head and arms to the heart.

Syncope: A temporary, insufficient blood supply to the brain which causes a loss of consciousness.

Systolic blood pressure: The highest blood pressure measured in the arteries. It occurs when the heart contracts with each heartbeat.

T

Tachycardia: Accelerated beating of the heart. Paroxysmal tachycardia is a particular form of rapid heart action, occurring in seizures that may last from a few seconds to several days.

Tachypnea: Rapid breathing.

Thallium-201 stress test: An x-ray study that follows the path of radioactive potassium carried by the blood into heart muscle. Damaged or dead muscle can be defined, as can the extent of narrowing in an artery.

Thrombolysis: The breaking up of a blood clot.

Glossary of Heart Terms

Thrombosis: A blood clot that forms inside the blood vessel or cavity of the heart.

Thrombolytic therapy: A drug that dissolves blood clots.

Thrombus: A blood clot.

Tissue plasminogen activator (TPA): A clot-dissolving drug used to treat heart attack patients.

Trans fat: Created when hydrogen is forced through an ordinary vegetable oil (hydrogenation), converting some polyunsaturates to monounsaturates, and some monounsaturates to saturates. Trans fat, like saturated fat, tends to raise LDL cholesterol levels, and, unlike saturated fat, trans fat also lowers HDL cholesterol levels at the same time.

Transesophageal echocardiography: A diagnostic test that analyzes sound waves bounced off the heart. The sound waves are sent through a tube-like device inserted in the mouth and passed down the esophagus (food pipe), which ends near the heart. This technique is useful in studying patients whose heart and vessels, for various reasons, are difficult to assess with standard echocardiography.

Transient ischemic attack (TIA): A temporary, stroke-like event that lasts for only a short time and is caused by a temporarily blocked blood vessel.

Transplantation: Replacing a defective organ with one from a donor.

Tricuspid valve: The structure that controls blood flow from the heart's right atrium (upper chamber) into the right ventricle (lower chamber).

Triglyceride: The most common fatty substance found in the blood; normally stored as an energy source in fat tissue. High triglyceride levels may thicken the blood and make a person more susceptible to clot formation. High triglyceride levels tend to accompany high cholesterol levels and other risk factors for heart disease such as obesity.

U

Ultrasound: High-frequency sound vibrations, not audible to the human ear, used in medical diagnosis.

V

Valvuloplasty: Reshaping of a heart valve with surgical or catheter techniques.

Varicose vein: Any vein that is abnormally dilated.

Vascular: Pertaining to the blood vessels.

Vasodilators: Any medication that dilates (widens) the arteries.

Vasopressors: Any medication that elevates blood pressure.

Vein: Any one of a series of blood vessels of the vascular system that carries blood from various parts of the body back to the heart; returns oxygen-depleted blood to the heart.

Ventricle (right and left): One of the two lower chambers of the heart.

Ventricular fibrillation: A condition in which the ventricles contract in a rapid, unsynchronized fashion. When fibrillation occurs, the ventricles cannot pump blood throughout the body.

Ventricular tachycardia: An arrhythmia (abnormal heartbeat) in the ventricle characterized by a very fast heartbeat.

Vertigo: A feeling of dizziness or spinning.

W

Wolff-Parkinson-White syndrome: A condition in which an extra electrical pathway connects the atria (two upper chambers) and the ventricles (two lower chambers). It may cause a rapid heartbeat.

X

X-ray: Form of radiation used to create a picture of internal body structures on film.

Chapter 64

Heart Healthy Cookbooks

American Heart Association Around the World Cookbook: Healthy Recipes with International Flavor
Published by Times Books, a division of Random House, Inc. (800) 793-2665.

The recipes featured in this cookbook offer international cuisine that is low in fat, cholesterol, and sodium.

American Heart Association Low-Fat, Low-Cholesterol Cookbook, Second Edition (1998)
Published by Times Books, a division of Random House, Inc. (800) 793-2665.

This spiral-bound hardcover cookbook presents a wide assortment of recipes, including breakfasts, soups, salads, appetizers, main dishes, and deserts. It also features tips, nutritional information, and color photos.

American Heart Association Low-Salt Cookbook
Published by Times Books, a division of Random House, Inc. (800) 793-2665.

This cookbook features 175 recipes for people who need to reduce their sodium intake. Also included are shopping tips, cooking techniques, and information about substituting ingredients.

Information in this chapter was compiled from various sources deemed reliable. This list is not intended to be comprehensive; inclusion does not constitute endorsement. Please check with your local library or bookstore, or contact the publisher for ordering information.

American Heart Association Kids' Cookbook
Published by Times Books, a division of Random House, Inc. (800) 793-2665.

The more than 30 recipes included in this book are intended for cooks aged eight to twelve. They are low in fat and cholesterol and feature kids' favorites like pizza and chicken nuggets.

American Heart Association Quick and Easy Cookbook (1998)
Published by Times Books, a division of Random House, Inc. (800) 793-2665.

From the American Heart Association, this cookbook presents more than 200 healthy recipes that can be made when time is limited.

Betty Crocker's New Low-Fat, Low-Cholesterol Cookbook (1996)
Published by IDG Books Worldwide (800) 434-3422.

This cookbook offers 185 low-fat, low-cholesterol recipes. The 1996 version is an update of the previous edition with 50 new recipes.

Choices for a Healthy Heart (1987)
Published by Workman Publishing (800) 722-7202.

This book is a companion volume to *Don't Eat Your Heart Out* (see below). It provides more than 200 additional recipes building on the concept of low-fat eating. It includes practical cooking tips and meal plans along with information about exercise, stress, smoking, and other lifestyle factors that impact health.

Delicious Heart Healthy Latino Recipes
Produced by the National Heart, Lung, and Blood Institute (NIH Pub. No. 96-4049); available online at: www.nhlbi.nih.gov/health/public/heart/other/sp_recip.htm

This publication of the National Heart, Lung, and Blood Institute includes heart-healthy versions of traditional Hispanic foods.

Don't Eat Your Heart Out Cookbook, Second Edition (1994)
Published by Workman Publishing (212) 254-5900.

This book is really two books in one: a guidebook to changing meal patterns and other habits in support of a healthier heart; and a cookbook of heart-healthy recipes.

Down Home Healthy: Family Recipes of Black American Chefs (1993)
Produced by the National Cancer Institute (NIH Pub. No. 93-3408); (800) 422-6237.

This cookbook gives recipes and cooking tips for low-fat meals, drawing on the New Orleans and Florida backgrounds of the authors, who are black American chefs. A bibliography is included.

Healthy Mexican Cooking: Authentic Low-Fat Recipes [Cocina mexicana saludable: Recetas autenticas con bajo contenido de grasa] (1995)
Published by Appletree Press (800) 322-5679.

This cookbook offers a collection of easy-to-prepare, low-fat Mexican recipes. Introductory chapters include information about heart disease and other disorders associated with eating habits, dietary guidelines, tips, and resources. Recipes include appetizers and salsas, soups and breads, salads, entrees, side dishes, and desserts. The cookbook is available in English or Spanish.

Healthy Snacks for Kids (1999)
Published by Bristol Publishing Enteprises.

The snack recipes presented in this 176-page cookbook include: Monkey Bars, Tomato Balloons, and Wiggle Sicles.

Heart-Healthy Cooking African American Style
Produced by the National Heart, Lung, and Blood Institute (NIH Pub. No. 97-3792); available at online at: www.nhlbi.gov/health/public/heart/other/chdblack/cooking.htm

This booklet offers 20 heart healthy recipes that are low in saturated fat, cholesterol, and salt, including cornbread, spicy southern barbecued chicken, and sweet potato pie.

The New American Heart Association Cookbook, 25th Anniversary Edition
Published by Times Books, a division of Random House, Inc. (800) 793-2665.

This cookbook, produced by the American Heart Association, contains more than 600 recipes, including healthy versions of classic recipes, quick recipes, one-dish recipes, and desserts.

Heart Diseases and Disorders Sourcebook, Second Edition

Stay Young at Heart: Cook the Heart-Healthy Way

Produced by the National Heart, Lung, and Blood Institute; available online at: www.nhlbi.nih.gov/health/public/heart/other/sayah/index.htm

This online cookbook features heart-healthy recipes for soups, entrees, vegetables, pasta, and desserts.

Chapter 65

Spanish Language Publications Available from the National Heart, Lung, and Blood Institute

The following publications are available from:

National Heart, Lung, and Blood Institute
31 Center Drive
MSC2470
Bethesda, MD 20892-2470
Voice: (301) 496-4236
Voice: (301) 592-8573 (Information Center)
Fax: (301) 582-8563 (Information Center)
Internet: www.nhlbi.nih.gov
E-Mail: NHLBIinfo@rover.nhlbi.nih.gov

¡Coma menos sal y sodio!
NIH Pub. No. 96-4042

Comer menos sal y sodio le ayuda a prevenir o bajar la presión alta.

¡Conozca su nivel de colesterol!
NIH Pub. No. 96-4043

Un nivel de colesterol de menos de 200 es deseable. ¡Mantenga su colesterol a un nivel menos de 200!

¡Cuide su peso!
NIH Pub. No 96-4047

Trate de lograr un peso saludable. Prepare las comidas de manera saludable. ¡Manténgase activo!

¡Manténgase activo y siéntase bien!
NIH Pub. No. 96-4046

Nunca es tarde para decidirse a tener un corazón y un cuerpo sano. Agregue actividad física a su vida y a la de su familia.

¡Póngase en acción—prevenga la alta presión!
NIH Pub. No. 96-4041.

La presión alta se conoce como "el asesino silencioso." Es una enfermedad que no da síntomas.

¡Proteja su corazón—baje su colesterol!
NIH Pub. No. 96-4044

¡Tome acción para bajar su colesterol en la sangre! Más vale prevenir que lamentar.

¡Reduzca la grasa—no el sabor!
NIH Pub. No. 96-4045

Proteja la salud de su corazón y el de su familia sirviendo alimentos bajos en grasa y grasa saturada.

¡Rompa con el hábito de fumar!
NIH Pub. No. 96-4048.

El humo de un cigarrillo deja en el aire más de 4.000 sustancias dañinas. Cuando fuma usted pone en peligro su salud y la de su familia. ¡Deje de fumar hoy!

Chapter 66

Directory of Resources for Heart Patients

American Alliance for Health, Physical Education, Recreation, and Dance
1900 Association Drive
Reston, VA 20191
Toll-free: (800) 213-7193
Voice: (703) 476-3400
E-mail: webmaster@aahperd.org
Internet: www.aahperd.org

The American Alliance for Health, Physical Education, and Dance is an organization of professionals involved in these specialties working to promote creative and healthy lifestyles.

American Dietetic Association
216 West Jackson Blvd.
Chicago, IL 60606-6995
Toll-free: (800) 0366-1655
Voice: (312) 899-0040
E-mail: cdr@eatright.org
Internet: www.eatright.org

The information in this chapter was compiled from various sources deemed accurate. All contact information was verified and updated in September 1999. Inclusion does not imply endorsement. This list is intended to serve as a starting point for information gathering; it is not comprehensive.

The American Dietetic Association promotes sound nutrition information by providing consumers and nutrition professionals with food and nutrition information.

American Heart Association
7272 Greenville Avenue
Dallas, TX 75231-4596
Toll-free: (800) 242-8721 (for local AHA offices)
Voice: (214) 706-1552
Fax: (214) 706-2139
Internet: www.amhrt.org

The American Heart Association, a nonprofit, voluntary health agency funded by private contributions, is dedicated to the reduction of death and disability from cardiovascular diseases, including heart diseases and stroke.

American Society of Hypertension
515 Madison Avenue, Suite 1212
New York, NY 10022
Voice: (212) 644-0650
Fax: (212) 644-0658
E-mail: ash@ash-us.org
Internet: www.ash-us.org

The American Society of Hypertension is a professional organization dedicated to hypertension and related cardiovascular diseases.

CARE (Cardiac Arrhythmias Research Education Foundation, Inc.)
2082 Michelson Drive, #301
Irvine, CA 92612
Toll-free: (800) 404-9500
Voice: (949) 752-2273
E-mail: care@longqt.org
Internet: www.longqt.org

CARE is involved with funding increased medical research in cardiac arrhythmias and working to promote physician education and public awareness of the unexpected, sudden death of children and young adults from this disorder.

Directory of Resources for Heart Patients

CHASER, Inc.
(Congenital Heart Anomalies Support, Education, and Resources, Inc.)
2112 North Wilkins Road
Swanton, OH 43558
Voice: (419) 825-5575
Fax: (419) 825-2880
E-mail: CHASER@compuserve.com
Internet: www.csun.edu/~hcmth011/chaser/hlhsflier.html

CHASER provides information to families of children born with heart defects, to adults with congenital heart defects, and to families of infants and children with acquired heart disease.

Children's Health Information Network
1561 Clark Drive
Yardley, PA 19067
Voice: (215) 493-3068
E-mail: mb@tchin.org
Internet: www.tchin.org

The Children's Health Information Network maintains the Congenital Heart Disease Information and Resources project, a web site that provides information and resources to families of children with congenital and acquired hart disease, adults with CHD, and the professionals who work with them.

Citizens for Public Action on Blood Pressure and Cholesterol
(Citizens for the Treatment of High Blood Pressure)
Box 30374
Bethesda, MD 20824
Voice: (301) 770-1711

Citizens for Public Action on Blood Pressure and Cholesterol is a non-profit, advocacy group for public policy and resources to prevent heart disease. Publications include a series of brochures related to blood pressure and cholesterol.

The Coronary Club, Inc.
9500 Euclid Avenue
Mail Code A42
Cleveland, OH 44195
Toll-free: 800 478-4255
Voice: (216) 444-3690

The Coronary Club, Inc, a nonprofit organization, was founded in 1968 to provide patients and their families with information on preventing heart attacks and adjusting to life with a heart condition.

Food and Nutrition Information Center
National Agricultural Library
Room 304
10301 Baltimore Boulevard
Beltsville, MD 20705-2351
Voice: (301) 504-5719
TTY: (301) 504-6856
Fax: (301) 504-6409
E-mail: fnic@nal.usda.gov
Internet: www.nalusda.gov/fnic

The Food and Nutrition Information Center, a program of the U.S. Department of Agriculture, provides print, audiovisual, and resource materials for consumers and bibliographies and resource guides for professionals on topics in human nutrition.

Healthfinder
Internet: www.healthfinder.gov

This gateway site offers links to more than 1,250 other sites to help consumers find information easily and quickly.

Heart Information Network
Internet: www.heartinfo.org

This website, produced by the Center for Cardiovascular Education, Inc., includes information on a wide variety of topics including heart attacks, hypertension, heart failure, valve abnormalities, and heart-healthy cooking.

HeartPoint
Internet: www.heartpoint.com

This website was created by medical professionals to provide information to cardiac patients.

Heart Surgery Forum
www.hsforum.com

This website offers an on-line cardiothoracic journal produced by the International Society for Minimally Invasive Cardiac Surgery.

Directory of Resources for Heart Patients

Indian Health Service
Communications Office
Parklawn Building, Room 6-35
5600 Fishers Lane
Rockville, MD 20857
Voice: (301) 443-3593
Fax: (301) 443-0507
Internet: www.ihs.gov/index.asp

The Indian Health Service provides a comprehensive health services delivery system for American Indians and Alaska Natives.

InteliHealth
Internet: www.intelihealth.com

A joint venture of Johns Hopkins University and Aetna U.S. Healthcare, this site offers a wide-ranging collection of consumer health information.

Johns Hopkins Bayview Medical Center
4940 Eastern Avenue
Baltimore, MD 21224
Voice: (410) 550-0100
Internet: www.jhbmc.jhu.edu

The website produced by Johns Hopkins Bayview Medical Center includes a page on cardiac rehabilitation and prevention at www.jhbmc.jhu.edu/cardiology/rehab/patientinfo.html.

Mayo Health Oasis
Internet: www. mayo.ivi.com

From the Mayo Clinic, this health information site provides user-friendly friendly features, including Newsstand, a weekly update, "Ask the Mayo Physician", interactive quizzes, and the Heart Center. "The Virtual Cookbook" lets you send in your favorite recipe and a Mayo dietitian will change it to cut fat, calories, salt, or cholesterol.

The Mended Hearts, Inc.
7272 Greenville Avenue
Dallas, TX 75231
Toll-free: (800) AHA-USA-1
Voice: (214) 706-1442

Fax: (214) 706-5231
E-mail: dbonham@heart.org
Internet: www.mendedhearts.org

The Mended Hearts, Inc. is a nonprofit self-help group for people suffering from heart disease. It operates through local chapters and is supported by local and national dues.

National Center for Chronic Disease Prevention and Health Promotion
4770 Buford Highway, NE
Mailstop K13
Atlanta, GA 30341
Voice: (770) 488-5080
Fax: (770) 488-5962
E-mail: ccdinfo@cdc.gov
Internet: www.cdc.gov/nccdphp/

This center, part of the Centers for Disease Control and Prevention (CDC), plans, directs and coordinates national programs for the prevention of premature mortality, morbidity, and disability due to chronic illnesses and conditions.

National Heart, Lung, and Blood Institute
31 Center Drive
MSC2470
Bethesda, MD 20892-2470
Voice: (301) 496-4236
Voice: (301) 592-8573 (Information Center)
Fax: (301) 592-8563 (Information Center)
Internet: www.nhlbi.nih.gov/nhlbi/nhlbi.htm

The National Heart, Lung, and Blood Institute's primary responsibility is the scientific investigation of heart, blood vessel, lung, and blood diseases. The Institute oversees resources and research, demonstration, prevention, education, control, and training activities in these fields. The program emphasizes the prevention and control of heart, lung, and blood diseases and the education concerning these diseases.

NIH Health Information
Internet: www.nih.gov/health

Directory of Resources for Heart Patients

This site gives consumers a single access point to the resources of the National Institutes of Health, including publications, clearinghouses, and the Combined Health Information Database.

Office of Minority Health Resource Center
Office of Minority Health
P.O. Box 37337
Washington, DC 20013-7337
Toll-free: (800) 444-6472
E-mail: lmosby@omhrc.gov
Internet: www.omhrc.gov

The Office of Minority Health Resource Center responds to requests on minority health. Activities concentrate on the minority health priority areas. Bilingual staff members are available to serve Spanish speaking requestors.

Office on Smoking and Health
National Center for Chronic Disease Prevention and Health Promotion
Centers for Disease Control and Prevention
Mail Stop K-50
4770 Buford Highway, NE
Atlanta, GA 30341-3724
Toll-free: (800) CDC-1311
Voice: (770) 488-5705
Fax: (770) 488-5939
E-mail: eecinfo@ccdod1.em.cdc.gov
Internet: www.cdc.gov/nccdphp/osh

The Office on Smoking and Health (OSH) is a division of the Centers for Disease Control and Prevention, National Center for Chronic Disease Prevention and Health promotion. Among its many functions, OSH develops and distributes the annual Surgeon General's report on smoking and health, coordinates a national public information and education program on tobacco use and health, and coordinates tobacco education research efforts within the Department of Health and Human Services (DHHS). Subjects such as smoking cessation, ETS/passive smoking, pregnancy/infants, and professional/technical information are among the many features of the publication list which is updated periodically and available upon request by calling.

Pulmonary Hypertension Association
Attn: Rino Aldrigheti
817 Silver Spring Avenue, Suite 303
Silver Spring, MD 20910
Toll free: (800) 748-7274 (between 10:00 a.m. and 6 p.m. CST)
E-mail: admin@phassociation.org
Internet: www.phassociation.org

Founded in 1990, the Pulmonary Hypertension Association, a nonprofit organization, serves patients with pulmonary hypertension. Regional support groups hold regular meetings and contact is maintained with distant members through phone and mail services.

Shape Up America!
6707 Democracy Blvd., Suite 306
Bethesda, MD 20817
E-mail: suainfo@shapeup.org
Internet: www.shapeup.org

The website posted by Shape Up America! seeks to provide information about physical fitness, weight management, and healthy eating. Their efforts are designed help Americans avoid problems associated with weight-related conditions, including obesity, heart disease, and Type II diabetes.

Texas Heart Institute
1011 Bates Avenue
P.O. Box 20345
Houston, TX 77030
Voice: (713) 791-4011
Internet: www.tmc.edu/thi/index.html

The Texas Heart Institute is a chartered, nonprofit organization located in St. Luke's Episcopal Hospital in the Texas Medical Center. The organization was founded in 1962 for the study and treatment of diseases of the heart and blood vessels.

YMCA of the USA
101 North Wacker Drive
Chicago, IL 60606
Voice: (312) 977-0031
Fax: (312) 977-9063

Directory of Resources for Heart Patients

E-mail: info@ymcausa.org
Internet: www.ymca.net

The YMCA of the USA is actively involved in improving spiritual, mental and physical health through its 2,000+ member associations. YMCA fitness and health programs are based on preventive health care activities designed to head off heart disease, stroke, and other afflictions before they begin to develop.

Index

Index

Page numbers followed by 'n' indicate a footnote. Page numbers in *italics* indicate a table or illustration.

A

Abben, Richard P. 472
abdominal aorta, defined 537
ablation, defined 537
Accupril (quinapril) 381, *415*
acebutolol *414*
ACE inhibitors *see* angiotensin converting enzyme (ACE) inhibitors
acetaminophen 257, 258
ACS *see* American Cancer Society (ACS)
Actron (ketoprofen) 258
Adalat (nifedipine) 384–85, *415*
adolescents
 blood cholesterol levels 92, 99
 exercise benefits 196–97
 sedentary lifestyle 189
Advice for the Patient: Drug Information in Lay Language (Micromedex) 381n
Advil Liquigels (solubilized ibuprofen) 258
AED *see* automatic external defibrillator (AED)

age factor
 angina 40
 blood cholesterol levels 78, 221
 cardiac rehabilitation 493
 cholesterol levels 503
 congestive heart failure *26*
 heart disease 76, 142–43, 155
 heart failure 316
 ischemic heart disease 16–19
Agency for Health Care Policy and Research (AHCPR)
 contact information 165, 488
 patient guideline 488
 publications clearinghouse 295
AHCPR *see* Agency for Health Care Policy and Research Center (AHCPR)
Air Force/Texas Coronary Atherosclerosis Prevention Study 224
Alabama, ischemic heart disease statistics 18
Alaska, ischemic heart disease statistics 18
alcohol dehydrogenase 118
alcohol use
 cardiac rehabilitation 493–94
 cholesterol levels 503
 digoxin 402
 heart disease 115–21, 146

573

alcohol use, continued
    high blood pressure 160
    hypertension 412
Aldactazide (spironolactone) 390, *416*
Aldactone (spironolactone) 389, *414*
Aldochlor (methyldopa) *416*
Aldomet (methyldopa) *414*
Aldoril (methyldopa) *416*
Aldrigheti, Rino 568
alexithymia 246
Aleve (naproxyn sodium) 258
alpha blockers, high blood pressure 162
Altace (ramipril) 381, *415*
alveoli, defined 537
American Alliance for Health, Physical Education, Recreation, and Dance, contact information 561
American Association of Cardiovascular and Pulmonary Rehabilitation, national program directory 488
American Cancer Society (ACS), contact information 165
American College of Obstetricians, moderate drinking advice 120
American College of Cardiology, chelation therapy 454
American Dietetic Association, contact information 561
American Heart Association
    aspirin a day 255, 259
    chain of survival 54–55
    chelation therapy 455
    contact information 57, 165, 239, 259, 294, 529, 562
    CPR classes information 533
    daily value for cholesterol 211
    death prevention 53
    gender in coronary artery disease 155
    heart arrhythmia 302
    heart healthy cookbooks 555, 556
    hospital rating 439
    patient education materials 488
    Step 1 diet 226
    ventricular arrhythmia 457, 459
    web site (Spanish lanuage) 346
American Heart Association Around the World Cookbook: Healthy Recipes with International Flavor 555

American Heart Association Kids' Cookbook 556
American Heart Association Low-Fat, Low-Cholesterol Cookbook, Second Edition 555
American Heart Association Low-Salt Cookbook 555
American Heart Association Quick and Easy Cookbook 556
American Lung Association
    contact information 165
    stop smoking 163
American Red Cross, CPR classes information 533
American Society of Hypertension, contact information 562
"America's Best Hospitals" *(U.S. News and World Report)* 151
amiloride 389–90, 391, *414*, *416*
amino acids, homocysteine 109–13
amiodarone 462
amlodipine *415*, *416*
aneurysm, defined 537
anger, heart disease 245–46
Anger Kills (Williams) 173
angina pectoris 340–41
    defined 537
    described 219
    diagnosis 274–75
    questions and answers 273–78
    treatment 275–76
    unstable 279–95
    visceral pain 40
    women 38
angiogram 134, 275
angiography, defined 537–38
angioplasty 443–45
    see also percutaneous transluminal coronary angioplasty (PTCA)
    aspirin 256
    defined 538
    laser 441
    statistics 193
    unstable angina 288–90
angiotensin converting enzyme (ACE) inhibitors
    congestive heart failure 28
    defined 323, 335
    digoxin 402–4

Index

angiotensin converting enzyme (ACE) inhibitors, continued
  heart attack 311–12
  heart failure 319, 320
  high blood pressure 161
  listed 381–83, *415*
animal research, congestive heart failure 30
annulus, defined 538
anticoagulants 405–9
  see also blood clots; clotting
  defined 538
anticonvulsives, alcohol use 119
antihypertensives 411–25
  defined 538
antioxidants 116
anxiety
  cardiac rehabilitation 496
  heart disease 243–44
aorta
  abdominal, defined 537
  ascending, defined 538
  defined 538
  depicted *63*
  described 71
aortic stenosis (AS) 347–48
aortic valve 64–65, 363
  defined 538
Apo-Chlorthalidone (chlorthalidone) 392
Apo-Diltiaz (diltiazem) 385
Apo-Furosemide (furosemide) 388
Apo-Hydro (hydrochlorothiazide) 392
Apo-ISDN (isosorbide dinitrate) 396
Apo-Nifed (nifedipine) 385
Apo-Triazide (triamterene) 390
Apo-Verap (verapamil) 385
Appletree Press, heart healthy cookbooks 557
Apresazide (hydralazine) *416*
Apresoline (hydralazine) *415*
Aquatensen (methyclothiazide) 391
Arizona, ischemic heart disease statistics 18
Arkansas, ischemic heart disease statistics 18
Arnstein, Paul M. 33n, 52
Aronow, Wilber 462

arrhythmias 297–305
  defined 323, 335, 538
  digoxin 401
  treatment 301–2, 457–64
  types, described 302–3
arteries
  see also aorta
  blockage removal 437–41
  defined 538
  described 69–71
arterioles
  defined 538
  described 71
arteriosclerosis
  defined 538
  depression 242
arteritis, defined 538
ascending aorta, defined 538
ASD *see* atrial septal defect (ASD)
ASH *see* asymmetrical septal hypertrophy (ASH)
aspirin 225
  alcohol use 119
  anticoagulants 406–7
  cardiovascular disease 255–59
  heart attack 311
  unstable angina 287
Aspirin Foundation of America, contact information 259
asymmetrical septal hypertrophy (ASH) *see* hypertrophic cardiomyopathy
atenolol 162, 311, 383, 384, *414*, *416*
atherectomy
  defined 538
  described 441
atherosclerosis 219, 339–40, 343–44
  angina 273
  chelation therapy 453–55
  defined 538
  described 75–76
  high blood pressure 158
  homocysteine levels 110
  rhythm disorders 458
  second-hand smoke 183–85
Atherosclerosis Risk in Communities (ARIC) study 184
atorvastatin 169, 223, 429

atria
 defined 539
 depicted *63*
 described 62–63
atrial fibrillation 303, 401
atrial flutter 303
atrial septal defect (ASD) 349
 defined 539
atrial septum, described 63
atrioventricular (AV) node
 arrhythmias 298
 defined 539
 described 65–66
atrioventricular canal defect 350–51
atrioventricular septal defect 350–51
atrium
 defined 539
 described 62–63
automatic external defibrillator (AED) 53–57
autonomic nervous system, sinus node control 66
Avapro (irbesartan) *415*
AV node *see* atrioventricular (AV) node

B

balloon angioplasty 256, 276
 depicted *289*
Baycol (cervastatin) 223
Bayer Corp., aspirin a day 255
benazepril 381, 382, *415*, *416*
bendroflumethiazide 383–84, 392–93
bepridil 385–86
beta blockers 462
 defined 335, 539
 dilated cardiomyopathy 328
 heart attack 311
 high blood pressure 162
 hypertrophic cardiomyopathy 331
 listed 383–84, *414*–16
 unstable angina 288
Betapace (sotalol) 462
betaxolol *414*
Betty Crocker's New Low-Fat, Low-Cholesterol Cookbook 556
bicuspid aortic valve 348

bile acid sequestrants 168
biopsy, defined 539
bisoprolol 383–84, *414*, *416*
Blalock-Taussig procedure, defined 539
Blocarden (timolol) *414*
blood, described 72–73
blood cholesterol levels 75–101
 average 77–79
 control 219–26
 heart disease 3–7
 test 123
blood clots
 see also anticoagulants; clotting
 defined 539
 homocysteine levels 110
blood plasma, described 73
blood pressure
 cuff *see* sphygmomanometer
 defined 539
 described 156–57, 227
 home monitoring 233–35
 testing 227–35
blood vessels *see* arteries; arterioles; capillaries; veins; venules
blue babies, defined 351, 539
Blue Cross/Blue Shield, transplant costs 478
Boston College University, Fellowship Program 52
Bowen, Debra 255, 259
bradycardia, defined 539
breast cancer, estrogen levels 117–18, 156
breast-feeding, alcohol use 120
Brewer, Camille 212, 213
Bristol Publishing Enterprise, heart healthy cookbooks 557
bumetanide 388–89, *414*
Bumex (bumetanide) 388, *414*
bundle-branch block, defined 539
Bureau of the Census *see* U.S. Brueau of the Census
Buselli, Elizabeth Florentino 33n, 52
bypass surgery *see* coronary artery bypass (CAB)

576

Index

C

CAB *see* coronary artery bypass (CAB)
Cacioppo, John T. 254
CAD *see* coronary artery disease (CAD)
Calan (verapamil) 384, *415*
calcium channel blockers
  defined 335, 540
  dilated cardiomyopathy 328
  high blood pressure 161
  hypertrophic cardiomyopathy 331
  listed 384–87, *416*
California, ischemic heart disease statistics 18
calories
  alcoholic beverages *121*
  comparison charts *94–98*
  exercise 175
  fats 80
capillaries
  defined 540
  depicted *72*
  described 72
Capoten (captopril) 311, 381, *415*
Capozide (captopril) *416*
captopril 161, 311, 381, 382, *415*, *416*
Cardene (nicardipine) 385, *415*
cardiac arrest
  defibrillation 53–57
  defined 335, 540
cardiac blood pool scan 136–37
cardiac catheterization 433–36
  angina pectoris 275
  defined 335, 540
  dilated cardiomyopathy 328
  heart murmur 369
  unstable angina 285
cardiac cycle, described 67
cardiac enzymes, defined 540
cardiac output
  defined 540
  described 62
Cardilate (erythrityl tetranitrate) 394–95, 396
cardiology, defined 540

cardiomyopathy 325–37
  defined 323, 335, 540
  dilated (congestive) 326–30
  hypertrophic 330–32
  nonischemic 325–26
  restrictive 332–34
cardiopulmonary bypass, defined 540
cardiopulmonary resuscitation (CPR) 533
  myocardial infarction 34
cardiovascular (CV), defined 540
cardiovascular disease (CVD), physical activity 187–98
cardioversion 301
  defined 540
Cardizem (diltiazem) 385, *415*
Cardura (doxazosin) *414*
CARE *see* Cholesterol and Recurrent Events (CARE study)
CARE (Cardiac Arrhythmias Research Education Foundation, Inc.), contact information 562
carotid artery, defined 541
carotid endarectomy 256
carteolol *414*
Carter, Ann 344
Cartrol (cartelol) *414*
carvedilol *415*
Catapres (clinidine) *414*
CDC *see* Centers for Disease Control and Prevention (CDC)
Center for Health Statistics, depression survey 242
Centers for Disease Control and Prevention (CDC)
  contact information 165
  moderate drinking 118
  Office on Smoking and Health (OSH), contact information 567
cerebral embolism, defined 541
cerebral hemorrhage, defined 541
cerebral thrombosis, defined 541
cerebrovascular, defined 541
cerebrovascular accident, defined 541
cerebrovascular occlusion, defined 541
cervastatin 223
chain of survival, described 54–55
chambers, described 62–63

Heart Diseases and Disorders Sourcebook, Second Edition

CHASER, Inc. (Congenital Heart Anomalies Support, Education, and Resources, Inc.), contact information 563
CHD *see* coronary heart disease (CHD)
chelation therapy 453–55
"Chest Pain Can Be an Emergency" 281, 284
CHF *see* congestive heart failure (CHF)
children
  aspirin 258
  blood cholesterol levels 90–92, 99, 527
  congenital heart disorders 345–56
  dilated cardiomyopathy 326
  exercise 192–93, 196–97
  obesity 189
Children's Health Information Network, contact information 563
chlorothiazide 161, 392–93
chlorthalidone 161, 392–93, *414*
Choices for a Healthy Heart 556
cholesterol 75–101, 166–69
  see also blood cholesterol levels
  "bad" *see* low density lipoprotein (LDL)
  cardiac rehabilitation 499–529
  comparison charts *94–98*
  control 219–26
  defined 77, 541
  food labels 210–12, 214
  "good" *see* high density lipoprotein (HDL)
  heart attack 308–9
  medications 427–31
  myocardial infarction 36–37
  test 123
Cholesterol and Recurrent Events (CARE study) 505
"Cholesterol-Lowering Drugs" (Mayo Clinic) 427n
cholestyramine 168, 224, 429
Chrousos, George C. 253
cigarette smoking *see* nicotine replacement therapy; smoking cessation; tobacco use
cineangiography, defined 541

Circulation 223
circulatory system 69–73
  see also vascular system
  defined 541
  high blood pressure 157
Citizens for Public Action on Blood Pressure and Cholesterol, contact information 563
Ciuchlor H (hydrochlorothiazide) 392
Clarke, Norman E., Sr. 454
claudication, defined 541
Clinical Practice Guideline on Cardiac Rehabilitation 488
Clinical Practice Guideline on Unstable Angina 295
Clinical Reference Systems, Ltd., coronary artery bypass surgery 447–51
clinical trials
  coenzyme Q10 264
  Dietary Approches to Stop Hypertension (DASH) 159
  Digitalis Investigation Group (DIG) 401–4
  postmenopausal estrogen/progestin interventions trial (PEPI) 265–69, 520
clonidine *414, 416*
"Clot Prevention: Anticoagulants to the Rescue" (Husten) 405n
clotting
  see also anticoagulants; blood clots
  aspirin 256–57
  cardiac X-rays 124–25
  described 73
  homocysteine levels 110
coarctation of the aorta (coarct) 348
coenzyme Q10 (ubiquinone) 261–64
cognitive-behavioral therapy 252
Colestid (colestipol) 224, 429
colestipol 168, 224, 429
collateral circulation, defined 541
Colorado, ischemic heart disease statistics 18
Columbia University, treating high blood cholesterol 223
¡Coma menos sal y sodio! 559
Combipres (clonidine) *416*
commissurotomy 365

Index

computed tomography (CT scan), defined 541
"The concepts of stress and stress system disorders" *(Journal of the American Medical Association)* 253
conduction system, defined 541
congenital, defined 542
congenital heart disorders 345–56
congenital heart failure, defined 542
congestion, defined 335
congestive cardiomyopathy *see* dilated cardiomyopathy
congestive heart failure (CHF) 341
   animal research 30
   defined 323, 542
   digoxin 401
   high blood pressure 158
   statistics 23–31
Connecticut, ischemic heart disease statistics 18
¡Conozca su nivel de colesterol! 559
Cooley, Denton A. 141, 142, 143, 145, 146, 147, 148, 151
Cordarone (amiodarone) 462
Coreg (carvedilol) *415*
Corgard (nadolol) *414*
coronary arteries
   damage process 39
   defined 542
   depicted *280, 282*
coronary artery bypass (CAB) 276, 311, 439–41, 447–51
   defined 542
   depicted *290*
   statistics 193
   unstable angina 291–92
coronary artery disease (CAD) 339–41
   defined 542
   high blood pressure 158
   prevention 44–45
   risk factors 142–43, 153–77
   unstable angina 279–95
The Coronary Club, Inc., contact information 563
coronary heart disease (CHD)
   blood cholesterol 75
   cholesterol levels 499–529
   defined 542
   risk factors 482–83, 506–7

coronary occlusion, defined 542
coronary thrombosis, defined 542
Coronex (isosorbide dinitrate) 396
Corzide (nadolol) 383, *416*
Coumadian (warfarin) 407
Covera (verapamil) *415*
Cozaar (losartan) *415*
CPK *see* creatinine phosphokinase (CPK)
CPR *see* cardiopulmonary resuscitation (CPR)
creatinine phosphokinase (CPK) 310
Crystodigin (digitoxin) 387
¡Cuide su peso! 559
Cummins, Richard 56
CVD *see* cardiovascular disease (CVD)
cyanosis, defined 542
cyanotic defects 351–55
   defined 351, 542
cyclosporine 473

D

daily intake levels, cholesterol 77
Daily Values 209–10, 213–15
DASH *see* Dietary Approches to Stop Hypertension (DASH)
death rates
   age adjusted, defined 542
   cardiovascular disease 34
   congestive heart failure *23, 28–29*
   heart disease 141
   ischemic heart disease *16, 18–19*
deep vein thrombosis, defined 542
defibrillation, early intervention 53–57
defibrillators
   see also automatic external defibrillator (AED)
   defined 543
   implantable 301, 463, 469–72
Delaware, ischemic heart disease statistics 18
Delicious Heart Healthy Latino Recipes 556
Demadex (torsemide) *414*
Demi-Regroton (reserpine) *416*
Denke, Margo 117

Department of Health and Human Services *see* U.S. Department of Health and Human Services (DHHS)
Deponit (nitroglycerin) 398
depression
 cardiac rehabilitation 495–98
 heart disease 241–43
Depression Is a Treatable Illness 488
DeRoin, Dee Ann 369
DHHS *see* U.S. Department of Health and Human Services (DHHS)
diabetes mellitus
 defined 543
 heart disease 76, 145, 171
 heart failure 316
 insulin resistance, heart disease 103–7
diastole
 depicted *315*
 described 67
diastolic blood pressure
 defined 543
 described 157–59, 228
diastolic heart failure
 defined 323
 described 314
Diazide (triamterene) *416*
diet and nutrition
 blood cholesterol levels 77–78, 80–101
 cardiac rehabilitation 485, 492
 cholesterol levels 502, 509–15
 heart disease 4–7, 145–46
 high blood pressure 229
 hypertension 412–13
Dietary Approches to Stop Hypertension (DASH) 159
Dietary Guidelines for Americans, alcohol use 118
dietitians 226, 522
Digitaline (digitoxin) 387
digitalis 319, 320
 defined 335
 dilated cardiomyopathy 328
 listed 387–88
Digitalis Investigation Group (DIG) 401–4
digitoxin 387

digoxin 387–88, 401–4
Dilacor (diltiazem) 385, *415*
dilatation, described 317
dilated cardiomyopathy 326–30
 defined 335
 depicted *320*
Dilatrate (isosorbide dinitrate) 394
diltiazem 161, 385–87,*415*, *416*
Diovan (valsartan) *415*
District of Columbia (Washington, DC), ischemic heart disease statistics 18
Diucardin (hydroflumethiazide) 391
Diulo (metolazone) 391
Diupres (reserpine) *416*
diuretics
 defined 335, 543
 dilated cardiomyopathy 328
 heart failure 319, 320, 402
 high blood pressure 161
 hypertrophic cardiomyopathy 331
 listed 383–84, 388–93, *414–16*
 restrictive cardiomyopathy 334
Diuril (chlorothiazide) 391
Don't Eat Your Heart Out Cookbook, Second Edition 556
Doppler ultrasound, defined 543
Down Home Healthy: Family Recipes of Black American Chefs 557
doxazosin 162, *414*
Duke University
 acute stress experiment 246
 survival rate 248
Duotrate (pentaerythritol tetranitrate) 394
Duretic (methyclothiazide) 392
Dyazide (triamterene) 390
DynaCirc (isradipine) 385, *415*
Dyrenium (triamterene) 389, *414*
dyspnea
 defined 323, 335, 543
 heart failure 316–17
dysrhythmia, defined 538

E

Ebstein's anomaly 349
ECG *see* electrocardiogram (ECG: EKG)

Index

echocardiogram
  fainting 376
  heart murmur 368
echocardiography 126–27, 318
  defined 323, 335, 543
  endoscopy 127–29
  hypertrophic cardiomyopathy 331
Edecrin (ethacrynic acid) 388, *414*
edema
  defined 323, 336, 543
  heart failure 317
EDTA 453
education, cardiac rehabilitation 484–85
EEG *see* electroencephalogram (EEG)
Eisenmenger's complex 350, 475
ejection fraction
  defined 543
  described 62
EKG *see* electrocardiogram (ECG: EKG)
electrocardiogram (ECG: EKG) 460–61
  angina pectoris 275
  arrhythmias 304–5
  defined 324, 336, 543
  depicted *304*
  described 129–30, 284
  fainting 376
  heart murmur 368
  hypertrophic cardiomyopathy 331
  myocardial infarction 44
electroencephalogram (EEG)
  defined 543
  fainting 376
electrophysiological study (EPS) 305
  defined 543–44
"Elevated blood pressure and personality: A meta-analytic review" *(Psychological Bulletin)* 253
embolism *see* embolus
embolus, defined 544
enalapril 161, 311, 381, 382, *415*, *416*
enalaprilat 381, 383
endarterectomy, defined 544
endocardial cusion defect 350–51
endocardium
  defined 544
  described 63

endocartitis 357–58
  defined 544
endothelium
  defined 544
  described 105–6
  diabete mellitus 103
Enduron (methyclothiazide) 391
enlarged heart, defined 544
environmental tobacco smoke (ETS) 184
enzymes
  cardiac 123
  defined 544
  heart attack 310
epicardium
  defined 544
  described 63
epinephrine 249
EPS *see* electrophysiological study (EPS)
Epstein, Andrew 460, 464
eritrityl tetranitrate 396
erythrityl tetranitrate 395–96, 396, 397, 398
erythrocytes, described 72
Esidrix (hydrochlorothiazide) 391, *414*
Esimil (guanethidine monosulfate) *416*
estrogen
  alcohol use 117–18
  clinical trial 265–69
  defined 544
  heart disease 142, 156
  high-density lipoprotein levels 156
estrogen replacement therapy
  coronary heart disease 37
  heart disease 156
ethacrynic acid 388–89, *414*
ETS *see* environmental tobacco smoke (ETS)
Everything You Need to Know about Medical Tests (Springhouse Corp.) 123n
exercise
  aerobic, described 12
  blood cholesterol levels 221
  blood pressure levels 156
  cardiac rehabilitation 484, 493

581

exercise, continued
  cholesterol levels 502
  heart disease 4, 11–13, 117
  heart rates 66
Exercise and Your Heart: A Guide to Physical Activity (NCEP) 528
exercise EKG *see* stress test
exercise electrocardiogram *see* stress test
exercise multiple-gated acquisition scan 134
exercise programs, doctor consultations 13
exercise stress test, defined 544
exercise tolerance test 285

F

Facts About Blood Cholesterol (NIH) 278
Facts About Coronary Heart Disease (NIH) 278
Facts About Heart Disease and Women: So You Have Heart Disease (NIH) 278
Facts About Heart Failure (NIH) 278
fainting, cardiac conditions 375–77
familial hypercholesterolemia
  defined 544
  heart disease 154
family issues
  angina 283
  cardiac rehabilitation 498
  physical activity 201
fats
  blood cholesterol levels 80, 86–87, 101, 427, 510–11
  comparison charts *94–98*
  defined 545
  food labels 210–12, 214
  heart disease 9–10
  monounsaturated, defined 547–48
  polyunsaturated, defined 549
  saturated, defined 550–51
  trans, defined 553
  triglycerides, defined 553
fatty acids, defined 545

FDA *see* U.S. Food and Drug Administration (FDA)
felodipine 385–86, *415*, *416*
femofibrate 225
fiber
  blood cholesterol levels 80, 511
  food labels 213
  high blood pressure 160
fibrates 519–20
fibric acid derivatives 225
fibrillation
  atrial 303
  defined 545
  ventricular 303
fibrin filaments, described 73
"first responders," defibrillation 55–56
flavonoids 116
Florida, ischemic heart disease statistics 18
flunarizine 385–86
flutter, defined 545
fluvastatin 169, 223, 429
folic acid, homocysteine levels 111, 155
Food and Drug Administration (FDA) *see* U.S. Food and Drug Administration
Food and Nutrition Information Center, contact information 564
food groups, blood cholesterol levels 82–87
food labels
  blood cholesterol levels 88, 99–101, 513–14
  heart disease prevention 209–17
fosinopril 382, 383, *415*
Framingham Heart Study, homocysteine levels 110
France, alcohol use 119–20
Frank, Catherine 253
free radicals, congestive heart disease 30
furosemide 388–89, *414*
Furoside (furosemide) 388

G

gated blood pool scan, defined 545
gated cardiac blood pool imaging 136

Index

Gathers, Hank 54
gemfibrozil 168, 225, 429
gender factor
  blood cholesterol levels 78, 221
  cardiac rehabilitation 493
  cholesterol levels 503
  congestive heart failure *24, 29*
  heart disease 33–52, 155–56
  ischemic heart disease 16–19
genetic engineering, congestive heart disease 30
genetic factors
  see also heredity
  cardiac rehabilitation 493
  congenital heart disorders 345–56
  heart disease 143
  high cholesterol levels 168
  homocysteine levels 110
Georgia, ischemic heart disease statistics 18
Gertz, Morie 454, 455
Gilbert, Linden 224
glucagon 104
glucose levels 104
  see also sugar
glyceryl trinitrate 393, 396
Gold, Philip W. 253
Goldberg, Rube 405
Grinkov, Sergei 457
guanabenz *414*
guanadrel *414*
guanethidine *414, 416*
guanfacine *414*
Gutman, Steven 221

H

hardening of the arteries *see* atherosclerosis
Harvard Health Letter
  coenzyme Q10 261, 262
  passive smoking and heart disease 183
Harvey, William 69
Hawaii, ischemic heart disease statistics 18
HDL cholesterol *see* high density lipoprotein (HDL)

Health and Human Services, *see* U.S. Department of Health and Human Services (DHHS)
health care teams
  cardiac rehabilitation 483–84, 522–23
  unstable angina 292–93
Healthfinder, web site 564
Health Resources and Services Administration (HRSA), Division of Transplantation, contact information 478
Healthy Mexican Cooking: Authentic Low-Fat Recipes 557
Healthy Snacks for Kids 557
heart
  depicted *63, 65*
  described 61–67
  electrical impulses 65–66
  parts, described 62–67
heart attack 307–12
  see also myocardial infarction (MI)
  causes 308–9
  coronary heart disease 75
  defined 545
  depression 242–43
  described 308
  diagnosis 309–10
  prevention 531–33
  symptoms 309
  treatment 310–11
  warning signs 528, 532
heartbeat, depicted *299*
heart block
  defined 545
  described 300
heart catheterization *see* cardiac catheterization
heart chambers, described 62–63
heart disease
  alcohol use 116–17
  homocysteine levels 109–10
  mental health 241–54
  prevention 141–269
  questions and answers 3–13
  red wine 115–16
  rehabilitation 481–533
heart failure 313–24
  see also congestive heart failure
  causes 315–16

Heart Diseases and Disorders Sourcebook, Second Edition

heart failure, continued
  defined 324, 336
  diagnosis 317–18
  statistics 314
  symptoms 316–17
  treatment 318–20
heart-health test 148–51
Heart-Healthy Cooking African American Style 557
heart-healthy living guidelines 79–90, 141–51
Heart Information Network, web site 564
heart-lung machine, defined 545
heart-lung transplantation 473–78
heart murmur 367–69
  defined 548
heart muscle disease *see* cardiomyopathy
heart palpitations 371–73
HeartPoint, web site 564
heart rates, average 66–67
"Hearts and Minds" *(Harvard Mental Health Letter)* 241n
heart scan 126–27
  see also echocardiography
  endoscopy 127–29
Heart Surgery Forum, web site 564
heart transplantation 473–78
  congestive heart failure 30
  defined 553
  dilated cardiomyopathy 329–30
  hypoplastic left heart syndrome 356
heart valves, described 64
hemoglobin, described 73
Henkel, John 226
Hennekens, Charles H. 183, 257, 258, 259, 406
heparin 310, 407, 409
heredity
  see also genetic factors
  blood cholesterol levels 4–7, 76, 78, 221
  cholesterol levels 502
  congenital heart disorders 345–46
  defined 545
  heart disease risk factor 154–55
  myocardial infarction 34–35

high blood pressure 227–28
  see also hypertension
  defined 545
  heart disease 3–7, 8, 156–62
  racial factor 154
High Blood Pressure and What You Can Do About It (NIH) 278
high density lipoprotein (HDL) 501–5
  alcohol use 117
  blood cholesterol levels 77–79, 220–21
  childhood levels 92
  coronary heart disease 36–37
  defined 545
  estrogen levels 142
  high cholesterol levels 166–67, 428
HMG-CoA reductase inhibitors 169
HOCM *see* hypertrophic obstructive cardiomyopathy (HOCM)
Hoffmann, Norbert 224, 225
Holter monitor 134–36, 304
  defined 545
homocysteine 109–13, 154
Honolulu Heart Study 116
hormone replacement therapy 268, 520
  see also estrogen replacement therapy
hospitalizations, congestive heart failure 24, *27–28*
"How to Be Heart Healthy" (Texas Heart Institute) 141n
HPA *see* hypothalamic pituitary axis (HPA)
HRSA *see* Health Resources and Services Administration (HRSA)
HRT *see* hormone replacement therapy (HRT)
Husten, Larry 405n
hydralazine 161, 319, 320, *415*, *416*
Hydro-chlor (hydrochlorothiazide) 392
hydrochlorothiazide 161, 383–84, 391, 392–93, *414*
Hydro-D (hydrochlorothiazide) 392
HydroDIURIL (hydrochlorothiazide) 392, *414*
hydroflumethiazide 392–93
Hydromox (quinethazone) 392

Index

Hydropres (reserpine) *416*
Hygroton (chlorthalidone) 392, *414*
Hylorel (guanadrel) *414*
hypercholesterolemia, familial
   defined 544
   heart disease 154
hypertension
   see also high blood pressure
   defined 546
   described 227
   heart disease 144–45
   heart failure 316
   resistant, described 425
   treatment 28, 411–25
     see also antihypertensives
hypertrophic cardiomyopathy 330–32
   defined 336, 546
   depicted *333*
hypertrophic obstructive cardiomyopathy (HOCM) *see* hypertrophic cardiomyopathy
hypertrophy, heart failure 317
hypoglycemia, defined 546
hypoplastic left heart syndrome 355–56
hypotension, defined 546
hypothalamic pituitary axis (HPA) 249
hypoxia, defined 546
Hytrin (terazosin) *414*
Hyzaar (losartan and hydrochlorothiazide) *416*

I

ibuprofen 257, 258
ICD-9 see International Classification of Diseases, Ninth Revision (ICD-9)
Idaho, ischemic heart disease statistics 18
IDDM *see* insulin-dependent diabetes mellitus (IDDM: Type I)
IDG Books, heart healthy cookbooks 556
idiopathic, defined 336
idiopathic hypertrophic subaortic stenosis (IHSS) *see* hypertrophic cardiomyopathy
IHD *see* ischemic heart disease (IHD)
IHSS *see* idiopathic hypertrophic subaortic stenosis (IHSS)
Illinois, ischemic heart disease statistics 18
IMDUR (isosorbide mononitrate) 394
immune system, heart disease 251
immunosuppressive medications, defined 546
impedance plethysmography, defined 546
"Implantable Defibrillator Can Aid People with Dangerously Irregular HEartbeats" (Cardiovascular Institute of the South) 469n
"Implanted Defibrillators Save More Lives than Drugs" (Mayo Foundation) 469n
indapamide *414*
Inderal (propranolol) *414*
Inderide (propranolol) 383, *416*
Indiana, ischemic heart disease statistics 18
Indian Health Service, contact information 565
infarct, defined 546
inferior vena cava
   defined 546
   depicted *63*
Informational Medical Systems
   heart catheterization 436
   pacemaker implantation 467
inotropic medications, defined 546
insulin, described 104
insulin-dependent diabetes mellitus (IDDM: Type I) 104
insulin resistance, heart disease 103–7
InteliHealth, web site 565
internal mammary graft 276
International Classification of Diseases, Ninth Revision (ICD-9)
   trends in heart disease 15
intravascular echocardiography, defined 546
Iowa, ischemic heart disease statistics 18
irbesartan *415*
ischemia
   angina pectoris 275
   defined 546
   silent, defined 551

ischemic heart disease (IHD)
defined 546
depression 242
statistics 15–21
Ismelin (guanethidine) *414*
ISMO (isosorbide mononitrate) 394
Iso-Bid (isosorbide dinitrate) 394
Isonate (isosorbide dinitrate) 394, 396
Isoptin (verapamil) 385, *415*
Isorbid (isosorbide dinitrate) 394, 396
Isordil (isosorbide dinitrate) 394–95, 396
isosorbide dinitrate 395–96, 397, 398
isosorbide mononitrate 395–96
Isotrate (isosorbide dinitrate) 394
isradipine 385–86, *415*

J

J-curve hypothesis 423
Johns Hopkins, depression-disease connection 496
Johns Hopkins Bayview Medical Center, contact information 565
Johnson, Blair T. 253
Jorgensen, Randall S. 253
jugular veins, defined 547

K

Kansas, ischemic heart disease statistics 18
Kentucky, ischemic heart disease statistics 18
Kerlone (betaxolol) *414*
Kessler, David A. 217
ketoprofen 257, 258
kidney failure, high blood pressure 158
Kiecolt-Glaser, Janice K. 254
Klavikordal (nitroglycerin) 394
Kolodziej, Monika E. 253
Kurtzweil, Paula 217
Kuter, David J. 408

L

labetalol *415*
Lanoxicaps (digoxin) 387
Lanoxin (digoxin) 387, 401
Lasix (furosemide) 388, *414*
LDL cholesterol *see* low density lipoprotein (LDL)
left ventricular assist device (LVAD) 30, 319, 330
defined 324, 336
Lescol (fluvastatin) 223, 429
lesions, defined 547
leukocytes, described 73
Levatol (penbutolol) *414*
Lexxel (felodipine) *416*
lifestyles
see also exercise; physical activity
cardiac rehabilitation 491–94
cholesterol levels 514–15
hypertension 412–13
myocardial infarction 35–36
sedentary 174–77, 189–90
Linden, W. 254
lipids 166, 522
see also fats
defined 547
Lipitor (atorvastatin) 223, 225, 429
lipoproteins 428, 501–5
see also high density lipoprotein (HDL); low density lipoprotein (LDL)
defined 547
described 77
lisinopril 161, 311, 382, 383, *415*, *416*
Living With Heart Disease: Is It Heart Failure? 488
Lonetin (minoxidil) *415*
Lopid (gemfibrozil) 168, 225, 429
Lopressor HCT (metoprolol and hydrochlorothiazide) 383
Lopressor (metoprolol) *414*, *416*
losartan 161, *415*, *416*
Lotensin (benazepril) 381, *415*, *416*
Lotrel (amlodipine and benazepril) *416*
Louisiana, ischemic heart disease statistics 18

Index

lovastatin 169, 223, 429
low blood pressure *see* hypotension
low density lipoprotein (LDL) 501–5
  blood cholesterol levels 77–79, 220–21, 508–9
  childhood levels 92
  coronary heart disease 36–37
  defined 547
  depression 242
  estrogen levels 142
  high cholesterol levels 166–67, 428
Loyola Marymount University, death of basketball star 54
Lozol (indapamide) *414*
lumen, defined 547
LVAD *see* left ventricular assist device (LVAD)

M

magnetic resonance imaging (MRI), defined 547
Maine, ischemic heart disease statistics 18
Managing Unstable Angina 488
¡Manténgase activo y siéntase bien! 560
Maryland, ischemic heart disease statistics 18
Massachusetts, ischemic heart disease statistics 18
Maurice, J. 254
Mavik (trandolapril) *415*
Maxide (triamterene) 390, *416*
Mayo Clinic
  anger and heart disease 245
  aspirin allergy 258
  Mayo Health Oasis, web site 565
mechanical heart devices, congestive heart disease 30
Medicaid, heart transplantion costs 478
medical history
  blood cholesterol levels 92
  functional health patterns 41–42
Medicare, heart transplantation costs 478

medications
  ACE inhibitors, listed 381–83, *415*
  angina pectoris 275–76
  arrhythmias 301
  beta blockers, listed 383–84, *414–16*
  calcium channel blockers, listed 384–87, *416*
  cholesterol-lowering 516–21
  digitalis, listed 387–88
  diuretics, listed 383–84, 388–93, *414–16*
  high blood pressure 160–62
  nitrates, listed 393–400
The Mended Hearts, Inc. 295
  contact information 565–66
mental health, heart health 241–54
Metahydrin (trichlormethiazide) 392
methyclothiazide 392–93
methyldopa *414*, *416*
metolazone 392–93, *414*
metoprolol 162, 311, 383–84, *414*, *416*
Mevacor (lovastatin) 223–24, 429
MI *see* myocardial infarction (MI)
mibefradil 225, *415*
Michigan, ischemic heart disease statistics 18
microvascular angina 278
Microzide (hydrochlorothiazide) 392, *414*
Midamor (amiloride) 389, *414*
Miller, Redonda 223, 225
Minipress (prazosin) *414*
Minitran (nitroglycerin) 398–99
Minizide (prazosin) *416*
Minnesota, ischemic heart disease statistics 18
Minnesota Multiphasic Personality Inventory (MMPI) 242
minoxidil 161, *415*
Mississippi, ischemic heart disease statistics 18
Missouri, ischemic heart disease statistics 18
mitral valve 64–65, 363
  defined 547
mitral valve prolapse, defined 547
MMPI *see* Minnesota Multiphasic Personality Inventory (MMPI)
Moduret (amiloride) 390

Moduretic (amiloride) 390, *416*
moexipril *415*
Monell Chemical Senses Center, drinking while breast-feeding 120
Monoket (isosorbide mononitrate) 394
Monopril (fosinopril) 381, *415*
monounsaturated fats, defined 547–48
Montana, ischemic heart disease statistics 18
Montreal Heart Institute, depression-disease connection 496
mortality
  see also death rates
  coronary heart disease 38–39
  defined 548
Moss, Arthur 463
MRI see magnetic resonance imaging (MRI)
MUGA see multiple-gated acquisition scan (MUGA)
multiple-gated acquisition scan (MUGA) 136
murmur 367–69
  defined 548
Mykrox (metolazone) 392, *414*
myocardial infarction (MI) 307–12
  see also heart attack
  co-morbidities 37
  congestive heart failure 25
  defined 548
  described 219
  diagnosis 43–44
  exercise 192
  prevention 34–38
  symptoms 40–41
myocardial ischemia 28
  defined 548
myocardium, defined 548
Myrosemide (furosemide) 388

N

nadolol 383–84, *414*, *416*
naproxen sodium 257, 258
Naqua (trichlormethiazide) 392
National Academy of Sciences, National Research Council 211

National Cancer Institute (NCI)
  contact information 165
  heart healthy cookbooks 557
National Center for Chronic Disease Prevention and Health Promotion, contact information 566
The National Center for Nutrition and Dietetics, Consumer Nutrition Hotline 529
National Cholesterol Education Program (NCEP) 81, 99, 212, 219, 225, 226, 528
National Health and Nutrition Examination Epidemiological Follow-up Study 242
National Heart, Lung, and Blood Institute (NHLBI)
  cardiomyopathy diagnosis and treatment 334
  contact information 226
  cholesterol treatment 222
  coenzyme Q10 263
  contact information 294, 302, 566
  depression-disease connection 497
  Digitalis Investigation Group (DIG) 403
  Family Heart Study 110
  heart arrhythmia 302
  heart failure research 322–23
  heart healthy cookbooks 556, 557, 558
  homocysteine link 109, 112
  implanted defibrillators 463
  incidence data 25
  incidence data research 29–31
  Information Center 31, 99, 113, 278, 336–37, 478, 529
  National Cholesterol Education Program (NCEP) 81, 219, 528
  patient education materials 488
  patient guideline 488
  Postmenopausal Estrogen/Progestin Interventions Trial (PEPI) 265
  Spanish language cookbooks 559–60
  Spanish language publications 559–60
  unstable angina 295
National Institute of Arthritis and Musculoskeletal and Skin Diseases, Postmenopausal Estrogen/Progestin Interventions Trial (PEPI) 266

Index

National Institute of Child Health and Human Development (NICHD), Postmenopausal Estrogen/Progestin Interventions Trial (PEPI) 266
National Institute of Diabetes and Digestive and Kidney Diseases (NIDDK), Postmenopausal Estrogen/Progestin Interventions Trial (PEPI) 266
National Institute of Nursing, research grant 52
National Institute on Aging (NIA), Postmenopausal Estrogen/Progestin Interventions Trial (PEPI) 265–68
National Institutes of Health (NIH)
  chelation therapy 454
  hormone replacement therapy (HRT) research 268
  implantable defibrillators 469, 470
  National Cholesterol Education Program (NCEP) 81, 212
  Postmenopausal Estrogen/Progestin Interventions Trial (PEPI) 265
  publications 278
  web site 566
National Library of Medicine, STAT electronic service 489
Naturetin (bendroflumethiazide) 392
NCI *see* National Cancer Institute (NCI)
Nebraska, ischemic heart disease statistics 18
necrosis, defined 548
Neo-Codema (hydrochlorothiazide) 392
Nevada, ischemic heart disease statistics 18
The New American Heart Association Cookbook, 25th Anniversary Edition 557
New England Journal of Medicine
  decline of heart disease deaths 220
  Digitalis Investigation Group (DIG) trial 403
New Hampshire, ischemic heart disease statistics 18
New Jersey, ischemic heart disease statistics 19

New Mexico, ischemic heart disease statistics 19
New York state, ischemic heart disease statistics 19
NHLBI *see* National Heart, Lung, and Blood Institute (NHLBI)
NIA *see* National Institute on Aging (NIA)
niacin 169, 224
nicardipine 385–86, *415*
NICHD *see* National Institute of Child Health and Human Development
nicotine replacement therapy 165–66, 181
  see also smoking cessation; tobacco use
nicotinic acid (niacin) 169, 224, 518–19
NIDDK *see* National Institute of Diabetes and Digestive and Kidney Diseases (NIDDK)
NIDDM *see* non-insulin-dependent diabetes mellitus (NIDDM: Type II)
nifedipine 161, 385–86, *415*
NIH *see* National Institutes of Health (NIH)
nimodipine 385–86
Nimotop (nimodipine) 385
Niong (nitroglycerin) 394
nisoldipine *415*
nitrates
  heart failure 320
  listed 393–400
  unstable angina 287–88
nitric oxide 105–6
Nitro-Bid (nitroglycerin) 398–99
Nitrocap (nitroglycerin) 394
Nitrodisc (nitroglycerin) 398
Nitro-Dur (nitroglycerin) 399
Nitrogard (nitroglycerin) 396
nitroglycerin 276, 395–400
  defined 548
  heart attack 310
Nitroglyn (nitroglycerin) 394
Nitrolingual (nitroglycerin) 393
Nitrol (nitroglycerin) 399
Nitronet (nitroglycerin) 394
Nitrong (nitroglycerin) 394–95, 399

Nitrospan (nitroglycerin) 394
Nitrostat (nitroglycerin) 396, 399
  alcohol use 118
nodes, heart *see* atrioventricular (AV) node; sinus node
non-insulin-dependent diabetes mellitus (NIDDM: Type II) 104
noninvasive procedures, defined 548
Nordenberg, Tamar 259
norepinephrine 249
Normodyne (labetalol) *415*
North Carolina, ischemic heart disease statistics 19
North Dakota, ischemic heart disease statistics 19
Norvasc (amlodipine) *415*
Notrolin (nitroglycerin) 394
Novo-Digoxin (digoxin) 387
Novo-Diltazem (diltiazem) 385
Novo-Hydrazide (hydrochlorothiazide) 392
Novo-Nifedin (nifedapine) 385
Novosemide (furosemide) 388
Novospiroton (spironolactone) 389
Novo-Spirozine (spironolactone) 390
Novo-Thalidone (chlorthalidone) 392
Novo-Triamzide (triamterene) 390
Novo-Veramil (verapamil) 385
Nu-Diltiaz (diltaizam) 385
Nu-nifed (nifedapine) 385
"Nutrition and Your Health: Dietary Guidelines for Americans" 113
Nutrition Labeling and Education Act (1990) 209
nutrition labels *see* food labels
Nu-Verap (verapamil) 385

O

obesity
  see also weight factor
  defined 548
  heart disease 3–7, 76, 169–70
  insulin resistance 105
obstruction defects 346–47
occluded artery, defined 548
Office of Minority Health Resource Center, contact information 567

Office on Smoking and Health (OSH), contact information 567
Ohio, ischemic heart disease statistics 19
Oklahoma, ischemic heart disease statistics 19
omega-3 fatty acids 83
open heart surgery, defined 549
oral contraceptives, heart disease 143–44
Oregon, ischemic heart disease statistics 19
Oretic (hydrochlorothiazide) 392
organ donation 474
Orloff, David 220, 223, 225
Ornato, Joseph P. 56
Orudis KT 258
OSH *see Office on* Smoking and Health (OSH)
oxygen
  angina pectoris 273
  blood tests 123–24
  capillaries 72
  unstable angina 279

P

PAC *see* premature atrial contractions (PAC)
pacemakers
  see also sinus node
  arrhythmias 301
  defined 549
  hypertrophic cardiomyopathy 331–32
  implantation 465–67
palpitations 371–73
  defined 549
pancreas, described 104
panic disorder, heart disease 243–44
paroxysmal atrial tachycardia (PAT) 303
passive smoking 183–85
PAT *see* paroxysmal atrial tachycardia (PAT)
patent ductus arteriosus (PDA) 346, 353–54
  defined 549

Index

Patlak, Margie 464
PDA *see* patent ductus arteriosus (PDA)
penbutolol sulfate *414*
Pennsylvania, ischemic heart disease statistics 19
pentaerythritol tetranitrate 395–96
Pentylan (pentaerythritol tetranitrate) 394
PEPI *see* postmenopausal estrogen/progestin interventions trial (PEPI)
percutaneous transluminal coronary angioplasty (PTCA) 193, 307, 437–39
pericardiocentesis, defined 549
pericarditis 359–61
  defined 549
pericardium
  defined 549
  described 63–64
Peritrate (pentaerythritol tetranitrate) 394–95
PET scan *see* positron emission tomography (PET scan)
phenols 116
phychotherapy, heart disease 251–53
physical activity 199–202
  see also exercise
  blood cholesterol levels 78, 89–91, 515
  cardiovascular health 187–98
  cholesterol levels 502
  heart disease 10–13, 76, 117
  high blood pressure 160
  hypertension 412
"Physical Activity and Cardiovascular Health" (NIH) 187n
"Physicians Health Study" 258
Physicians' Health Study (Harvard), homocysteine levels 110, 154
pindolol 383–84, *414*
plaques 219
  angina pectoris 340–41
  cholesterol levels 503–4
  defined 549
  heart attack 308–9
platelets (thrombocytes) 73
  defined 549
  heart attack 310

Plendil (felodipine) 385, *415*
polythiazide 392–93
polyunsaturated fats, defined 549
¡Póngase en acción - prevenga la alta presión! 560
Posicor (mibefradil) 225, *415*
positron emission tomography (PET scan), defined 549–50
postmenopausal estrogen/progestin interventions trial (PEPI) 265–69, 520
potassium channel blockers 462
Pravachol (pravastatin) 223–24, 429
pravastatin 169, 223, 429
prazosin *414, 416*
pregnancy
  alcohol use 120
  cardiac X-rays 125
  Holter monitoring 137
premature atrial contractions (PAC) 303
premature supraventricular contractions 303
premature ventricular complexes (PVC) 303
prevalence, defined 550
Prinivil (lisinopril) 311, 381, *415*
Prinzide (lisinopril) *416*
Prinzmetal's angina 277
procainamide 462
Procan 462
Procanbid (procainamide) 462
Procardia (nifedipine) 385, *415*
progestin, clinical trial 265–69
Pronestyl 462
propranolol 162, 311, 383–84, *414, 416*
prostaglandins 256
¡Proteja su corazón - baje su colesterol! 560
prothrombin clotting time test 124, 408
PS *see* pulmonary stenosis (PS)
psychosocial factors, heart disease 37–38
"Psychosocial intervention for patients with coronary artery disease" *(Archives of Internal Medicine)* 254
PTCA *see* percutaneous transluminal coronary angioplasty (PTCA)

591

pulmonary, defined 550
pulmonary artery, depicted 63
pulmonary atresia 353–54
pulmonary congestion, defined 324, 336
Pulmonary Hypertension Association, contact information 568
pulmonary stenosis (PS) 347
pulmonary valve 64–65, 363
  defined 550
pulmonary veins 62
  defined 550
  depicted 63
PVC see premature ventricular complexes (PVC)

Q

Q10 (ubiquinone) 261–64
"Questions and Answers About Chelation Therapy" (American Heart Association) 455
Questran (cholestyramine) 224–25, 429
Quinaglute 462
quinapril 382, 383, 415
quinethazone 392–93
Quinidex 462

R

racial factor
  angina 38
  blood pressure levels 227
  congestive heart failure 29
  heart disease 154
  ischemic heart disease 16–19
  myocardial infarction 34–35
radionuclide ventriculography
  defined 550
  dilated cardiomyopathy 328
  hypertrophic cardiomyopathy 331
ramipril 382, 383, 415
Random House, Inc., heart healthy cookbooks 556, 557
Rankin, Sally H. 33n, 52
RDV see recommended daily value (RDV)
recommended daily value (RDV), vitamins 111–12
red blood cells (erythrocytes) 72

¡Reduzca la grasa - no el sabor! 560
regurgitation, defined 550
rehabilitation
  cardiac 481–89
  myocardial infarction 45–46
"The relationship between social support and physiological processes" (Psychological Bulletin) 254
relaxation therapy 252
  high blood pressure 160
renal, defined 550
Renedil (felodipine) 385
Renese (polythiazide) 392
reperfusion, described 310
reserpine 414, 416
resins 224–25, 429, 518
restrictive cardiomyopathy 332–34
  defined 336
  depicted 333
revascularization, described 437
rheumatic fever, defined 550
Rhode Island, ischemic heart disease statistics 19
rhythm disorders 297–305
  treatment 457–64
Rimm, Eric 116, 119
risk factors
  defined 550
  heart disease 3–7, 75–76, 142–48
  identification 153–77
Rolfe, Ann 52
¡Rompa con el hábito de fumar! 560
rubella, defined 550

S

salt see sodium
Saluron (hydroflumethiazide) 392
saphenous vein 276
saturated fats
  blood cholesterol 77, 509–10
  comparison charts 94–98
  defined 550–51
  food labels 214
  recommended daily intake levels 101
Scandinavian Simvastatin Survival Study 223, 504

Index

Scarbrough, Ed 210
Schreer, George E. 253
scintillation camera 136, 137
second-hand smoke *see* passive smoking
Sectral (acebutolol) *414*
septal defects 349-51
  defined 551
septum
  defined 336, 551
  described 63
Ser-Ap-Es (reserpine) *416*
Serpasil (reserpine) *414*
Shape Up America!, contact information 568
shock, defined 551
shunt, defined 551
Sibelium (flunarizine) 385
sick sinus syndrome 303
  defined 551
silent ischemia, defined 551
simvastatin 169, 223, 429, 504
sinus arrhythmia 302
sinus node 65, 298-300
  defined 551
  rhythm disorders 458
sinus tachycardia 303
Smith, Stephen 253
smoking *see* tobacco use
smoking cessation 179-82
  see also nicotine replacement therapy; tobacco use
  cardiac rehabilitation 486
  ischemic heart disease 20
  programs 164-65
sodium
  cholesterol levels 511
  comparison charts *94-98*
  defined 551
  heart disease 5, 7
  high blood pressure 159-60, 229
  hypertension 412
  racial factor 154
sodium channel blockers 462
Sopko, George 257, 259
Sorbitrate (isosorbide dinitrate) 394, 396
sotalol 462
South Carolina, ischemic heart disease statistics 19

South Dakota, ischemic heart disease statistics 19
So You Have High Blood Cholesterol (NIH) 278
Spanish language publications, heart information 559-60
sphygmomanometer
  blood pressure home monitoring 233
  defined 551
  described 157
spironolactone 389-90, 391, *414*, *416*
Spirozide (spironolactone) 390
St. Luke's Episcopal Hospital, Texas Heart Institute 151
Stanford University, group therapy 252
Stanton, Marshall S. 470
statins 169, 223, 429, 517-18
Stay Young at Heart: Cook the Heart-Healthy Way 558
stenosis, defined 551
stents 439
  defined 551
Step by Step: Eating to Lower Your High Blood Cholesterol (NIH) 278, 528
sternum, defined 552
stethoscope
  blood pressure home monitoring 233
  blood pressure levels 157
  defined 551
Stossel, C. 254
streptococcal infection, defined 551
streptokinase 310
  defined 552
stress
  blood cholesterol levels 221
  cardiac rehabilitation 494
  cholesterol levels 503
  defined 552
  described 237
  heart disease 146-47, 171-74, 246-47
  smoking cessation 181
"Stress and the heart: Biobehavioral aspects of sudden cardiac death" *(Psychosomatics)* 253

593

stress management 173–74, 237–39
stress test 131–34, 275, 304, 312, 544
stroke
    defined 552
    high blood pressure 158
    risk factors 3–7
subarachnoid hemorrhage, defined 552
subartic stenosis 348–49
sudden cardiac arrest *see* cardiac arrest
sudden cardiac death
    defined 324
    exercise 192
    rhythm disorders 457
sudden death
    defined 336, 552
    hypertrophic cardiomyopathy 330–31
sugar
    blood cholesterol levels 87
    heart disease 9–10
    insulin resistance, heart disease 103–7
Sular (nisoldipine) *415*
superior vena cava
    defined 552
    depicted *63*
supraventricular tachycardia (SVT) 303
surgical procedures
    arrhythmias 302
    coronary artery bypass 193, 276, *290,* 291–92, 311, 542
    hypertrophic cardiomyopathy 331–32
    open heart surgery 549
SVT *see* supraventricular tachycardia (SVT)
syncope, defined 552
Syn-Diltiazem (diltiazem) 385
systole
    depicted *315*
    described 67
systolic blood pressure
    defined 552
    described 156–58, 228
systolic heart failure
    defined 324
    described 314

T

tachycardia 303, 459–60
    defined 552
tachypnea, defined 552
Tarka (verapamil) *416*
technetium 136
Teczem (diltiazem) *416*
Tenex (guanfacine) *414*
Tennessee, ischemic heart disease statistics 19
Tenoretic (atenolol) 383, *416*
Tenormin (atenolol) *414*
terazosin 162, *414*
tests, described
    see also *individual tests*
    angiogram 285
    blood tests
        cardiac enzymes 123
        cholesterol levels 123
        oxygen content 123–24
        prothrombin time 124
        thryoid 124
    cardiac blood pool scan 136–37
    cardiac catheterization 285, 433–36
    cardiac X-rays 124–25
    echocardiogram 126–27
    endoscopy 127–29
    echocardiograph 543, 546, 553
    exercise stress test 544
    heart scan 126–27
    endoscopy 127–29
    Holter monitor 134–36, 304
    intravascular echocardiography 546
    stress test 131–34, 284–85, 304
    thallium-201 stress test 552
    transesophageal echocardiography 553
tetralogy of Fallot 351–52
Texas, ischemic heart disease statistics 19
Texas Heart Institute
    contact information 568
    "Glossary" 537n
    heart-health test 148
    "The Texas Heart Institute Heart-Health Test" 141n

594

Index

Texas Heart Institute, continued
  top ten cardiology center 151
  web site 149
Thalitone (chlorthalidone) 392
thallium scan 134, 275
thallium-201 stress test, defined 552
thrombocytes, described 73
thrombolysis, defined 552
thrombolytic therapy, defined 553
thrombosis
  cerebral, defined 541
  coronary, defined 542
  deep vein, defined 542
  defined 553
thrombotic function 190
thrombus defined 553
thyroid test 124
TIA *see* transient ischemic attack (TIA)
Tiazac (diltiazem) *415*
Timolide (timolol) 383, *416*
timolol 311, 383–84, *414*, *416*
tissue plasminogen activator (TPA) 310
  defined 553
tobacco use
  see also nicotine replacement therapy; passive smoking; smoking cessation
  cardiac rehabilitation 494
  heart disease 4–7, 143–44, 876
  heart disease prevention 162–66
  high blood pressure 159
  hypertension 413
  second-hand smoke 183–85
Toprol-XL (metoprolol) *414*
torsemide *414*
total anomalous pulmonary venous connection 354–55
total blood cholesterol *see* blood cholesterol levels
To Your Health: Two Physicians Explore the Health Benefits of Wine 120
TPA *see* tissue plasminogen activator (TPA)
Trandate (labetalol) *415*
trandolapril *415*
Transderm-Nitro (nitroglycerin) 399

transesophageal echocardiography
  defined 553
  described 128
trans fat 86–87
  defined 553
transient ischemic attack (TIA)
  defined 553
transposition of the great arteries 352–53
triamterene 389–90, 391, *414*, *416*
Trichlorex (trichlormethiazide) 392
trichlormethiazide 392–93
Tricor (fenofibrate) 225
tricuspid atresia 353
tricuspid valve 64–65, 363
  defined 553
triglycerides 166–69, 428, 501–5
  defined 553
  described 93
Tromso Study (Norway), homocysteine levels 110
truncus ariteriosus 354
Tylenol (acetaminophen) 258
Type A personality 244–45

U

ubiquinone (coenzyme Q10) 261–64
Uchino, Bert N. 254
ultrasound
  defined 553
  Doppler, defined 543
"Uncorking the Facts about Alcohol and Your Health" (Tufts University) 115n
United Network for Organ Sharing (UNOS)
  donor organs 475
  transplant costs 477, 478
units of blood, described 72
Univasc (moexipril) *415*
UNOS *see* United Network for Organ Sharing (UNOS)
unstable angina 279–95
  treatment 286–92
Uridon (chlorthalidone) 392
Uritol (furosemide) 388
Urozide (hydrochlorothiazide) 392

U.S. Bureau of the Census, trends in heart disease 15
U.S. Department of Agriculture (USDA)
  daily value for fiber 213
  Nutrition Labeling and Education Act of 1990 209, 211
U.S. Department of Health and Human Services (DHHS), web site 113
U.S. Department of Transportation, National Highway Traffic Safety Administration First Responder... 55
U.S. Food and Drug Administration (FDA)
  addition of folic acid 112
  alcohol warning 258
  aspirin a day 255, 256
  chelation therapy 454, 455
  coenzyme Q10 263
  daily value for fiber 213
  defibrillator approval 460
  Digitalis Investigation Group (DIG) 401
  gemfibrozil therapy 520
  health claims 216
  laser angioplasty 441
  lipid-lowering drugs 430
  Nutrition Labeling and Education Act of 1990 209, 211
  percutaneous transluminal coronary angioplasty (PTCA) 437
  statin drugs approval 220
  ventricular arrhythmia 457, 462, 464
USDA *see* U.S. Department of Agriculture (USDA)
Utah, ischemic heart disease statistics 19

V

valsartan 161, *415*
valve disease 363–65
valve replacement 365
valves
  defined 324
  described 64
  heart failure 316

valvular heart disease 28
valvuloplasty 365
  defined 554
variant angina 277
varicose veins, defined 554
Vascor (bepridil) 385
vascular, defined 554
vascular system 69–73
  see also circulatory system
  depicted *70*
Vaseretic (enalapril maleate) *416*
vasodilators 402
  defined 554
  dilated cardiomyopathy 328
  high blood pressure 161
vasopressors, defined 554
Vasotec (enalapril) 311, 381, *415*
vein folds, described 71
veins
  defined 554
  described 71
vena cava, described 71
  see also inferior vena cava; superior vena cava
ventricles
  defined 336, 554
  depicted *63*
  described 62–63
ventricular fibrillation (VF) 54, 303, 457, 460
  defined 336, 554
  described 250
ventricular septal defect (VSD) 349–50
ventricular septum, described 63
ventricular tachycardia 303
  defined 554
venules, described 71
verapamil 161, 385–87, *415*, *416*
Verelan (verapamil) 385, *415*
Vermont, ischemic heart disease statistics 19
vertigo, defined 554
Veterans Affairs Cooperative Studies Program, Digitalis Investigation Group (DIG) 403
VF *see* ventricular fibrillation (VF)
Virginia, ischemic heart disease statistics 19

Index

Viskazide (pindolol) 383
Visken (pindolol) *414*
vitamin K 408
vitamins
  homocysteine 109
  homocysteine levels 111–12
VSD *see* ventricular septal defect (VSD)

W

walking, heart disease 12
warfarin 407–9
Washington, DC *see* District of Columbia
Washington state, ischemic heart disease statistics 19
weight factor
  see also obesity
  blood cholesterol levels 78, 90, 221, 515–16
  cardiac rehabilitation 492–93
  chart *170, 206*
  cholesterol levels 502
  food servings table *205*
  heart disease 7–10, 144
  high blood pressure 159
  smoking cessation 182
  weight loss hints 203–7
West Virginia, ischemic heart disease statistics 19
white blood cells (leukocytes) 73
Willett, Walter C. 183
Williams, Louise 268
Williams, Redford 173
Wisconsin, ischemic heart disease statistics 19
Wolff-Parkinson-White syndrome 303

women
  see also gender factor
  heart attack symptoms 40–41
  heart disease 142
  high blood pressure 156
  moderate alcohol use 118–19
  "Women and Heart Attacks: Prevention, Diagnosis, and Care" (Arnstein et al.) 33n
Workman Publishing, heart healthy cookbooks 556
Wyoming, ischemic heart disease statistics 19
Wytensin (Guanabenz acetate) *414*

X

xenotransplantation, described 30
X-rays
  cardiac 124–25
  defined 554
  heart murmur 368

Y

Yale University, survival rates 248
YMCA
  cardiac rehabilitation services 484
  contact information 568–69

Z

Zaroxolyn (metolazone) 392, *414*
Zebeta (bisoprolol) *414*
Zestoretic (lisinopril) *416*
Zestril (lisinopril) 311, 381, *415*
Ziac (bisoprolol) 383, *416*
Zocor (simvastatin) 223–24, 429

Health Reference Series
COMPLETE CATALOG

AIDS Sourcebook, 1st Edition

Basic Information about AIDS and HIV Infection, Featuring Historical and Statistical Data, Current Research, Prevention, and Other Special Topics of Interest for Persons Living with AIDS

Along with Source Listings for Further Assistance

Edited by Karen Bellenir and Peter D. Dresser. 831 pages. 1995. 0-7808-0031-1. $78.

"One strength of this book is its practical emphasis. The intended audience is the lay reader . . . useful as an educational tool for health care providers who work with AIDS patients. Recommended for public libraries as well as hospital or academic libraries that collect consumer materials."
— *Bulletin of the Medical Library Association, Jan '96*

"This is the most comprehensive volume of its kind on an important medical topic. Highly recommended for all libraries." — *Reference Book Review, '96*

"Very useful reference for all libraries."
— *Choice, Association of College and Research Libraries, Oct '95*

"There is a wealth of information here that can provide much educational assistance. It is a must book for all libraries and should be on the desk of each and every congressional leader. Highly recommended."
— *AIDS Book Review Journal, Aug '95*

"Recommended for most collections."
— *Library Journal, Jul '95*

■

AIDS Sourcebook, 2nd Edition

Basic Consumer Health Information about Acquired Immune Deficiency Syndrome (AIDS) and Human Immunodeficiency Virus (HIV) Infection, Featuring Updated Statistical Data, Reports on Recent Research and Prevention Initiatives, and Other Special Topics of Interest for Persons Living with AIDS, Including New Antiretroviral Treatment Options, Strategies for Combating Opportunistic Infections, Information about Clinical Trials, and More

Along with a Glossary of Important Terms and Resource Listings for Further Help and Information

Edited by Karen Bellenir. 751 pages. 1999. 0-7808-0225-X. $78.

"Recommended reference source."
— *Booklist, American Library Association, Dec '99*

"A solid text for college-level health libraries."
— *The Bookwatch, Aug '99*

Cited in *Reference Sources for Small and Medium-Sized Libraries, American Library Association, 1999*

Alcoholism Sourcebook

Basic Consumer Health Information about the Physical and Mental Consequences of Alcohol Abuse, Including Liver Disease, Pancreatitis, Wernicke-Korsakoff Syndrome (Alcoholic Dementia), Fetal Alcohol Syndrome, Heart Disease, Kidney Disorders, Gastrointestinal Problems, and Immune System Compromise and Featuring Facts about Addiction, Detoxification, Alcohol Withdrawal, Recovery, and the Maintenance of Sobriety

Along with a Glossary and Directories of Resources for Further Help and Information

Edited by Karen Bellenir. 650 pages. 2000. 0-7808-0325-6. $78.

SEE ALSO *Drug Abuse Sourcebook, Substance Abuse Sourcebook*

■

Allergies Sourcebook

Basic Information about Major Forms and Mechanisms of Common Allergic Reactions, Sensitivities, and Intolerances, Including Anaphylaxis, Asthma, Hives and Other Dermatologic Symptoms, Rhinitis, and Sinusitis

Along with Their Usual Triggers Like Animal Fur, Chemicals, Drugs, Dust, Foods, Insects, Latex, Pollen, and Poison Ivy, Oak, and Sumac; Plus Information on Prevention, Identification, and Treatment

Edited by Allan R. Cook. 611 pages. 1997. 0-7808-0036-2. $78.

■

Alternative Medicine Sourcebook

Basic Consumer Health Information about Alternatives to Conventional Medicine, Including Acupressure, Acupuncture, Aromatherapy, Ayurveda, Bioelectromagnetics, Environmental Medicine, Essence Therapy, Food and Nutrition Therapy, Herbal Therapy, Homeopathy, Imaging, Massage, Naturopathy, Reflexology, Relaxation and Meditation, Sound Therapy, Vitamin and Mineral Therapy, and Yoga, and More

Edited by Allan R. Cook. 737 pages. 1999. 0-7808-0200-4. $78.

■

Alzheimer's, Stroke & 29 Other Neurological Disorders Sourcebook, 1st Edition

Basic Information for the Layperson on 31 Diseases or Disorders Affecting the Brain and Nervous System, First Describing the Illness, Then Listing Symptoms, Diagnostic Methods, and Treatment Options, and Including Statistics on Incidences and Causes

Edited by Frank E. Bair. 579 pages. 1993. 1-55888-748-2. $78.

"Nontechnical reference book that provides reader-friendly information."
— *Family Caregiver Alliance Update, Winter '96*

"Should be included in any library's patient education section." — *American Reference Books Annual, 1994*

"Written in an approachable and accessible style. Recommended for patient education and consumer health collections in health science center and public libraries." — *Academic Library Book Review, Dec '93*

"It is very handy to have information on more than thirty neurological disorders under one cover, and there is no recent source like it." — *Reference Quarterly, Reference and User Services Association, Fall '93*

SEE ALSO *Brain Disorders Sourcebook*

Alzheimer's Disease Sourcebook, 2nd Edition

Basic Consumer Health Information about Alzheimer's Disease, Related Disorders, and Other Dementias, Including Multi-Infarct Dementia, AIDS-Related Dementia, Alcoholic Dementia, Huntington's Disease, Delirium, and Confusional States

Along with Reports Detailing Current Research Efforts in Prevention and Treatment, Long-Term Care Issues, and Listings of Sources for Additional Help and Information

Edited by Karen Bellenir. 524 pages. 1999. 0-7808-0223-3. $78.

"Recommended reference source."
—*Booklist, American Library Association, Oct '99*

Arthritis Sourcebook

Basic Consumer Health Information about Specific Forms of Arthritis and Related Disorders, Including Rheumatoid Arthritis, Osteoarthritis, Gout, Polymyalgia Rheumatica, Psoriatic Arthritis, Spondyloarthropathies, Juvenile Rheumatoid Arthritis, and Juvenile Ankylosing Spondylitis

Along with Information about Medical, Surgical, and Alternative Treatment Options, and Including Strategies for Coping with Pain, Fatigue, and Stress

Edited by Allan R. Cook. 550 pages. 1998. 0-7808-0201-2. $78.

". . . accessible to the layperson."
—*Reference and Research Book News, Feb '99*

Asthma Sourcebook

Basic Consumer Health Information about Asthma, Including Symptoms, Traditional and Nontraditional Remedies, Treatment Advances, Quality-of-Life Aids, Medical Research Updates, and the Role of Allergies, Exercise, Age, the Environment, and Genetics in the Development of Asthma

Along with Statistical Data, a Glossary, and Directories of Support Groups and Other Resources for Further Information

Edited by Annemarie S. Muth. 650 pages. 2000. 0-7808-0381-7. $78.

Back & Neck Disorders Sourcebook

Basic Information about Disorders and Injuries of the Spinal Cord and Vertebrae, Including Facts on Chiropractic Treatment, Surgical Interventions, Paralysis, and Rehabilitation

Along with Advice for Preventing Back Trouble

Edited by Karen Bellenir. 548 pages. 1997. 0-7808-0202-0. $78.

"The strength of this work is its basic, easy-to-read format. Recommended."
—*Reference and User Services Quarterly, American Library Association, Winter '97*

Blood & Circulatory Disorders Sourcebook

Basic Information about Blood and Its Components, Anemias, Leukemias, Bleeding Disorders, and Circulatory Disorders, Including Aplastic Anemia, Thalassemia, Sickle-Cell Disease, Hemochromatosis, Hemophilia, Von Willebrand Disease, and Vascular Diseases

Along with a Special Section on Blood Transfusions and Blood Supply Safety, a Glossary, and Source Listings for Further Help and Information

Edited by Karen Bellenir and Linda M. Shin. 554 pages. 1998. 0-7808-0203-9. $78.

"Recommended reference source."
—*Booklist, American Library Association, Feb '99*

"An important reference sourcebook written in simple language for everyday, non-technical users."
—*Reviewer's Bookwatch, Jan '99*

Brain Disorders Sourcebook

Basic Consumer Health Information about Strokes, Epilepsy, Amyotrophic Lateral Sclerosis (ALS/Lou Gehrig's Disease), Parkinson's Disease, Brain Tumors, Cerebral Palsy, Headache, Tourette Syndrome, and More

Along with Statistical Data, Treatment and Rehabilitation Options, Coping Strategies, Reports on Current Research Initiatives, a Glossary, and Resource Listings for Additional Help and Information

Edited by Karen Bellenir. 481 pages. 1999. 0-7808-0229-2. $78.

"Recommended reference source."
—*Booklist, American Library Association, Oct '99*

SEE ALSO *Alzheimer's, Stroke & 29 Other Neurological Disorders Sourcebook, 1st Edition*

Breast Cancer Sourcebook

Basic Consumer Health Information about Breast Cancer, Including Diagnostic Methods, Treatment Options, Alternative Therapies, Help and Self-Help Information, Related Health Concerns, Statistical and Demographic Data, and Facts for Men with Breast Cancer

Along with Reports on Current Research Initiatives, a Glossary of Related Medical Terms, and a Directory of Sources for Further Help and Information

Edited by Edward J. Prucha. 600 pages. 2000. 0-7808-0244-6. $78.

SEE ALSO *Cancer Sourcebook for Women, 1st and 2nd Editions, Women's Health Concerns Sourcebook*

■

Burns Sourcebook

Basic Consumer Health Information about Various Types of Burns and Scalds, Including Flame, Heat, Cold, Electrical, Chemical, and Sun Burns

Along with Information on Short-Term and Long-Term Treatments, Tissue Reconstruction, Plastic Surgery, Prevention Suggestions, and First Aid

Edited by Allan R. Cook. 604 pages. 1999. 0-7808-0204-7. $78.

"Recommended reference source."
—*Booklist, American Library Association, Dec '99*

SEE ALSO *Skin Disorders Sourcebook*

■

Cancer Sourcebook, 1st Edition

Basic Information on Cancer Types, Symptoms, Diagnostic Methods, and Treatments, Including Statistics on Cancer Occurrences Worldwide and the Risks Associated with Known Carcinogens and Activities

Edited by Frank E. Bair. 932 pages. 1990. 1-55888-888-8. $78.

Cited in *Reference Sources for Small and Medium-Sized Libraries*, American Library Association, 1999

"Written in nontechnical language. Useful for patients, their families, medical professionals, and librarians."
—*Guide to Reference Books, 1996*

"Designed with the non-medical professional in mind. Libraries and medical facilities interested in patient education should certainly consider adding the *Cancer Sourcebook* to their holdings. This compact collection of reliable information . . . is an invaluable tool for helping patients and patients' families and friends to take the first steps in coping with the many difficulties of cancer."
—*Medical Reference Services Quarterly, Winter '91*

"Specifically created for the nontechnical reader . . . an important resource for the general reader trying to understand the complexities of cancer."
—*American Reference Books Annual, 1991*

"This publication's nontechnical nature and very comprehensive format make it useful for both the general public and undergraduate students." —*Choice, Association of College and Research Libraries, Oct '90*

New Cancer Sourcebook, 2nd Edition

Basic Information about Major Forms and Stages of Cancer, Featuring Facts about Primary and Secondary Tumors of the Respiratory, Nervous, Lymphatic, Circulatory, Skeletal, and Gastrointestinal Systems, and Specific Organs; Statistical and Demographic Data; Treatment Options; and Strategies for Coping

Edited by Allan R. Cook. 1,313 pages. 1996. 0-7808-0041-9. $78.

"An excellent resource for patients with newly diagnosed cancer and their families. The dialogue is simple, direct, and comprehensive. Highly recommended for patients and families to aid in their understanding of cancer and its treatment." —*Booklist Health Sciences Supplement, American Library Association, Oct '97*

"The amount of factual and useful information is extensive. The writing is very clear, geared to general readers. Recommended for all levels." —*Choice, Association of College and Research Libraries, Jan '97*

■

Cancer Sourcebook, 3rd Edition

Basic Consumer Health Information about Major Forms and Stages of Cancer, Featuring Facts about Primary and Secondary Tumors of the Respiratory, Nervous, Lymphatic, Circulatory, Skeletal, and Gastrointestinal Systems, and Specific Organs

Along with Statistical and Demographic Data, Treatment Options, Strategies for Coping, a Glossary, and a Directory of Sources for Additional Help and Information

Edited by Edward J. Prucha. 1,100 pages. 2000. 0-7808-0227-6. $78.

■

Cancer Sourcebook for Women, 1st Edition

Basic Information about Specific Forms of Cancer That Affect Women, Featuring Facts about Breast Cancer, Cervical Cancer, Ovarian Cancer, Cancer of the Uterus and Uterine Sarcoma, Cancer of the Vagina, and Cancer of the Vulva; Statistical and Demographic Data; Treatments, Self-Help Management Suggestions, and Current Research Initiatives

Edited by Allan R. Cook and Peter D. Dresser. 524 pages. 1996. 0-7808-0076-1. $78.

". . . written in easily understandable, non-technical language. Recommended for public libraries or hospital and academic libraries that collect patient education or consumer health materials."
—*Medical Reference Services Quarterly, Spring '97*

"Would be of value in a consumer health library. . . . written with the health care consumer in mind. Medical jargon is at a minimum, and medical terms are explained in clear, understandable sentences."
—*Bulletin of the Medical Library Association, Oct '96*

601

"The availability under one cover of all these pertinent publications, grouped under cohesive headings, makes this certainly a most useful sourcebook."
— *Choice, Association of College and Research Libraries, Jun '96*

"Presents a comprehensive knowledge base for general readers. Men and women both benefit from the gold mine of information nestled between the two covers of this book. Recommended."
—*Academic Library Book Review, Summer '96*

"This timely book is highly recommended for consumer health and patient education collections in all libraries." — *Library Journal, Apr '96*

SEE ALSO *Breast Cancer Sourcebook, Women's Health Concerns Sourcebook*

Cancer Sourcebook for Women, 2nd Edition

Basic Consumer Health Information about Specific Forms of Cancer That Affect Women, Including Cervical Cancer, Ovarian Cancer, Endometrial Cancer, Uterine Sarcoma, Vaginal Cancer, Vulvar Cancer, and Gestational Trophoblastic Tumor; and Featuring Statistical Information, Facts about Tests and Treatments, a Glossary of Cancer Terms, and an Extensive List of Additional Resources

Edited by Edward J. Prucha. 600 pages. 2000. 0-7808-0226-8. $78.

SEE ALSO *Breast Cancer Sourcebook, Women's Health Concerns Sourcebook*

Cardiovascular Diseases & Disorders Sourcebook, 1st Edition

Basic Information about Cardiovascular Diseases and Disorders, Featuring Facts about the Cardiovascular System, Demographic and Statistical Data, Descriptions of Pharmacological and Surgical Interventions, Lifestyle Modifications, and a Special Section Focusing on Heart Disorders in Children

Edited by Karen Bellenir and Peter D. Dresser. 683 pages. 1995. 0-7808-0032-X. $78.

". . . comprehensive format provides an extensive overview on this subject."
—*Choice, Association of College and Research Libraries, Jun '96*

". . . an easily understood, complete, up-to-date resource. This well executed public health tool will make valuable information available to those that need it most, patients and their families. The typeface, sturdy non-reflective paper, and library binding add a feel of quality found wanting in other publications. Highly recommended for academic and general libraries. "
—*Academic Library Book Review, Summer '96*

SEE ALSO *Healthy Heart Sourcebook for Women, Heart Diseases & Disorders Sourcebook, 2nd Edition*

Communication Disorders Sourcebook

Basic Information about Deafness and Hearing Loss, Speech and Language Disorders, Voice Disorders, Balance and Vestibular Disorders, and Disorders of Smell, Taste, and Touch

Edited by Linda M. Ross. 533 pages. 1996. 0-7808-0077-X. $78.

"This is skillfully edited and is a welcome resource for the layperson. It should be found in every public and medical library." — *Booklist Health Sciences Supplement, American Library Association, Oct '97*

Congenital Disorders Sourcebook

Basic Information about Disorders Acquired during Gestation, Including Spina Bifida, Hydrocephalus, Cerebral Palsy, Heart Defects, Craniofacial Abnormalities, Fetal Alcohol Syndrome, and More

Along with Current Treatment Options and Statistical Data

Edited by Karen Bellenir. 607 pages. 1997. 0-7808-0205-5. $78.

"Recommended reference source."
— *Booklist, American Library Association, Oct '97*

SEE ALSO *Pregnancy & Birth Sourcebook*

Consumer Issues in Health Care Sourcebook

Basic Information about Health Care Fundamentals and Related Consumer Issues, Including Exams and Screening Tests, Physician Specialties, Choosing a Doctor, Using Prescription and Over-the-Counter Medications Safely, Avoiding Health Scams, Managing Common Health Risks in the Home. Care Options for Chronically or Terminally Ill Patients, and a List of Resources for Obtaining Help and Further Information

Edited by Karen Bellenir. 618 pages. 1998. 0-7808-0221-7. $78.

"The editor has researched the literature from government agencies and others, saving readers the time and effort of having to do the research themselves. Recommended for public libraries."
— *Reference and User Services Quarterly, American Library Association, Spring '99*

"Recommended reference source."
— *Booklist, American Library Association, Dec '98*

Contagious & Non-Contagious Infectious Diseases Sourcebook

Basic Information about Contagious Diseases like Measles, Polio, Hepatitis B, and Infectious Mononucleosis, and Non-Contagious Infectious Diseases like Tetanus and Toxic Shock Syndrome, and Diseases Occurring as Secondary Infections Such as Shingles and Reye Syndrome

Along with Vaccination, Prevention, and Treatment Information, and a Section Describing Emerging Infectious Disease Threats

Edited by Karen Bellenir and Peter D. Dresser. 566 pages. 1996. 0-7808-0075-3. $78.

Death & Dying Sourcebook

Basic Consumer Health Information for the Layperson about End-of-Life Care and Related Ethical and Legal Issues, Including Chief Causes of Death, Autopsies, Pain Management for the Terminally Ill, Life Support Systems, Insurance, Euthanasia, Assisted Suicide, Hospice Programs, Living Wills, Funeral Planning, Counseling, Mourning, Organ Donation, and Physician Training

Along with Statistical Data, a Glossary, and Listings of Sources for Further Help and Information

Edited by Annemarie S. Muth. 641 pages. 1999. 0-7808-0230-6. $78.

Diabetes Sourcebook, 1st Edition

Basic Information about Insulin-Dependent and Non-insulin-Dependent Diabetes Mellitus, Gestational Diabetes, and Diabetic Complications, Symptoms, Treatment, and Research Results, Including Statistics on Prevalence, Morbidity, and Mortality

Along with Source Listings for Further Help and Information

Edited by Karen Bellenir and Peter D. Dresser. 827 pages. 1994. 1-55888-751-2. $78.

". . . very informative and understandable for the layperson without being simplistic. It provides a comprehensive overview for laypersons who want a general understanding of the disease or who want to focus on various aspects of the disease."
— *Bulletin of the Medical Library Association, Jan '96*

Diabetes Sourcebook, 2nd Edition

Basic Consumer Health Information about Type 1 Diabetes (Insulin-Dependent or Juvenile-Onset Diabetes), Type 2 (Noninsulin-Dependent or Adult-Onset Diabetes), Gestational Diabetes, and Related Disorders, Including Diabetes Prevalence Data, Management Issues, the Role of Diet and Exercise in Controlling Diabetes, Insulin and Other Diabetes Medicines, and Complications of Diabetes Such as Eye Diseases, Periodontal Disease, Amputation, and End-Stage Renal Disease

Along with Reports on Current Research Initiatives, a Glossary, and Resource Listings for Further Help and Information

Edited by Karen Bellenir. 688 pages. 1998. 0-7808-0224-1. $78.

"Recommended reference source."
— *Booklist, American Library Association, Feb '99*

". . . provides reliable mainstream medical information . . . belongs on the shelves of any library with a consumer health collection." — *E-Streams, Sep '99*

"Provides useful information for the general public."
— *Healthlines, University of Michigan Health Management Research Center, Sep/Oct '99*

Diet & Nutrition Sourcebook, 1st Edition

Basic Information about Nutrition, Including the Dietary Guidelines for Americans, the Food Guide Pyramid, and Their Applications in Daily Diet, Nutritional Advice for Specific Age Groups, Current Nutritional Issues and Controversies, the New Food Label and How to Use It to Promote Healthy Eating, and Recent Developments in Nutritional Research

Edited by Dan R. Harris. 662 pages. 1996. 0-7808-0084-2. $78.

"Useful reference as a food and nutrition sourcebook for the general consumer."
— *Booklist Health Sciences Supplement, American Library Association, Oct '97*

"Recommended for public libraries and medical libraries that receive general information requests on nutrition. It is readable and will appeal to those interested in learning more about healthy dietary practices."
— *Medical Reference Services Quarterly, Fall '97*

"An abundance of medical and social statistics is translated into readable information geared toward the general reader." — *Bookwatch, Mar '97*

"With dozens of questionable diet books on the market, it is so refreshing to find a reliable and factual reference book. Recommended to aspiring professionals, librarians, and others seeking and giving reliable dietary advice. An excellent compilation."
— *Choice, Association of College and Research Libraries, Feb '97*

SEE ALSO *Digestive Diseases & Disorders Sourcebook, Gastrointestinal Diseases & Disorders Sourcebook*

Diet & Nutrition Sourcebook, 2nd Edition

Basic Consumer Health Information about Dietary Guidelines, Recommended Daily Intake Values, Vitamins, Minerals, Fiber, Fat, Weight Control, Dietary Supplements, and Food Additives

Along with Special Sections on Nutrition Needs throughout Life and Nutrition for People with Such Specific Medical Concerns as Allergies, High Blood Cholesterol, Hypertension, Diabetes, Celiac Disease, Seizure Disorders, Phenylketonuria (PKU), Cancer, and Eating Disorders, and Including Reports on Current Nutrition Research and Source Listings for Additional Help and Information

Edited by Karen Bellenir. 650 pages. 1999. 0-7808-0228-4. $78.

"Recommended reference source."
—*Booklist, American Library Association*, Dec '99

SEE ALSO *Digestive Diseases & Disorders Sourcebook, Gastrointestinal Diseases & Disorders Sourcebook*

Digestive Diseases & Disorders Sourcebook

Basic Consumer Health Information about Diseases and Disorders that Impact the Upper and Lower Digestive System, Including Celiac Disease, Constipation, Crohn's Disease, Cyclic Vomiting Syndrome, Diarrhea, Diverticulosis and Diverticulitis, Gallstones, Heartburn, Hemorrhoids, Hernias, Indigestion (Dyspepsia), Irritable Bowel Syndrome, Lactose Intolerance, Ulcers, and More

Along with Information about Medications and Other Treatments, Tips for Maintaining a Healthy Digestive Tract, a Glossary, and Directory of Digestive Diseases Organizations

Edited by Karen Bellenir. 335 pages. 1999. 0-7808-0327-2. $48.

SEE ALSO *Diet & Nutrition Sourcebook, 1st and 2nd Editions, Gastrointestinal Diseases & Disorders Sourcebook*

Disabilities Sourcebook

Basic Consumer Health Information about Physical and Psychiatric Disabilities, Including Descriptions of Major Causes of Disability, Assistive and Adaptive Aids, Workplace Issues, and Accessibility Concerns

Along with Information about the Americans with Disabilities Act, a Glossary, and Resources for Additional Help and Information

Edited by Dawn D. Matthews. 600 pages. 2000. 0-7808-0389-2. $78.

Domestic Violence & Child Abuse Sourcebook

Basic Information about Spousal/Partner, Child, and Elder Physical, Emotional, and Sexual Abuse, Teen Dating Violence, and Stalking, Including Information about Hotlines, Safe Houses, Safety Plans, and Other Resources for Support and Assistance, Community Initiatives, and Reports on Current Directions in Research and Treatment

Along with a Glossary, Sources for Further Reading, and Governmental and Non-Governmental Organizations Contact Information

Edited by Helene Henderson. 600 pages. 2000. 0-7808-0235-7. $78.

Drug Abuse Sourcebook

Basic Consumer Health Information about Illicit Substances of Abuse and the Diversion of Prescription Medications, Including Depressants, Hallucinogens, Inhalants, Marijuana, Narcotics, Stimulants, and Anabolic Steroids

Along with Facts about Related Health Risks, Treatment Issues, and Substance Abuse Prevention Programs, a Glossary of Terms, Statistical Data, and Directories of Hotline Services, Self-Help Groups, and Organizations Able to Provide Further Information

Edited by Karen Bellenir. 600 pages. 2000. 0-7808-0242-X. $78.

SEE ALSO *Alcoholism Sourcebook, Substance Abuse Sourcebook*

Ear, Nose & Throat Disorders Sourcebook

Basic Information about Disorders of the Ears, Nose, Sinus Cavities, Pharynx, and Larynx, Including Ear Infections, Tinnitus, Vestibular Disorders, Allergic and Non-Allergic Rhinitis, Sore Throats, Tonsillitis, and Cancers That Affect the Ears, Nose, Sinuses, and Throat

Along with Reports on Current Research Initiatives, a Glossary of Related Medical Terms, and a Directory of Sources for Further Help and Information

Edited by Karen Bellenir and Linda M. Shin. 576 pages. 1998. 0-7808-0206-3. $78.

"Overall, this sourcebook is helpful for the consumer seeking information on ENT issues. It is recommended for public libraries."
—*American Reference Books Annual*, 1999

"Recommended reference source."
—*Booklist, American Library Association*, Dec '98

Endocrine & Metabolic Disorders Sourcebook

Basic Information for the Layperson about Pancreatic and Insulin-Related Disorders Such as Pancreatitis, Diabetes, and Hypoglycemia; Adrenal Gland Disorders Such as Cushing's Syndrome, Addison's Disease, and Congenital Adrenal Hyperplasia; Pituitary Gland Disorders Such as Growth Hormone Deficiency, Acromegaly, and Pituitary Tumors; Thyroid Disorders Such as Hypothyroidism, Graves' Disease, Hashimoto's Disease, and Goiter; Hyperparathyroidism; and Other Diseases and Syndromes of Hormone Imbalance or Metabolic Dysfunction

Along with Reports on Current Research Initiatives

Edited by Linda M. Shin. 574 pages. 1998. 0-7808-0207-1. $78.

"Recommended reference source."
— *Booklist, American Library Association, Dec '98*

Environmentally Induced Disorders Sourcebook

Basic Information about Diseases and Syndromes Linked to Exposure to Pollutants and Other Substances in Outdoor and Indoor Environments Such as Lead, Asbestos, Formaldehyde, Mercury, Emissions, Noise, and More

Edited by Allan R. Cook. 620 pages. 1997. 0-7808-0083-4. $78.

"Recommended reference source."
— *Booklist, American Library Association, Sep '98*

"This book will be a useful addition to anyone's library." — *Choice Health Sciences Supplement, Association of College and Research Libraries, May '98*

". . . a good survey of numerous environmentally induced physical disorders . . . a useful addition to anyone's library."
— *Doody's Health Sciences Book Reviews, Jan '98*

". . . provide[s] introductory information from the best authorities around. Since this volume covers topics that potentially affect everyone, it will surely be one of the most frequently consulted volumes in the Health Reference Series." — *Rettig on Reference, Nov '97*

Ethical Issues in Medicine Sourcebook

Basic Information about Controversial Treatment Issues, Genetic Research, Reproductive Technologies, and End-of-Life Decisions, Including Topics Such as Cloning, Abortion, Fertility Management, Organ Transplantation, Health Care Rationing, Advance Directives, Living Wills, Physician-Assisted Suicide, Euthanasia, and More; Along with a Glossary and Resources for Additional Information

Edited by Helene Henderson. 600 pages. 2000. 0-7808-0237-3. $78.

Family Planning Sourcebook

Basic Information about Planning for Pregnancy and Contraception, Including Traditional Methods, Barrier Methods, Hormonal Methods, Permanent Methods, Future Methods, Emergency Contraception, Birth Control Choices for Women at Each Stage of Life, and Men's Role in Family Planning

Along with Statistics, Glossary, and Sources of Additional Information

Edited by Amy Marcaccio Keyzer. 600 pages. 2000. 0-7808-0379-5. $78.

SEE ALSO *Pregnancy & Birth Sourcebook*

Fitness & Exercise Sourcebook

Basic Information on Fitness and Exercise, Including Fitness Activities for Specific Age Groups, Exercise for People with Specific Medical Conditions, How to Begin a Fitness Program in Running, Walking, Swimming, Cycling, and Other Athletic Activities, and Recent Research in Fitness and Exercise

Edited by Dan R. Harris. 663 pages. 1996. 0-7808-0186-5. $78.

"A good resource for general readers."
— *Choice, Association of College and Research Libraries, Nov '97*

"The perennial popularity of the topic . . . make this an appealing selection for public libraries."
— *Rettig on Reference, Jun/Jul '97*

Food & Animal Borne Diseases Sourcebook

Basic Information about Diseases That Can Be Spread to Humans through the Ingestion of Contaminated Food or Water or by Contact with Infected Animals and Insects, Such as Botulism, E. Coli, Hepatitis A, Trichinosis, Lyme Disease, and Rabies

Along with Information Regarding Prevention and Treatment Methods, and Including a Special Section for International Travelers Describing Diseases Such as Cholera, Malaria, Travelers' Diarrhea, and Yellow Fever, and Offering Recommendations for Avoiding Illness

Edited by Karen Bellenir and Peter D. Dresser. 535 pages. 1995. 0-7808-0033-8. $78.

"Targeting general readers and providing them with a single, comprehensive source of information on selected topics, this book continues, with the excellent caliber of its predecessors, to catalog topical information on health matters of general interest. Readable and thorough, this valuable resource is highly recommended for all libraries."
— *Academic Library Book Review, Summer '96*

"A comprehensive collection of authoritative information." — *Emergency Medical Services, Oct '95*

Food Safety Sourcebook

Basic Consumer Health Information about the Safe Handling of Meat, Poultry, Seafood, Eggs, Fruit Juices, and Other Food Items, and Facts about Pesticides, Drinking Water, Food Safety Overseas, and the Onset, Duration, and Symptoms of Foodborne Illnesses, Including Types of Pathogenic Bacteria, Parasitic Protozoa, Worms, Viruses, and Natural Toxins

Along with the Role of the Consumer, the Food Handler, and the Government in Food Safety; a Glossary, and Resources for Additional Help and Information

Edited by Dawn D. Matthews. 339 pages. 1999. 0-7808-0326-4. $48.

Forensic Medicine Sourcebook

Basic Consumer Information for the Layperson about Forensic Medicine, Including Crime Scene Investigation, Evidence Collection and Analysis, Expert Testimony, Computer-Aided Criminal Identification, Digital Imaging in the Courtroom, DNA Profiling, Accident Reconstruction, Autopsies, Ballistics, Drugs and Explosives Detection, Latent Fingerprints, Product Tampering, and Questioned Document Examination

Along with Statistical Data, a Glossary of Forensics Terminology, and Listings of Sources for Further Help and Information

Edited by Annemarie S. Muth. 574 pages. 1999. 0-7808-0232-2. $78.

"A wealth of information, useful statistics, references are up-to-date and extremely complete. This wonderful collection of data will help students who are interested in a career in any type of forensic field. It is a great resource for attorneys who need information about types of expert witnesses needed in a particular case. It also offers useful information for fiction and nonfiction writers whose work involves a crime. A fascinating compilation. All levels."
— Choice, Association of College and Research Libraries, Jan 2000

Gastrointestinal Diseases & Disorders Sourcebook

Basic Information about Gastroesophageal Reflux Disease (Heartburn), Ulcers, Diverticulosis, Irritable Bowel Syndrome, Crohn's Disease, Ulcerative Colitis, Diarrhea, Constipation, Lactose Intolerance, Hemorrhoids, Hepatitis, Cirrhosis, and Other Digestive Problems, Featuring Statistics, Descriptions of Symptoms, and Current Treatment Methods of Interest for Persons Living with Upper and Lower Gastrointestinal Maladies

Edited by Linda M. Ross. 413 pages. 1996. 0-7808-0078-8. $78.

"... very readable form. The successful editorial work that brought this material together into a useful and understandable reference makes accessible to all readers information that can help them more effectively understand and obtain help for digestive tract problems."
— Choice, Association of College and Research Libraries, Feb '97

SEE ALSO Diet & Nutrition Sourcebook, 1st and 2nd Editions, Digestive Diseases & Disorders Sourcebook

Genetic Disorders Sourcebook

Basic Information about Heritable Diseases and Disorders Such as Down Syndrome, PKU, Hemophilia, Von Willebrand Disease, Gaucher Disease, Tay-Sachs Disease, and Sickle-Cell Disease, Along with Information about Genetic Screening, Gene Therapy, Home Care, and Including Source Listings for Further Help and Information on More Than 300 Disorders

Edited by Karen Bellenir. 642 pages. 1996. 0-7808-0034-6. $78.

"Recommended for undergraduate libraries or libraries that serve the public."
— Science & Technology Libraries, Vol. 18, No. 1, '99

"Provides essential medical information to both the general public and those diagnosed with a serious or fatal genetic disease or disorder."
—Choice, Association of College and Research Libraries, Jan '97

"Geared toward the lay public. It would be well placed in all public libraries and in those hospital and medical libraries in which access to genetic references is limited." — Doody's Health Sciences Book Review, Oct '96

Head Trauma Sourcebook

Basic Information for the Layperson about Open-Head and Closed-Head Injuries, Treatment Advances, Recovery, and Rehabilitation

Along with Reports on Current Research Initiatives

Edited by Karen Bellenir. 414 pages. 1997. 0-7808-0208-X. $78.

Health Insurance Sourcebook

Basic Information about Managed Care Organizations, Traditional Fee-for-Service Insurance, Insurance Portability and Pre-Existing Conditions Clauses, Medicare, Medicaid, Social Security, and Military Health Care

Along with Information about Insurance Fraud

Edited by Wendy Wilcox. 530 pages. 1997. 0-7808-0222-5. $78.

"Particularly useful because it brings much of this information together in one volume. This book will be a handy reference source in the health sciences library, hospital library, college and university library, and medium to large public library."
— Medical Reference Services Quarterly, Fall '98

Awarded "Books of the Year Award"
by the American Journal of Nursing, 1997

"The layout of the book is particularly helpful as it provides easy access to reference material. A most useful addition to the vast amount of information about health insurance. The use of data from U.S. government agencies is most commendable. Useful in a library or learning center for healthcare professional students."
— *Doody's Health Sciences Book Reviews, Nov '97*

Health Resources Sourcebook

Basic Consumer Health Information about Sources of Medical Assistance, Featuring an Annotated Directory of Private and Public Consumer Health Organizations and Listings of Other Resources, Including Hospitals, Hospices, and State Medical Associations

Along with Guidelines for Locating and Evaluating Health Information

Edited by Dawn D. Matthews. 500 pages. 2000. 0-7808-0328-0. $78.

Healthy Aging Sourcebook

Basic Consumer Health Information about Maintaining Health through the Aging Process, Including Advice on Nutrition, Exercise, and Sleep, Help in Making Decisions about Midlife Issues and Retirement, and Guidance Concerning Practical and Informed Choices in Health Consumerism

Along with Data Concerning the Theories of Aging, Different Experiences in Aging by Minority Groups, and Facts about Aging Now and Aging in the Future; and Featuring a Glossary, a Guide to Consumer Help, Additional Suggested Reading, and Practical Resource Directory

Edited by Jenifer Swanson. 536 pages. 1999. 0-7808-0390-6. $78.

SEE ALSO *Physical & Mental Issues in Aging Sourcebook*

Healthy Heart Sourcebook for Women

Basic Consumer Health Information about Cardiac Issues Specific to Women, Including Facts about Major Risk Factors and Prevention, Treatment and Control Strategies, and Important Dietary Issues

Along with a Special Section Regarding the Pros and Cons of Hormone Replacement Therapy and Its Impact on Heart Health, and Additional Help, Including Recipes, a Glossary, and a Directory of Resources

Edited by Dawn D. Matthews. 400 pages. 2000. 0-7808-0329-9. $48.

SEE ALSO *Cardiovascular Diseases & Disorders Sourcebook, 1st Edition, Heart Diseases & Disorders Sourcebook, 2nd Edition, Women's Health Concerns Sourcebook*

Heart Diseases & Disorders Sourcebook, 2nd edition

Basic Consumer Health Information about Heart Attacks, Angina, Rhythm Disorders, Heart Failure, Valve Disease, Congenital Heart Disorders, and More, Including Descriptions of Surgical Procedures and Other Interventions, Medications, Cardiac Rehabilitation, Risk Identification, and Prevention Tips

Along with Statistical Data, Reports on Current Research Initiatives, a Glossary of Cardiovascular Terms, and Resource Directory

Edited by Karen Bellenir. 600 pages. 2000. 0-7808-0238-1. $78.

SEE ALSO *Cardiovascular Diseases & Disorders Sourcebook, 1st Edition, Healthy Heart Sourcebook for Women*

Immune System Disorders Sourcebook

Basic Information about Lupus, Multiple Sclerosis, Guillain-Barré Syndrome, Chronic Granulomatous Disease, and More

Along with Statistical and Demographic Data and Reports on Current Research Initiatives

Edited by Allan R. Cook. 608 pages. 1997. 0-7808-0209-8. $78.

Infant & Toddler Health Sourcebook

Basic Consumer Health Information about the Physical and Mental Development of Newborns, Infants, and Toddlers, Including Neonatal Concerns, Nutritional Recommendations, Immunization Schedules, Common Pediatric Disorders, Assessments and Milestones, Safety Tips, and Advice for Parents and Other Caregivers

Along with a Glossary of Terms and Resource Listings for Additional Help

Edited by Jenifer Swanson. 600 pages. 2000. 0-7808-0246-2. $78.

Kidney & Urinary Tract Diseases & Disorders Sourcebook

Basic Information about Kidney Stones, Urinary Incontinence, Bladder Disease, End Stage Renal Disease, Dialysis, and More

Along with Statistical and Demographic Data and Reports on Current Research Initiatives

Edited by Linda M. Ross. 602 pages. 1997. 0-7808-0079-6. $78.

Learning Disabilities Sourcebook

Basic Information about Disorders Such as Dyslexia, Visual and Auditory Processing Deficits, Attention Deficit/Hyperactivity Disorder, and Autism

Along with Statistical and Demographic Data, Reports on Current Research Initiatives, an Explanation of the Assessment Process, and a Special Section for Adults with Learning Disabilities

Edited by Linda M. Shin. 579 pages. 1998. 0-7808-0210-1. $78.

"Readable . . . provides a solid base of information regarding successful techniques used with individuals who have learning disabilities, as well as practical suggestions for educators and family members. Clear language, concise descriptions, and pertinent information for contacting multiple resources add to the strength of this book as a useful tool."
—Choice, Association of College and Research Libraries, Feb '99

"Recommended reference source."
—Booklist, American Library Association, Sep '98

"This is a useful resource for libraries and for those who don't have the time to identify and locate the individual publications."
—Disability Resources Monthly, Sep '98

Liver Disorders Sourcebook

Basic Consumer Health Information about the Liver and How It Works; Liver Diseases, Including Cancer, Cirrhosis, Hepatitis, and Toxic and Drug Related Diseases; Tips for Maintaining a Healthy Liver; Laboratory Tests, Radiology Tests, and Facts about Liver Transplantation

Along with a Section on Support Groups, a Glossary, and Resource Listings

Edited by Joyce Brennfleck Shannon. 591 pages. 2000. 0-7808-0383-3. $78.

Medical Tests Sourcebook

Basic Consumer Health Information about Medical Tests, Including Periodic Health Exams, General Screening Tests, Tests You Can Do at Home, Findings of the U.S. Preventive Services Task Force, X-ray and Radiology Tests, Electrical Tests, Tests of Blood and Other Body Fluids and Tissues, Scope Tests, Lung Tests, Genetic Tests, Pregnancy Tests, Newborn Screening Tests, Sexually Transmitted Disease Tests, and Computer Aided Diagnoses

Along with a Section on Paying for Medical Tests, a Glossary, and Resource Listings

Edited by Joyce Brennfleck Shannon. 691 pages. 1999. 0-7808-0243-8. $78.

"This is an overall excellent reference with a wealth of general knowledge that may aid those who are reluctant to get vital tests performed."
—Today's Librarian, Jan 2000

Men's Health Concerns Sourcebook

Basic Information about Health Issues That Affect Men, Featuring Facts about the Top Causes of Death in Men, Including Heart Disease, Stroke, Cancers, Prostate Disorders, Chronic Obstructive Pulmonary Disease, Pneumonia and Influenza, Human Immunodeficiency Virus and Acquired Immune Deficiency Syndrome, Diabetes Mellitus, Stress, Suicide, Accidents and Homicides; and Facts about Common Concerns for Men, Including Impotence, Contraception, Circumcision, Sleep Disorders, Snoring, Hair Loss, Diet, Nutrition, Exercise, Kidney and Urological Disorders, and Backaches

Edited by Allan R. Cook. 738 pages. 1998. 0-7808-0212-8. $78.

"Recommended reference source."
—Booklist, American Library Association, Dec '98

Mental Health Disorders Sourcebook, 1st Edition

Basic Information about Schizophrenia, Depression, Bipolar Disorder, Panic Disorder, Obsessive-Compulsive Disorder, Phobias and Other Anxiety Disorders, Paranoia and Other Personality Disorders, Eating Disorders, and Sleep Disorders

Along with Information about Treatment and Therapies

Edited by Karen Bellenir. 548 pages. 1995. 0-7808-0040-0. $78.

"This is an excellent new book . . . written in easy-to-understand language." —Booklist Health Sciences Supplement, American Library Association, Oct '97

". . . useful for public and academic libraries and consumer health collections."
—Medical Reference Services Quarterly, Spring '97

"The great strengths of the book are its readability and its inclusion of places to find more information. Especially recommended." —Reference Quarterly, Reference and User Services Association, Winter '96

". . . a good resource for a consumer health library."
—Bulletin of the Medical Library Association, Oct '96

"The information is data-based and couched in brief, concise language that avoids jargon. . . . a useful reference source." —Readings, Sep '96

"The text is well organized and adequately written for its target audience."
—Choice, Association of College and Research Libraries, Jun '96

". . . provides information on a wide range of mental disorders, presented in nontechnical language."
—Exceptional Child Education Resources, Spring '96

"Recommended for public and academic libraries."
—Reference Book Review, 1996

Mental Health Disorders Sourcebook, 2nd Edition

Basic Consumer Health Information about Anxiety Disorders, Depression and Other Mood Disorders, Eating Disorders, Personality Disorders, Schizophrenia, and More, Including Disease Descriptions, Treatment Options, and Reports on Current Research Initiatives

Along with Statistical Data, Tips for Maintaining Mental Health, a Glossary, and Directory of Sources for Additional Help and Information

Edited by Karen Bellenir. 605 pages. 2000. 0-7808-0240-3. $78.

Mental Retardation Sourcebook

Basic Consumer Health Information about Mental Retardation and Its Causes, Including Down Syndrome, Fetal Alcohol Syndrome, Fragile X Syndrome, Genetic Conditions, Injury, and Environmental Sources

Along with Preventive Strategies, Parenting Issues, Educational Implications, Health Care Needs, Employment and Economic Matters, Legal Issues, a Glossary, and a Resource Listing for Additional Help and Information

Edited by Joyce Brennfleck Shannon. 600 pages. 2000. 0-7808-0377-9. $78.

Ophthalmic Disorders Sourcebook

Basic Information about Glaucoma, Cataracts, Macular Degeneration, Strabismus, Refractive Disorders, and More

Along with Statistical and Demographic Data and Reports on Current Research Initiatives

Edited by Linda M. Ross. 631 pages. 1996. 0-7808-0081-8. $78.

Oral Health Sourcebook

Basic Information about Diseases and Conditions Affecting Oral Health, Including Cavities, Gum Disease, Dry Mouth, Oral Cancers, Fever Blisters, Canker Sores, Oral Thrush, Bad Breath, Temporomandibular Disorders, and other Craniofacial Syndromes

Along with Statistical Data on the Oral Health of Americans, Oral Hygiene, Emergency First Aid, Information on Treatment Procedures and Methods of Replacing Lost Teeth

Edited by Allan R. Cook. 558 pages. 1997. 0-7808-0082-6. $78.

"Unique source which will fill a gap in dental sources for patients and the lay public. A valuable reference tool even in a library with thousands of books on dentistry. Comprehensive, clear, inexpensive, and easy to read and use. It fills an enormous gap in the health care literature." — *Reference and User Services Quarterly, American Library Association, Summer '98*

"Recommended reference source."
— *Booklist, American Library Association, Dec '97*

Osteoporosis Sourcebook

Basic Consumer Health Information about Primary and Secondary Osteoporosis, Juvenile Osteoporosis, Related Conditions, and Other Such Bone Disorders as Fibrous Dysplasia, Myeloma, Osteogenesis Imperfecta, Osteopetrosis, and Paget's Disease

Along with Information about Risk Factors, Treatments, Traditional and Non-Traditional Pain Management, and Including a Glossary and Resource Directory

Edited by Allan R. Cook. 600 pages. 2000. 0-7808-0239-X. $78.

SEE ALSO *Women's Health Concerns Sourcebook*

Pain Sourcebook

Basic Information about Specific Forms of Acute and Chronic Pain, Including Headaches, Back Pain, Muscular Pain, Neuralgia, Surgical Pain, and Cancer Pain

Along with Pain Relief Options Such as Analgesics, Narcotics, Nerve Blocks, Transcutaneous Nerve Stimulation, and Alternative Forms of Pain Control, Including Biofeedback, Imaging, Behavior Modification, and Relaxation Techniques

Edited by Allan R. Cook. 667 pages. 1997. 0-7808-0213-6. $78.

"The text is readable, easily understood, and well indexed. This excellent volume belongs in all patient education libraries, consumer health sections of public libraries, and many personal collections."
— *American Reference Books Annual, 1999*

"A beneficial reference." — *Booklist Health Sciences Supplement, American Library Association, Oct '98*

"The information is basic in terms of scholarship and is appropriate for general readers. Written in journalistic style... intended for non-professionals. Quite thorough in its coverage of different pain conditions and summarizes the latest clinical information regarding pain treatment."
— *Choice, Association of College and Research Libraries, Jun '98*

"Recommended reference source."
— *Booklist, American Library Association, Mar '98*

Pediatric Cancer Sourcebook

Basic Consumer Health Information about Leukemias, Brain Tumors, Sarcomas, Lymphomas, and Other Cancers in Infants, Children, and Adolescents, Including Descriptions of Cancers, Treatments, and Coping Strategies

Along with Suggestions for Parents, Caregivers, and Concerned Relatives, a Glossary of Cancer Terms, and Resource Listings

Edited by Edward J. Prucha. 587 pages. 1999. 0-7808-0245-4. $78.

Physical & Mental Issues in Aging Sourcebook

Basic Consumer Health Information on Physical and Mental Disorders Associated with the Aging Process, Including Concerns about Cardiovascular Disease, Pulmonary Disease, Oral Health, Digestive Disorders, Musculoskeletal and Skin Disorders, Metabolic Changes, Sexual and Reproductive Issues, and Changes in Vision, Hearing, and Other Senses

Along with Data about Longevity and Causes of Death, Information on Acute and Chronic Pain, Descriptions of Mental Concerns, a Glossary of Terms, and Resource Listings for Additional Help

Edited by Jenifer Swanson. 660 pages. 1999. 0-7808-0233-0. $78.

"Recommended reference source."
— Booklist, American Library Association, Oct '99

SEE ALSO Healthy Aging Sourcebook

Plastic Surgery Sourcebook

Basic Consumer Health Information on Cosmetic and Reconstructive Plastic Surgery, Including Statistical Information about Different Surgical Procedures, Things to Consider Prior to Surgery, Plastic Surgery Techniques and Tools, Emotional and Psychological Considerations, and Procedure-Specific Information

Along with a Glossary of Terms and a Listing of Resources for Additional Help and Information

Edited by M. Lisa Weatherford. 400 pages. 2000. 0-7808-0214-4. $48.

Pregnancy & Birth Sourcebook

Basic Information about Planning for Pregnancy, Maternal Health, Fetal Growth and Development, Labor and Delivery, Postpartum and Perinatal Care, Pregnancy in Mothers with Special Concerns, and Disorders of Pregnancy, Including Genetic Counseling, Nutrition and Exercise, Obstetrical Tests, Pregnancy Discomfort, Multiple Births, Cesarean Sections, Medical Testing of Newborns, Breastfeeding, Gestational Diabetes, and Ectopic Pregnancy

Edited by Heather E. Aldred. 737 pages. 1997. 0-7808-0216-0. $78.

"A well-organized handbook. Recommended."
— Choice, Association of College and Research Libraries, Apr '98

"Reecommended reference source."
— Booklist, American Library Association, Mar '98

"Recommended for public libraries."
— American Reference Books Annual, 1998

SEE ALSO Congenital Disorders Sourcebook, Family Planning Sourcebook

Public Health Sourcebook

Basic Information about Government Health Agencies, Including National Health Statistics and Trends, Healthy People 2000 Program Goals and Objectives, the Centers for Disease Control and Prevention, the Food and Drug Administration, and the National Institutes of Health

Along with Full Contact Information for Each Agency

Edited by Wendy Wilcox. 698 pages. 1998. 0-7808-0220-9. $78.

"Recommended reference source."
— Booklist, American Library Association, Sep '98

"This consumer guide provides welcome assistance in navigating the maze of federal health agencies and their data on public health concerns."
— SciTech Book News, Sep '98

Rehabilitation Sourcebook

Basic Consumer Health Information about Rehabilitation for People Recovering from Heart Surgery, Spinal Cord Injury, Stroke, Orthopedic Impairments, Amputation, Pulmonary Impairments, Traumatic Injury, and More, Including Physical Therapy, Occupational Therapy, Speech/Language Therapy, Massage Therapy, Dance Therapy, Art Therapy, and Recreational Therapy

Along with Information on Assistive and Adaptive Devices, a Glossary, and Resources for Additional Help and Information

Edited by Dawn D. Matthews. 531 pages. 1999. 0-7808-0236-5. $78.

Respiratory Diseases & Disorders Sourcebook

Basic Information about Respiratory Diseases and Disorders, Including Asthma, Cystic Fibrosis, Pneumonia, the Common Cold, Influenza, and Others, Featuring Facts about the Respiratory System, Statistical and Demographic Data, Treatments, Self-Help Management Suggestions, and Current Research Initiatives

Edited by Allan R. Cook and Peter D. Dresser. 771 pages. 1995. 0-7808-0037-0. $78.

"Designed for the layperson and for patients and their families coping with respiratory illness. . . . an extensive array of information on diagnosis, treatment, management, and prevention of respiratory illnesses for the general reader."
— Choice, Association of College and Research Libraries, Jun '96

"A highly recommended text for all collections. It is a comforting reminder of the power of knowledge that good books carry between their covers."
— Academic Library Book Review, Spring '96

"A comprehensive collection of authoritative information presented in a nontechnical, humanitarian style for patients, families, and caregivers."
— Association of Operating Room Nurses, Sep/Oct '95

Sexually Transmitted Diseases Sourcebook

Basic Information about Herpes, Chlamydia, Gonorrhea, Hepatitis, Nongonoccocal Urethritis, Pelvic Inflammatory Disease, Syphilis, AIDS, and More

Along with Current Data on Treatments and Preventions

Edited by Linda M. Ross. 550 pages. 1997. 0-7808-0217-9. $78.

Skin Disorders Sourcebook

Basic Information about Common Skin and Scalp Conditions Caused by Aging, Allergies, Immune Reactions, Sun Exposure, Infectious Organisms, Parasites, Cosmetics, and Skin Traumas, Including Abrasions, Cuts, and Pressure Sores

Along with Information on Prevention and Treatment

Edited by Allan R. Cook. 647 pages. 1997. 0-7808-0080-X. $78.

"... comprehensive, easily read reference book."
— *Doody's Health Sciences Book Reviews, Oct '97*

SEE ALSO Burns Sourcebook

Sleep Disorders Sourcebook

Basic Consumer Health Information about Sleep and Its Disorders, Including Insomnia, Sleepwalking, Sleep Apnea, Restless Leg Syndrome, and Narcolepsy

Along with Data about Shiftwork and Its Effects, Information on the Societal Costs of Sleep Deprivation, Descriptions of Treatment Options, a Glossary of Terms, and Resource Listings for Additional Help

Edited by Jenifer Swanson. 439 pages. 1998. 0-7808-0234-9. $78.

"Recommended reference source."
— *Booklist, American Library Association, Feb '99*

"A useful resource that provides accurate, relevant, and accessible information on sleep to the general public. Health care providers who deal with sleep disorders patients may also find it helpful in being prepared to answer some of the questions patients ask."
— *Respiratory Care, Jul '99*

Sports Injuries Sourcebook

Basic Consumer Health Information about Common Sports Injuries, Prevention of Injury in Specific Sports, Tips for Training, and Rehabilitation from Injury

Along with Information about Special Concerns for Children, Young Girls in Athletic Training Programs, Senior Athletes, and Women Athletes, and a Directory of Resources for Further Help and Information

Edited by Heather E. Aldred. 624 pages. 1999. 0-7808-0218-7. $78.

Substance Abuse Sourcebook

Basic Health-Related Information about the Abuse of Legal and Illegal Substances Such as Alcohol, Tobacco, Prescription Drugs, Marijuana, Cocaine, and Heroin; and Including Facts about Substance Abuse Prevention Strategies, Intervention Methods, Treatment and Recovery Programs, and a Section Addressing the Special Problems Related to Substance Abuse during Pregnancy

Edited by Karen Bellenir. 573 pages. 1996. 0-7808-0038-9. $78.

"A valuable addition to any health reference section. Highly recommended."
— *The Book Report, Mar/Apr '97*

"... a comprehensive collection of substance abuse information that's both highly readable and compact. Families and caregivers of substance abusers will find the information enlightening and helpful, while teachers, social workers and journalists should benefit from the concise format. Recommended."
— *Drug Abuse Update, Winter '96/'97*

SEE ALSO Alcoholism Sourcebook, Drug Abuse Sourcebook

Traveler's Health Sourcebook

Basic Consumer Health Information for Travelers, Including Physical and Medical Preparations, Transportation Health and Safety, Essential Information about Food, Water, Sun Exposure, Insect and Snake Bites, Camping and Wilderness Medicine, and Travel with Physical or Medical Disabilities

Along with International Travel Tips, Vaccination Recommendations, Geographical Health Issues, Disease Risks, a Glossary, and a Listing of Additional Resources

Edited by Joyce Brennfleck Shannon. 650 pages. 2000. 0-7808-0384-1. $78.

Women's Health Concerns Sourcebook

Basic Information about Health Issues That Affect Women, Featuring Facts about Menstruation and Other Gynecological Concerns, Including Endometriosis, Fibroids, Menopause, and Vaginitis; Reproductive Concerns, Including Birth Control, Infertility, and Abortion; and Facts about Additional Physical, Emotional, and Mental Health Concerns Prevalent among Women Such as Osteoporosis, Urinary Tract Disorders, Eating Disorders, and Depression

Along with Tips for Maintaining a Healthy Lifestyle

Edited by Heather E. Aldred. 567 pages. 1997. 0-7808-0219-5. $78.

"Handy compilation. There is an impressive range of diseases, devices, disorders, procedures, and other physical and emotional issues covered ... well organized, illustrated, and indexed."
— *Choice, Association of College and Research Libraries, Jan '98*

SEE ALSO Breast Cancer Sourcebook, Cancer Sourcebook for Women, 1st and 2nd Editions, Healthy Heart Sourcebook for Women, Osteoporosis Sourcebook

Workplace Health & Safety Sourcebook

Basic Information about Musculoskeletal Injuries, Cumulative Trauma Disorders, Occupational Carcinogens and Other Toxic Materials, Child Labor, Workplace Violence, Histoplasmosis, Transmission of HIV and Hepatitis-B Viruses, and Occupational Hazards Associated with Various Industries, Including Mining, Confined Spaces, Agriculture, Construction, Electrical Work, and the Medical Professions, with Information on Mortality and Other Statistical Data, Preventative Measures, Reproductive Risks, Reducing Stress for Shiftworkers, Noise Hazards, Industrial Back Belts, Reducing Contamination at Home, Preventing Allergic Reactions to Rubber Latex, and More

Along with Public and Private Programs and Initiatives, a Glossary, and Sources for Additional Help and Information

Edited by Chad Kimball. 600 pages. 2000. 0-7808-0231-4. $78.

Health Reference Series Cumulative Index, 1st Edition

A Comprehensive Index to the Health Reference Series, 1990-1999

1,500 pages. 2000. 0-7808-0382-5. $78.